THE TECHNIQUE OF
TOTAL KNEE ARTHROPLASTY
SECOND EDITION

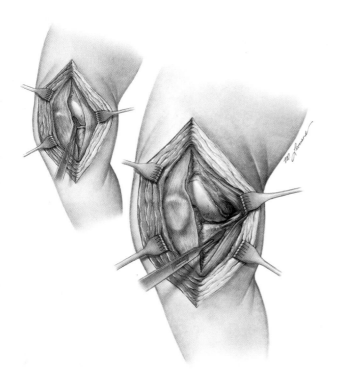

WILLIAM M. MIHALKO
MD, PhD

Campbell Clinic
Department of Orthopaedic Surgery &
Biomedical Engineering
Professor & JR Hyde Chair of Excellence
Chair Joint Graduate Program in
Biomedical Engineering
University of Tennessee Health Science Center

MICHAEL A. MONT
MD

Orthopaedic Attending
Rubin Institute for Advanced Orthopedics
Center for Joint Preservation and Replacement
Sinai Hospital of Baltimore

KENNETH A. KRACKOW
MD

Professor, Department of Orthopaedics
Jacobs School of Medicine & Biomedical Sciences
Statue University at Buffalo
Buffalo, NY

THE TECHNIQUE OF
TOTAL KNEE ARTHROPLASTY

SECOND EDITION

ELSEVIER

Elsevier
1600 John F. Kennedy Blvd.
Ste 1800
Philadelphia, PA 19103-2899

THE TECHNIQUE OF TOTAL KNEE ARTHROPLASTY, SECOND EDITION   ISBN: 978-0-323713023

Previous edition copyrighted 1990.

Content Strategist: Belinda Kuhn
Content Development Specialist: Kevin Travers
Content Development Manager: Meghan Andress
Publishing Services Manager: Deepthi Unni
Project Manager: Radhika Sivalingam
Design Direction: Brian Salisbury

Printed in India

Last digit is the print number: 9 8 7 6 5 4 3 2 1

CONTRIBUTORS

Jose Carlos Alcerro, MD
Adult Joint Reconstruction
Orthopedic Surgery
Instituto hondurreño de Seguridad Social, Tegucigalpa
Francisco Morazan
Honduras

Zhongming Chen, MD
Research Fellow
Department of Orthopaedics
Rubin Institute for Advanced Orthopedics
Center for Joint Preservation and Replacement
Sinai Hospital of Baltimore
Baltimore, MD
United States

Joseph Cline, MD
Orthopaedic Surgery Resident
University of Tennessee Health Science Center
Campbell Clinic Department of Orthopaedic Surgery
    and Biomedical Engineering
Memphis, TN
United States

Evgeny Dyskin, MD, PhD
Assistant Professor
Orthopedic Surgery
Erie County Medical Center, Buffalo
Assistant Professor
Orthopaedic Surgery
Buffalo General Medical Center
Buffalo, NY
United States

Travis Eason, MD
Orthopaedic Surgery Resident
University of Tennessee Health Science Center
Campbell Clinic Department of Orthopaedic Surgery
    and Biomedical Engineering
Memphis, TN
United States

Michael M. Katz, MD
Orthopedic Surgery Specialist
Dallas, TX
United States

Carlos J. Lavernia, MD, FAAOS
Adjunct Professor
Biomedical Engineering
University of Miami
Miami, FL
United States

Kenneth B. Mathis, MD
Associate professor
Orthopedic Surgery
McGovern Medical School at the University of Texas
    Health Science Center-Houston
Houston, TX
United States

William M. Mihalko, MD, PhD
Professor
Campbell Clinic Department of Orthopaedic Surgery
    and Biomedical Engineering
University of Tennessee
Memphis, TN
United States

Curtis Miller, MD
Orthopaedic Surgeon
Canyon
OrthoArizona, Phoenix
Team Physician-Spring Training
Chicago White Sox
Glendale, AZ
United States

Michael Mont, MD
Clinical Trials Director
Department of Orthopaedics
Northwell Health
New York, NY
United States
Orthopaedic Surgeon
Department of Orthopaedics
Rubin Institute of Advanced Orthopedics
Center for Joint Preservation and Replacement
Sinai Hospital of Baltimore
Baltimore, MD
United States

Arun Mullaji, FRCS Ed, MCh Orth, MS Orth, DNB Orth, D Orth
Consultant Orthopaedic Surgeon
Orthopaedics
Breach Candy Hospital
Director
Mullaji Knee Clinic
Mumbai, India

Ananya Munjal, MS
Carver College of Medicine Class of 2023
University of Iowa
Iowa City, IA
United States

Sandeep Munjal, MD, FAAOS
Chairman
Department of Orthopedics
Physicians Clinic of Iowa
Cedar Rapids, IA
United States

Philip Noble, PhD
Adjunct Professor
Orthopedic Surgery
UTHealth
Houston, TX
United States

Matthew Phillips, MD, FAAOS
Chief
Orthopaedics
Kaleida Health
Buffalo, NY
United States
Assistant Professor
Orthopaedics
The Jacobs School of Medicine and Biomedical
    Sciences
Buffalo, NY
United States

Karisankappa Puttaswamy, MBBS, MS Orthopedics
Senior Consultant
Orthopedics Care Health
Fortis Hospital, Bangalore
Karnataka
India

Sridhar Rachala, MD
Clinical Assistant Professor
Orthopaedic Surgery
University of Buffalo
Buffalo General Hospital
Buffalo, NY
United States

John M. Tarazi, MD
Research Fellow
Department of Orthopaedics
Northwell Health
Huntington, NY
United States

Patrick Toy, MD
Associate Professor
University of Tennessee Health Science Center
Campbell Clinic Department of Orthopaedic Surgery
    and Biomedical Engineering
Memphis, TN
United States

Audrey M. Tsao, MD
Department of Orthopedic Surgery
Mid-Atlantic Permanente Medical Group
Rockville, MD
United States

It has now been over 25 years since Dr. Kenneth A. Krackow wrote the first edition of *The Technique of Total Knee Arthroplasty*. The first edition quickly became a go to textbook for residents, fellows, and arthroplasty surgeons around the world. The first edition paid close attention to detail concerning not just the surgical procedure, but assessing the difficulty of each individual case and teaching the surgeon attention to detail concerning the level of difficulty to expect in the operating room for a given operative case. It was one of the best sources for describing and categorizing different levels of deformity and how to approach correction in the operating room with specifics on soft tissue balancing. In this second edition Michael A. Mont, MD, and I (William M. Mihalko, MD, PhD), who were both protégés and residents/fellows of Dr. Krackow, have updated this iconic textbook on total knee arthroplasty (TKA) that covers patient optimization, pain management, and blood management techniques, while adding updated chapters on considerations for outpatient or ambulatory surgery–based TKA along with a chapter on new technologies and robotics.

Dr. Krackow was a pioneer when it came to computer-navigated knee arthroplasty surgery and he performed the first procedure in the United States with a system that he and Dr. Mont and myself built in the laboratory over a 3-year period starting in a research postdoc year and then throughout my residency. The system was based on software that was written to program an electromagnetic tracking system that was used to perform multiple cadaveric studies to objectively measure the effects of soft tissue releases in extension and flexion. This system eventually evolved into the Stryker navigation system.

Dr. Krackow was often referred to around Buffalo General Hospital as the "Hand Surgeon of Hip and Knee Arthroplasty." This was because his attention to the most minute detail was so intense in the operating room and his handling of soft tissue during any procedure was so exceptional. Our approach to this second edition was to keep in mind this relentless attention to detail from how he examined the patient in the office to the preoperative workup and planning, to the operative and perioperative technique, to making certain the postoperative course was one that gave the patient the best chance.

Michael Mont and I have edited this second edition in Dr. Krackow's honor and are donating proceeds to the Alzheimer's Foundation of America.

In **Chapter 1** Dr. Matthew Phillips (University at Buffalo Resident 1991 to 1996, Fellow 1997, and Partner since 1997) covers the topic of: **Patient Considerations: Comorbidities and Optimization**. It is important today with well-informed patients from the internet that the proper discussion of the risks and alternatives to the procedure be addressed.

Dr. Sandeep Munjal (University at Buffalo Fellow 1998 and Resident 1999 to 2002) covers issues with some of the most common modifiable comorbidities we deal with as arthroplasty surgeons today in **Chapter 2: Modify What's Modifiable: Smoking, Obesity, Opioid Dependence, and Nutrition Deficiencies**. We have realized now the importance of these comorbidities and their effect on the risk of major complications. Knowing how to convey these issues to the patient and the importance of handling these comorbidities before undergoing the procedure is paramount.

In **Chapter 3** Dr. Sridhar Rachala (University at Buffalo Resident 2004, Partner on staff) discusses other comorbidities that may or may not be modifiable: **Optimizing Important Comorbidities: Diabetes, Rheumatoid Arthritis, Peripheral Vascular Disease, Cardiac Disease**. Compared with when the first edition of this book was published, we now know the importance of diabetic control and new measures that can help determine whether a patient is an optimal candidate for the procedure. Rheumatoid arthritis drugs are now far superior to those from two decades ago and at this point, the percentage of patients who have the diagnosis that we see in our offices with end-stage disease is markedly lower. When a patient does present with end-stage disease, however, it is important to understand how to handle their disease-modifying antirheumatological medications to decrease the risk of an infection or wound healing issues. Cardiovascular disease is a major issue in the United States today and making sure that certain patients are able to survive the procedure and do not have circulatory compromise that will affect their surgical outcome is extremely important.

Dr. Curtis Miller (University at Buffalo Fellow 1996) covers the topic of assessing surgical difficulty in **Chapter 4**. This is a topic that anyone who trained with Dr. Krackow knows he took seriously and he prepared for each and every case on an individual basis. Realizing how to prepare for severe deformity cases, bone loss, poor bone quality, and soft tissue balancing, as well as soft tissue insufficiencies, is important to make certain everything you may need to complete a case is present on the day of surgery, but also it gives the surgeon a better chance at having the operative procedure go as smoothly as possible.

In Chapter 5 Dr. Carlos Lavernia, et al. (Johns Hopkins Fellow 1991 to 1992) discuss the topic of **Preoperative Planning From Medical Issues To Implants**. An extension of Chapter 4, this topic makes certain that planning is complete and all possibilities are covered for what you might need in the operating room if a first plan does not work.

Chapter 6 (William M. Mihalko, MD, PhD, Postdoc 1995, Resident 1999, and Partner 2002 to 2006) covers this newest topic: **Setting Up an Outpatient or Same Day Discharge TKA Program**. When the first edition was published, it was routine for patients to be admitted the night before the procedure and stay for 4 or more days afterward. These days are long gone, because we now focus on the economic effect of our care and have determined ways to make certain that cost is reduced without compromising quality. Most institutions now have a same-day or ambulatory surgery program setup for knee arthroplasty and Medicare has now taken the procedure off of the inpatient only list.

In **Chapters 7 and 8** Dr. Audrey Tsao (Johns Hopkins Fellowship 1992) covers the surgical technique in the manner of precision that Dr. Krackow always strove for in a relentless fashion. The added chapter on bone cutting technique covers issues that Dr. Krackow would discuss with all trainees: from choosing a saw blade to understanding the "throw" of the sagittal saw and issues with bone cutting accuracy due to cutting transitions from softer to more sclerotic bone, along with making sure that certain surrounding structures were kept safe.

Chapter 9 covers soft tissue balancing procedures by Dr. Arhun Mulaji, who considered Dr. Krackow one of his mentors. He describes deformity and soft tissue balancing in a stepwise detailed approach.

New technologies in knee arthroplasty surgery are covered in **Chapter 10** by Dr. Philip C. Noble, et al.

From navigation to robotics to sensor technology, we now have many tools that were not available when the first edition was published. Although navigation was not popularized in the manner Dr. Krackow thought it would be, he was a proponent of new technology and was a test surgeon for ROBODOC at the Buffalo General Hospital. This chapter discusses all the newer technologies and their possible advantages.

Chapter 11 William M. Mihalko, et al. highlight cement techniques in knee arthroplasty. This portion of the procedure was one that Dr. Krackow would spend the most time on to make certain it was performed in a routine, established manner, with the surgical team being well versed in how the procedure would be performed. The latest generation cement techniques and considerations in the operating room are covered to make certain that this is not the weakest part of the procedure.

In **Chapter 12** Dr. Evengy Dyskin (University of Buffalo Fellowship 2010, University of Buffalo staff 2016 to present) covers the topics of avoiding peri- and post-operative complications.

Dr. Puttaswamy (University of Buffalo Fellowship 2012) in **Chapter 13** discusses the evidence basis of knee arthroplasty outcomes and what we should discuss with our patients concerning what they should expect after the procedure is performed. A discussion of how to treat patients in the postoperative period is also covered to help avoid long-term issues.

It has been an honor for the two of us to coedit the second edition of this iconic textbook. We thank all of our authors for their hard work, expertise, and all of the attention to detail that Ken was well known for in our field. We have all dedicated our time to this project on Ken's behalf and have donated the proceeds to the Alzheimer's Foundation of America in his name.

AUTHOR'S TRIBUTES TO DR. KENNETH A. KRACKOW

I first met Dr. Krackow when I interviewed for a research fellowship/postdoc at his home in 1993. I had matched into the orthopedic surgery program at Virginia Commonwealth University, but both my parents became ill/disabled and, being from Buffalo, I wanted to transfer into the local residency program. Dr. Krackow offered me a research year to transition into the orthopedic program at Buffalo. My PhD work on knee kinematics allowed him to use my talents to have multiple cadaveric studies published with him on soft tissue balancing. My research year was very productive, and ultimately, over my 5 years of fellowship and residency that I spent with Dr. Krackow, I published over a dozen laboratory-based manuscripts and then with his help was off to an adult reconstructive surgery fellowship with Dr. Leo Whiteside. I am in debt to Dr. Krackow for giving me the opportunity that allowed me to be close to my parents during a difficult time. I remember vividly the day during my residency when Dr. Krackow signed my copy of the first edition of *The Technique of Total Knee Arthroplasty*. During my residency, the electromagnetic kinematic tracking system we used to perform the cadaveric studies was turned into a prototype for the first computer navigation platform for knee arthroplasty in the United States, which would later become the Stryker navigation platform. He entrenched the need for precision and attention to detail into not just operative technique and patient care but also into life in general. I would later become Dr. Krackow's partner at the University at Buffalo in 2002 and would further benefit from his mentorship and his sponsorship into The Knee Society in 2008. I enjoyed the transition over the years from being his resident to being his partner, friend, and colleague.

—William M. Mihalko, MD, PhD
(Postdoc Research Fellow 1995,
Resident 1999, Partner 2002 to 2006)

I did my fellowship at Johns Hopkins with Dr. Krackow and David Hungerford from 1989 to 1990. While finishing the year and interviewing at over 10 places for a permanent job, Dr. Krackow took me out to lunch and said to me: "Why don't you simply stay on as my partner?" I was absolutely flabbergasted—what an honor to be partners with someone who I idolized as a surgeon, teacher, and personal mentor. I had about 2 years as his direct partner until he went to Buffalo. During this time, my entire life was influenced positively by him. I quote his teachings every day, even today 30 years later, on a daily basis in the operating room. I may be teaching the Krackow suture on the hip, using the intramedullary goniometer on a knee, or showing his meticulous surgical techniques in so many ways. He taught me patient care in an exemplary manner. What I personally note the most was through his great friendship and paying attention to my life and his invaluable advice to me on so many important topics.

—Michael A. Mont
(Fellow 1990, Partner 1990 to 1992)

Dr. Kenneth Krackow is one of the most incredible men I have ever met in my life. He is an innovator, scientist, and surgeon and was as eager to learn as he was to teach. Dr. Krackow always prided himself on good patient outcomes, and nothing brought him more satisfaction than the joy of a job well done. His soft tissue handling was impeccable, and he used to say that knee replacement is predominantly surgery of the soft tissue. He knew better than anyone that optimizing the modifiable factors affecting soft tissue led to the best postsurgical outcomes, and he was always thinking about how to improve and be even better. Dr. Krackow is not only a phenomenal physician and mentor, but he is also able to humanize his patients and clearly see the person under the knife, not just the joint. Surgery itself is a modifiable factor, and a large part of my chapter centers on having conversations with patients, encouraging them, and meeting them where they are at—something Dr. Krackow encouraged wholeheartedly throughout his career. He cared genuinely for the people he healed, and I still recall him creating multiple recordings of every surgery for his patients to listen to after speaking with him so that they could go home and explain their consults with their families and loved ones. I remember his impeccable dressing and his love for watches and infamous monologues on shaving amused us all. I am where I am today thanks to the teaching and wisdom of Dr. Ken Krackow.

—Sandeep Munjal, MD
(Fellow 1998, Resident 2004)

I first met Dr. Krackow on a gloomy Buffalo morning in February for a fellowship interview. His name sounded familiar, because I had used a stitch named after him during my orthopedic surgery career in Russia. Once regular interview sessions were over, we went to a nearby restaurant to enjoy the local cuisine. To my surprise, traditional silverware was replaced by a pair of Kocher clamps when the food arrived! We must have been perceived as a very odd couple, eating wings and french fries with surgical instruments and wearing chest napkins hung around our necks with old dental metal chains as the Food Channel was filming their show next to us. I did my best with the Kochers; however, a few wings still escaped to the floor. It turned out that I was unknowingly taking a test for dexterity and courage. The evaluation was completed and I got the job. Dr. Krackow opened the door to American academic medicine to me. I will always remember and thank him for that.

—Evgeny Dyskin
(Fellow 2010, Partner 2016 to present)

During the winter of 1994, I was almost done serving in the United States Air Force as a General Orthopaedic Surgeon. With less than 6 months remaining in my commitment, I was in the process of looking for a "real" job in the civilian world. One night, thumbing through the job advertisements at the end of the most recent *Journal of Bone and Joint Surgery* and contemplating my future, I came across an advertisement that Ken Krackow, MD, was looking to fill the position of his "very first" clinical fellow in Buffalo (Bill Mihalko, our editor, was his first research fellow). I quickly called a friend and former Air Force orthopedist, who had done his residency at Johns Hopkins and had trained under Dr. Krackow, to see what he thought of the idea of me applying for the fellowship. You see, for 3 years, as we served together in the United States Air Force, my friend almost daily would quote Dr. Krackow or point out that "this is how Dr. Krackow would do it!" The Orthopaedic Department at Johns Hopkins had many famous attendings at the time. Yet my colleague always seemed to do things "the Krackow Way." While I had never met Dr. Krackow before 1994, I felt my 3 years with his former resident had been a "mini-fellowship." Trying to decide whether to start my civilian career, with considerably higher income, or spend another year in training on a fellow's salary along with the prospect of doing a fellowship after being a junior attending might have been a difficult decision for many. However, the opportunity to train under one of the world's best joint replacement doctors made the decision to move my young family from Arizona to New York an easy one. It was the best career decision I have ever made. I learned more from Dr. Krackow in that year than I had in 5 years of residency. He was technically the best surgeon I have ever met! While he is well known for, among many things, helping to design the first size-specific total knee cutting blocks for the former company Howmedica and for designing Stryker's first computer navigation system for total knee replacement, I am fully convinced that he did those things to help the community orthopedists who did 10 joints a year, because Dr. Krackow could easily do a total joint surgery with little more than a scalpel, a saw, and some suture (as

long as he had his intramedullary goniometer!). The most lasting lesson that I learned from Dr. Krackow was "attention to detail matters!" Being a "Krackow fellow" caries some gravitas, not because of anything I have accomplished, but only because of the reputation of Ken Krackow. I will be forever grateful for the year I spent with Ken. I am extremely lucky to have absorbed just a little bit of his knowledge. It has made me a better person, a better physician, and a much better surgeon. Thank you Ken from the bottom of my heart.

—Curtis Miller
(Fellow 1996)

Kenneth A. Krackow was already one of the most well-known and well-respected arthroplasty surgeons in the world when he joined The State University of New York at Buffalo Department of Orthopaedics in 1992 after having distinguished himself at the Johns Hopkins University Medical Institutions. As a PGY-2 in an orthopedics residency, I was initially in awe. I quickly learned that Ken was a tireless and meticulous surgeon, a patient advocate, a researcher, an inventor, and a great teacher and mentor. Both inside and outside of medicine, he was an extremely generous man who gave of himself both professionally and financially. He was a tremendous asset to our program and our community. His decision to come to Buffalo was certainly life changing for me. Ken started an arthroplasty fellowship in Buffalo and I was his second fellow. Six months into the fellowship, he asked me to join him in practice and I became his junior partner. For 21 years, I had the honor of being his partner and, along the way, he became my brother-in-law. My initial awe never really went away. His operative skills, patient care, and academic prowess are sorely missed by our community and our department.

—Matthew Phillips
(Resident 1996, Fellow 1997, Partner 1998 to present)

Dr. Kenneth Krackow was not only a great surgeon but was also a great philosopher who influenced many careers including mine. He always believed in the philosophy of picking a fellow based on whose career he would have the greatest effect on. By using this method he was able to make a huge effect on many careers. Some of the thoughts reflected in my chapter are based on some of those teachings I inherited from him.

—Sridhar R. Rachala
(Resident 2004, Partner)

CONTENTS

THE TECHNIQUE OF
TOTAL KNEE ARTHROPLASTY
SECOND EDITION

Preoperative Considerations

1

Patient Considerations: Comorbidities and Optimization

Matthew J. Phillips, MD, FAAOS and Scott R. Nodzo, MD, FAAOS

Total knee arthroplasty (TKA) continues to be one of the most reliable methods for treating end-stage arthritis when nonoperative management has failed. Choosing which patients would benefit the most from this procedure is paramount to maximize subjective outcomes. Alternative surgical procedures to TKA may also be indicated, and they should be explored with the patient in select scenarios. This chapter focuses on the preoperative steps that should be undertaken in evaluating patients for TKA and discusses alternative nonarthroplasty options.

PATIENT HISTORY

In general, the indications for a TKA include knee pain, mechanical instability, decreased range of motion secondary to pain, and the decreased ability to perform activities of daily living. Knee pain and the amount of knee pain during daily activities should be the primary consideration for TKA, with an improvement in function being a secondary consideration.[1,2] Additionally, each insurance carrier may have a unique set of criteria that the patient must fulfill in the nonoperative setting before TKA. One should be wary of the patient who is considering a TKA mainly for improvements in range of motion or in the ability to perform a recreational event but who does not have marked pain with daily activities.[1-3] The majority of patients will experience pain reduction after TKA with considerable improvement in knee function; however, an expectation of improved pain, but not necessarily completely resolved pain, should remain the main point of discussion with the patient in the preoperative period. Setting a preoperative expectation of improved pain relief, but possibly not complete resolution of pain, is important as many

patients will still have some periods of discomfort that come and go postoperatively.

A description of the patient's preoperative pain symptoms should be thoroughly recorded. This includes the severity of pain at rest and with activities such as stair use and the distance the patient is able to walk without pain. The use of preoperative narcotics or alternate analgesics, the use of an assistive device for ambulation, and pain that keeps the patient up at night or awakens them in the middle of the night are all important factors in determining the severity of a patient's symptoms and whether a knee arthroplasty is a reasonable consideration. An accurate description of the changes in severity of the pain throughout daily activities can help the surgeon better understand provocative activities that cause pain. Severe pain and what activities provoke this severe pain should always be investigated thoroughly. In rare instances patients can be in constant and severe pain; additional sources of pain generation should be considered in those patients who have unrelenting and severe pain.

In addition to pain at rest the pain during specific activities should be evaluated. It is important to document what activities cause pain and what activities are unable to be performed because of pain. Identifying the activities the patient used to perform and the activities they would like to return to performing will guide preoperative expectation counseling. Delineation of pain during activities of daily living versus during sporting events or primarily recreational activities will help guide the preoperative discussion of pain relief. One of the most reliable indications for TKA is pain with simple daily activities that is interfering with quality of life. The expectation to return to normal daily activities is a reasonable one versus the expectation to return to high-level sporting performance that the patient may or may not be able to do after TKA.[4] Symptoms that do not correlate with radiographic findings should be further evaluated, and caution should be considered when offering these patients the option of TKA.

A patient's occupation should also be considered before performing a TKA.[5] Patients whose occupation requires constant kneeling and climbing may not be well-suited for TKA.[4] In this scenario counseling should be provided about the possibility of the patient not being able to return to the exact occupation or job description that they currently hold. The patient should also consider the option of job retraining or a less manually strenuous aspect of their current occupation, although many people under the age of 60 years will return to their previous occupation after TKA.[6] The amount of time needed for postoperative recovery can be discussed at this time. A return to work 4 to 6 weeks postoperatively may be reasonable for patients who have a more sedentary job, whereas return to work at 8 to 12 weeks may be more realistic for patients who have strenuous jobs that allow for minimal breaks in the workday.[7] This discussion will allow patients to plan their sick leave or time off from work with their employer. If the patient is near retirement age, they may elect to delay surgery until after retirement so as to not exhaust all sick leave and vacation time. Ultimately, the timeframe for return to work will be patient- and occupation-specific and variable based on the postoperative recovery process.[6,7] Return to driving is another important consideration after TKA. Previous work suggests that reaction time to braking may return to normal around the 4- to 6-week postoperative time point, and this can be used as a guideline for resumption of driving.[8,9]

Another important aspect of the patient's history is their response to and frequency of intraarticular injections, physical therapy, bracing, and nonsteroidal analgesics.[10] These nonoperative treatment modalities should be tried in most, if not all, patients before surgery. The length of pain relief obtained from intraarticular injections should be carefully documented. If a local anesthetic is included in the injection, the pain relief from the injection should be noted before the patient leaving the office. If marked pain relief is not obtained in the near immediate time frame after injection, alternate pain sources should be evaluated before consideration of TKA. Identifying which nonoperative treatment options have been successful and which have not is important to

ensure that the surgeon does not recommend treatment options that have been tried and failed. This can frustrate the patient.

The use of preoperative narcotics must also be carefully considered.[11] Preoperative narcotic use has been shown to decrease subjective postoperative outcomes, and these patients are more likely to continue narcotic use a year after surgery.[11-13] Although literature suggests a decline in subjective outcomes with preoperative opioid use, it remains debatable whether or not to counsel patients about this to temper their postoperative expectations. Cessation of preoperative narcotic use is ideal and mandatory in some practices, but this may not be possible in all patients. One approach in counseling these patients is to clearly describe in layman's terms the effects that chronic opioid use has on pain tolerance and perceived pain in the postoperative period in order to appropriately set postoperative expectations. The topic of opioid use is covered in more detail in the next chapter.

The patient's medical history must be considered before surgery. Comorbidities that can be optimized should be identified. More specific recommendations on perioperative medical management will be discussed later in this book. It is important to understand the medical history when counseling patients on their perioperative risks of cardiac events, deep vein thromboses, unexpected pulmonary events, periprosthetic joint infections, anesthetic complications, and even death. Although perioperative outcomes after TKA have dramatically improved from the 1970s to 2020, the possibility of perioperative risks must be considered and thoroughly discussed with the patient during the preoperative discussion.

PHYSICAL EXAMINATION

The physical examination begins with an initial observation of the patient's gait and their ability to transfer from chair to standing and to climb onto an examining table. The amount of pain and dysfunction observed during these activities can be helpful adjuncts to the oral history. Observation of a varus or valgus thrust, recurvatum or hyperflexibility, quadriceps inhibition, or a fixed flexion contracture can additionally give insight into the expected complexity of the case.[14,15]

Routine assessment of passive and active range of motion, the ability to correct the deformity, crepitus, and peripheral circulation is important. In a varus knee tenderness along both the medial joint line and posterior lateral soft tissues is often observed because of the stretching of the lateral tissues as the varus deformity progresses. With the leg in full extension, an anterior to posterior pressure applied to the patella and palpation of the medial and lateral facets of the patella with medial and lateral patellar tilt maneuvers may elicit pain. This finding gives insight into the sensitivity of the patellofemoral joint, which may influence the surgical decision-making process.

Evaluation of the skin and any previous skin incisions that will influence the surgical approach should be documented. In general, the oldest incision should be used if it does not result in an undo strain on the surgical approach. Otherwise, the oldest and most laterally based incision should be used because of the main blood supply of the cutaneous tissues originating from the medial aspect of the limb. Careful examination of the foot and lower leg should also be performed. Findings of open ulcers, severe lymphedema, or chronic cellulitis need to be addressed prior to any elective TKA because of the increased risk of periprosthetic joint infection in patients who have these conditions. These conditions should be considered contraindications to surgery until resolved or optimized.[16] Additionally, patients with decreased sensation in their feet, or a history of decreased sensation, without a known diagnosis of diabetes should be screened with a hemoglobin A1c test.[17] These issues will be discussed further in subsequent chapters (Chapters 2 and 3).

A hip examination should always be performed because of the possibility of referred knee pain. Branches of the obturator nerve and femoral nerve innervate the anterior hip capsule.[18] In patients who have hip arthritis or hip pathology this nerve can become inflamed and result in referred pain to the knee. Knee pain with range of motion of the hip and minimal knee pain when knee motion is isolated should alert the surgeon to the possibility of a referred pain phenomenon.[19]

The overreaction of the patient to perceived pain and pain out of proportion to provocative maneuvers should carefully be evaluated for either a secondary gain purpose or alternate sources of pain. Hyperanalgesia of the skin or noted skin changes may represent a complex regional pain type syndrome that may be exacerbated by TKA. History of depression or anxiety noted on the oral history may correlate with an overly anxious patient during the physical examination. Patients who have pain out of proportion to radiographic and physical examination findings may have poor subjective satisfaction after knee arthroplasty surgery.[20,21]

RADIOGRAPHIC EXAMINATION

Routine radiographs include weight-bearing anteroposterior (AP), lateral, and patellofemoral views and a notch or tunnel view. Long-standing radiographs are an additional and helpful adjunct to isolated knee radiographs. The long-standing films allow for an assessment of overall limb alignment, any proximal tibial or distal femoral remodeling that has occurred secondary to the arthritic process, the presence of hardware that may influence the surgery, and the presence of femoral or tibial shaft bowing that may influence intramedullary guides. It also gives a screening shot of the pelvis for hip joint pathology.[22] The preoperative deformity noted on radiographs, along with the correctability of the deformity on examination, will give a good preoperative estimate of the soft tissue releases that may or may not be necessary during surgery.[23] Additionally, if conventional instrumentation is being used, the measured angle between the femoral shaft axis and the femoral mechanical axis can be measured and used for determining the angle of the distal femoral cut. This angle may not always equal 6 degrees, which is the traditionally noted resection angle for the distal femoral cut. A more patient-oriented approach with a variable distal angle measurement based on this preoperatively measured angle may be indicated and has been shown to improve patient outcomes.[24,25]

General bone quality can be observed on the radiographs, along with osteophyte formation, evidence of joint effusion, and any periarticular erosions that may indicate an inflammatory rather than routine osteoarthritic joint. Sclerotic changes on one side of the joint with relative decreased mineralization on the opposite side of the joint may indicate asymmetrical loading of the joint. Observation of the size and relative position of the bony anatomy, including medial femoral overgrowth or lateral femoral hypoplasia in the valgus knee, should also be noted. It is also important to identify the rotational alignment of the knee joint with the patella facing forward in the radiography. A knee with tibia vara remodeling and relative rotation can be recognized by an increasingly overlapped position of the fibula on the tibia. This can alert the surgeon that additional surgical considerations may be needed to properly balance the knee through component positioning and soft tissue balancing. Additionally, subluxation of the tibia laterally on a standing view may indicate ligamentous stretching or an incompetent anterior cruciate ligament (ACL).

On the lateral view, evaluation of the wear pattern in the medial and lateral joint lines is important to note. The medial tibial plateau is seen as a subtle concavity, whereas the lateral plateau is relatively flat. The lateral femoral condyle can best be identified by finding the linea terminalis, which is the delineation of the patellofemoral joint from the lateral tibiofemoral joint and has an observed subtle flattening on the condyle.[26] A wear pattern on the posterior aspect of the tibia indicates a relative flexion contracture that may also be observed on physical examination. Joint effusions are best observed on the lateral radiograph and can be identified as an increased density or haziness in the suprapatellar pouch where a clear or black region would normally be located.

The standing tunnel view adds additional information about the knee joint space, especially in knees with seemingly mild arthritic changes on routine standing AP radiographs. Using the Rosenberg technique, the standing tunnel view is a posterior to anterior projection with the knee in approximately 45 degrees of flexion.[27] This view allows visualization of the arthritic changes, specifically joint space narrowing, in partial flexion that may be more pronounced in the valgus knee. This more impressive joint space narrowing seen on the partial flexion standing tunnel view may also be identified in some patients who have varus deformity and otherwise mild arthritic changes seen on the routine standing AP radiograph. The addition of this view may increase the detection of arthritic changes that may otherwise go undetected in a subset of the population.[28]

A thorough history and physical examination can aid the surgeon in appropriate selection of TKA candidates and identify patients whose comorbidities require optimization to maximize patient outcomes and decrease the risk of postoperative complications. Patients may be divided into two distinct groups: (1) those whose symptoms can be explained by physical and radiographic findings and (2) those who have symptoms out of proportion to the examination findings. In these latter patients alternate sources of pain generation should be evaluated, including a synovial disease process such as pigmented villonodular synovitis; bony pathology including routine bone bruising, nondisplaced fractures, or tumors; isolated articular cartilage or meniscal pathology; a regional pain syndrome; lumbar spine pathology; and sources of referred pain. Advanced imaging such as CT scan or MRI can identify many of these subtle pathologies, and in rare cases a diagnostic arthroscopy may be indicated.

TREATMENT ALTERNATIVES TO ARTHROPLASTY

TKA provides reliable improvements in function and pain relief by resurfacing the articular surfaces and improving overall limb alignment. When the articular surface remains intact with minimal wear patterns or damage, alternate procedures may be indicated to improve symptoms resulting from limb malalignment or overloading of the medial or lateral compartments. These procedures may include distal femoral osteotomy, proximal tibial osteotomy, or patellar realignment surgery. Limb realignment and joint preservation procedures may be indicated in the very young and active patient who does not have an inflammatory arthritic condition and with mild to moderate wear of one compartment of the knee.

Distal Femoral and Proximal Tibial Osteotomy

The goal of the osteotomy procedure is to unload the affected side of the knee joint and to load the relatively unaffected side of the joint by realigning the distal femur or tibia to change the overall mechanical axis of the limb and redistribute the forces through the knee during weightbearing. One of the first steps in determining whether an osteotomy is prudent is identifying where the main source of the limb deformity is occurring.[29,30]

In the valgus knee the overall limb deformity tends to occur in the distal femur, and a varus-producing medial distal femoral closing wedge osteotomy just proximal to the adductor tubercle may be performed to correct this deformity.[31,32] This allows for good bone-to-bone contact and improved healing potential at the osteotomy site. Closing wedge osteotomy, however, may be more technically challenging because the wedge resection needs to be carefully calculated preoperatively. Over- or underresection of the wedge is difficult to correct intraoperatively. An alternative to medial closing wedge varus osteotomy is an opening lateral wedge osteotomy with bone grafting of the osteotomy site. The opening wedge allows for a more controlled titration of the limb deformity correction. The tradeoff is an increased risk of nonunion postoperatively because of the need to bone graft the osteotomy site.[33]

In the varus knee the anatomical deformity often arises from the proximal tibia resulting in relative tibia vara.[34] A valgus-producing medial opening tibial wedge osteotomy is often performed in this setting and can provide satisfactory limb alignment correction. Just as in the distal femur, a proximal tibia lateral closing wedge osteotomy is an alternative to the medial opening wedge. This tends to be technically more demanding, introduces the need to address the proximal fibula, and can lead to more infrapatellar scarring with patella baja and a more distorted joint line for future knee arthroplasty.[35,36] In some cases the overall contribution of limb deformity will be from both the distal femur and the proximal tibia, and a combined osteotomy may be indicated.[37]

An osteotomy may be considered if there is relative isolation of the arthritic process in one aspect of the joint with minimal or mild arthritic changes in the opposite compartment, which will ultimately see increased loads and stress after the osteotomy procedure. Additional factors to consider include:

1. Life expectancy. Young patients who would be expected to outlive their knee prosthesis may consider an osteotomy to bridge them to a knee arthroplasty surgery or, in some scenarios, help them avoid this procedure. In young patients both loosening of the implant and wear of the polyethylene need to be considered.
2. Activity level. Patients who desire to perform very high-impact activities postoperatively may not be suitable candidates for TKA. The risk of periprosthetic fracture and rapid polyethylene wear in these patients may not outweigh the benefits of arthroplasty surgery.

Factors that are not necessarily contraindications to an osteotomy procedure include:

1. Mild patellofemoral disease or the presence of patellar osteophytes especially with minimal joint space narrowing. Some patients will have radiographic findings of patellofemoral arthritis but have minimal sensitivity or pain from the compartment, and they may still be indicated for an osteotomy procedure. A careful clinical examination to determine how much, if any, pain is coming from the patellofemoral joint should be performed.
2. The presence of mild arthritic changes in the opposite compartment. In the very young patient

the benefits of osteotomy may still outweigh the risks of progression of the arthritic process in the compartment that is not being loaded during weightbearing. Preoperative counseling about the longevity of the osteotomy procedure and the potential for incomplete pain relief is imperative. The notion that this procedure may be a bridge to a knee arthroplasty later in life should be conveyed to the patient.

Knee instability factors must also be considered before an osteotomy.

1. A positive pivot shift or Lachman test may indicate ACL deficiency that may need to be addressed at the time of the osteotomy. In young active patients who have arthritis isolated to one compartment and symptomatic ACL instability an extraarticular ACL reconstruction may be indicated at the time of the osteotomy procedure. Modern intraarticular ACL reconstruction may also be considered as a staged procedure.
2. Patients who have a lax or damaged medial collateral ligament (MCL) in need of an osteotomy also pose a marked challenge. Reconstruction of the MCL with allograft or autograft may be indicated at time of the osteotomy. In some instances the resulting change in tension of the medial-sided tissues, if a lateral closing or medial opening wedge proximal tibial osteotomy is performed, may provide enough stability.
3. Intraarticular pathology such as meniscal damage or chondral defects can also be addressed at the time of surgery either in open fashion or arthroscopically. Multiple options are available as cartilage restoration procedures, and they should be done in conjunction with the osteotomy if indicated.

Several factors are clear contraindications to an osteotomy.

1. Advanced age where a prosthesis would likely last the remainder of the patient's lifetime is one contraindication.
2. Patients who have limited range of motion and marked flexion contracture preoperatively will likely not obtain the clinical success of patients with satisfactory preoperative range of motion.
3. Arthritis secondary to an inflammatory disease process or marked synovial disease process should preclude patients from osteotomy consideration.
4. Uncorrectable knee instability due to ligamentous, capsular, and surrounding soft tissue injury is a

contraindication. Additionally, alternative options should be considered for rough or a severely worn articular surface that results in a depressed joint surface.

These contraindications may lead many surgeons to consider arthroplasty options versus an osteotomy, especially with the improved success of unicompartmental knee arthroplasty (UKA) and cementless TKA.[38] However, in patients in their 30s or early 40s an osteotomy should be considered and discussed prior to undertaking an irreversible procedure such as a UKA or TKA. Any discussion about osteotomy must include the facts that, in general, osteotomy is less predictable than TKA, may lead to incomplete pain relief, and may be a bridge to a TKA later in life. Also, it is important to consider the increased planning and possible difficulty of a future TKA after a periarticular osteotomy is performed.

Arthrodesis

Currently, the most common indication for knee arthrodesis is a patient who has failed multiple treatments and surgeries for periprosthetic joint infection. Although not a common procedure in modern practice, it may be the most reliable option in certain patient populations. Patients who have nonreconstructible extensor mechanism disruption or a paralytic condition of the femoral nerve may still benefit from this option.[39]

When considering knee fusion, there must be a notion that the joint is so unreconstructible that a knee arthroplasty would not be a reliable option or that failure of the prosthesis (including a hinge or distal femoral replacing prosthesis) would be so imminent or catastrophic that a fusion would be a more reliable treatment option. Fusion after TKA is often more technically challenging than a primary knee arthrodesis because of the bone loss from a multiply revised knee. This may result in marked shortening of the limb or bone grafting of the defect. Internal fusion nails and external fixation devices are effective and should be used in this clinical scenario.

Ultimately, this option should be considered the final option for the treatment of knee pathology. Conversion of a knee arthrodesis to a TKA in the future is a technically difficult procedure with limited success and is usually not a viable option for most patients who have a fusion.[40] Patients must understand there is obligatory shortening of the fused side of at least three-fourths of an inch to allow for adequate swing through of the limb and push off on the opposite side. This shortening may be even more severe if there is bone loss at the time of fusion surgery. They must also understand that fusion is performed mainly for pain relief and to obtain a stable knee rather than to provide a high-performing limb postoperatively.

INFORMED CONSENT

Informed consent starts with the formation of a relationship with the patient and family to create an environment in which an open dialog can occur. Patient participation in the treatment decision-making process is paramount. The surgeon should offer guidance through discussion of the risks and benefits of the most reliable treatment options. Patient education packets and knee models in the office can help patients make an informed decision. A description of a TKA as a resurfacing of the knee joint surface rather than a complete replacement of all the bones in the knee is helpful. As not all patients learn in the same manner, information for patients to take home are often necessary.[41]

As with any elective procedure, the surgeon should never pressure or urge patients to get a joint arthroplasty but rather should create a dialog that allows the patients to determine whether a knee arthroplasty is the correct procedure for them. The patient is the only one who knows how much pain they are in on a daily basis and can decide whether major surgery is worth the risks of the procedure. There is a fundamental difference between "offering surgery" and "recommending surgery" to patients.

It is important to describe a knee arthroplasty as a procedure that should markedly decrease knee pain but may not result in a "perfect" knee. The resulting knee kinematics after TKA do not recreate the normal knee kinematics of the native knee no matter what knee implant design or advanced technology is used.[42-45] TKA should be offered as a reliable option to treat debilitating pain. It also generally affords good functional outcomes for performing daily activities. Although there is a subset of patients who are able to perform a higher level of recreational activities, this should not be guaranteed to the patient, and they must understand that they may have to give up certain recreational sporting activities postoperatively.[4] A brief discussion of prosthesis longevity should also be undertaken, especially in the younger patient population.[46,47] This may bring into consideration alternate nonarthroplasty surgical options or simply a continuance of nonoperative management of the arthritic process.

Although knee arthroplasty has come a long way in terms of rapid patient discharge, it still should be conveyed to patients that this is a major surgical procedure and appropriate risks and benefits should be discussed. A careful discussion of the risk of periprosthetic joint infection and what this would entail in regard to further surgical procedures and medical management should be had with the patient. Helping patients to understand the effects that diabetes, obesity, and smoking have on their risk of infection may help persuade patients to work on the medical comorbidities that are modifiable for them to be optimized before surgery. Additionally, other complications that could markedly affect postoperative recovery such as deep vein thromboses, cardiac events, and significant stiffness in the form of arthrofibrosis should be discussed with the patient. Although rare, a special discussion of peroneal nerve palsy should be had with all patients with valgus knee deformity.[48] Additionally, patients should understand that full knee recovery may take 12 to 18 months and that they will notice changes in strength and function up to a year after the surgical procedure.[49]

Ultimately, the final decision to undergo TKA must come from the patient. They must be comfortable with this decision and be both mentally and physically prepared for the procedure and its recovery. They should be comfortable that they have exhausted all other nonoperative options and that TKA is the next most reliable option to treat their long-standing chronic knee pain.

REFERENCES

1. Van Manen MD, Nace J, Mont MA. Management of primary knee osteoarthritis and indications for total knee arthroplasty for general practitioners. *J Am Osteopath Assoc*. 2012;112(11):709–715.
2. Mancuso CA, Ranawat CS, Esdaile JM, Johanson NA, Charlson ME. Indications for total hip and total knee arthroplasties. Results of orthopaedic surveys. *J Arthroplasty*. 1996;11(1):34–46.
3. Cross 3rd WW, Saleh KJ, Wilt TJ, Kane RL. Agreement about indications for total knee arthroplasty. *Clin Orthop Relat Res*. 2006;446:34–39.
4. Parvizi J, Nunley RM, Berend KR, et al. High level of residual symptoms in young patients after total knee arthroplasty. *Clin Orthop Relat Res*. 2014;472(1):133–137.
5. Foote JA, Smith HK, Jonas SC, Greenwood R, Weale AE. Return to work following knee arthroplasty. *Knee*. 2010;17(1):19–22.
6. Lombardi AV Jr, Nunley RM, Berend KR, et al. Do patients return to work after total knee arthroplasty? *Clin Orthop Relat Res*. 2014;472(1):138–146.
7. Tilbury C, Schaasberg W, Plevier JW, Fiocco M, Nelissen RG, Vliet Vlieland TP. Return to work after total hip and knee arthroplasty: a systematic review. *Rheumatology (Oxford)*. 2014;53(3):512–525.
8. Dalury DF, Tucker KK, Kelley TC. When can I drive?: brake response times after contemporary total knee arthroplasty. *Clin Orthop Relat Res*. 2011;469(1):82–86.
9. Jordan M, Hofmann UK, Rondak I, Gotze M, Kluba T, Ipach I. Brake response time is significantly impaired after total knee arthroplasty: investigation of performing an emergency stop while driving a car. *Am J Phys Med Rehabil*. 2015;94(9):665–676.
10. Brown GA. AAOS Clinical Practice Guideline: treatment of osteoarthritis of the knee: evidence-based guideline, 2nd edition. *J Am Acad Orthop Surg*. 2013;21(9):577–579.
11. Cancienne JM, Patel KJ, Browne JA, Werner BC. Narcotic use and total knee arthroplasty. *J Arthroplasty*. 2018;33(1):113–118.
12. Bedard NA, Pugely AJ, Westermann RW, Duchman KR, Glass NA, Callaghan JJ. Opioid use after total knee arthroplasty: trends and risk factors for prolonged use. *J Arthroplasty*. 2017;32(8):2390–2394.
13. Rozell JC, Courtney PM, Dattilo JR, Wu CH, Lee GC. Preoperative opiate use independently predicts narcotic consumption and complications after total joint arthroplasty. *J Arthroplasty*. 2017;32(9):2658–2662.
14. Chang AH, Chmiel JS, Moisio KC, et al. Varus thrust and knee frontal plane dynamic motion in persons with knee osteoarthritis. *Osteoarthritis Cartilage*. 2013;21(11):1668–1673.
15. Chang A, Hochberg M, Song J, et al. Frequency of varus and valgus thrust and factors associated with thrust presence in persons with or at higher risk of developing knee osteoarthritis. *Arthritis Rheum*. 2010;62(5):1403–1411.
16. Alamanda VK, Springer BD. Perioperative and modifiable risk factors for periprosthetic joint infections (PJI) and recommended guidelines. *Curr Rev Musculoskelet Med*. 2018;11(3):325–331.
17. Adams OP, Herbert JR, Howitt C, Unwin N. The prevalence of peripheral neuropathy severe enough to cause a loss of protective sensation in a population-based sample of people with known and newly detected

diabetes in Barbados: a cross-sectional study. *Diabet Med.* 2019;36(12):1629–1636.

18. Birnbaum K, Prescher A, Hessler S, Heller KD. The sensory innervation of the hip joint-an anatomical study. *Surg Radiol Anat.* 1997;19(6):371–375.

19. Dibra FF, Prieto HA, Gray CF, Parvataneni HK. Don't forget the hip! Hip arthritis masquerading as knee pain. *Arthroplast Today.* 2018;4(1):118–124.

20. Halawi MJ, Cote MP, Singh H, et al. The effect of depression on patient-reported outcomes after total joint arthroplasty is modulated by baseline mental health: a registry study. *J Bone Joint Surg Am.* 2018;100(20): 1735–1741.

21. Gold HT, Slover JD, Joo L, Bosco J, Iorio R, Oh C. Association of depression with 90-day hospital readmission after total joint arthroplasty. *J Arthroplasty.* 2016;31(11):2385–2388.

22. van Raaij TM, Brouwer RW, Reijman M, Bierma-Zeinstra SM, Verhaar JA. Conventional knee films hamper accurate knee alignment determination in patients with varus osteoarthritis of the knee. *Knee.* 2009;16(2): 109–111.

23. Hohman Jr. DW, Nodzo SR, Phillips M, Fitz W. The implications of mechanical alignment on soft tissue balancing in total knee arthroplasty. *Knee Surg Sports Traumatol Arthrosc.* 2015;23(12):3632–3636.

24. Nam D, Maher PA, Robles A, McLawhorn AS, Mayman DJ. Variability in the relationship between the distal femoral mechanical and anatomical axes in patients undergoing primary total knee arthroplasty. *J Arthroplasty.* 2013;28(5):798–801.

25. Mihalko WM, Boyle J, Clark LD, Krackow KA. The variability of intramedullary alignment of the femoral component during total knee arthroplasty. *J Arthroplasty.* 2005;20(1):25–28.

26. Rehder U. Morphometrical studies on the symmetry of the human knee joint: femoral condyles. *J Biomech.* 1983;16(5):351–361.

27. Rosenberg TD, Paulos LE, Parker RD, Coward DB, Scott SM. The forty-five-degree posteroanterior flexion weight-bearing radiograph of the knee. *J Bone Joint Surg Am.* 1988;70(10):1479–1483.

28. Babatunde OM, Danoff JR, Patrick DA Jr, Lee JH, Kazam JK, Macaulay W. The combination of the tunnel view and weight-bearing anteroposterior radiographs improves the detection of knee. *Arthritis.* 2016:2016:9786924.

29. Phillips MJ, Krackow KA. High tibial osteotomy and distal femoral osteotomy for valgus or varus deformity around the knee. *Instr Course Lect.* 1998;47:429–436.

30. Mihalko WM, Krackow KA. Preoperative planning for lower extremity osteotomies: an analysis using

4 different methods and 3 different osteotomy techniques. *J Arthroplasty.* 2001;16(3):322–329.

31. Matsuda S, Miura H, Nagamine R, et al. Anatomical analysis of the femoral condyle in normal and osteoarthritic knees. *J Orthop Res.* 2004;22(1):104–109.

32. Terry GC, Cimino PM. Distal femoral osteotomy for valgus deformity of the knee. *Orthopedics.* 1992;15(11):1283–1289. discussion 1289–1290.

33. Phillips MI, Krackow KA. Distal femoral varus osteotomy: indications and surgical technique. *Instr Course Lect.* 1999;48:125–129.

34. Marti RK, Verhagen RA, Kerkhoffs GM, Moojen TM. Proximal tibial varus osteotomy. Indications, technique, and five to twenty-one-year results. *J Bone Joint Surg Am.* 2001;83(2):164–170.

35. Ranawat AS, Nwachukwu BU, Pearle AD, Zuiderbaan HA, Weeks KD, Khamaisy S. Comparison of lateral closing-wedge versus medial opening-wedge high tibial osteotomy on knee joint alignment and kinematics in the ACL-deficient knee. *Am J Sports Med.* 2016;44(12): 3103–3110.

36. Closkey RF, Windsor RE. Alterations in the patella after a high tibial or distal femoral osteotomy. *Clin Orthop Relat Res.* 2001;389:51–56.

37. Saragaglia D, Sigwalt L, Rubens-Duval B, Chedal-Bornu B, Pailhe R. Concept of combined femoral and tibial osteotomies. *J Knee Surg.* 2017;30(8):756–763.

38. Zuiderbaan HA, van der List JP, Khamaisy S, et al. Unicompartmental knee arthroplasty versus total knee arthroplasty: which type of artificial joint do patients forget? *Knee Surg Sports Traumatol Arthrosc.* 2017;25(3): 681–686.

39. Somayaji HS, Tsaggerides P, Ware HE, Dowd GS. Knee arthrodesis-a review. *Knee.* 2008;15(4):247–254.

40. Cho SH, Jeong ST, Park HB, Hwang SC, Kim DH. Two-stage conversion of fused knee to total knee arthroplasty. *J Arthroplasty.* 2008;23(3):476–479.

41. Johnson MR, Singh JA, Stewart T, Gioe TJ. Patient understanding and satisfaction in informed consent for total knee arthroplasty: a randomized study. *Arthritis Care Res (Hoboken).* 2011;63(7):1048–1054.

42. Stiehl JB, Komistek RD, Dennis DA, Paxson RD, Hoff WA. Fluoroscopic analysis of kinematics after posterior-cruciate-retaining knee arthroplasty. *J Bone Joint Surg Br.* 1995;77(6):884–889.

43. Lutzner J, Kirschner S, Gunther KP, Harman MK. Patients with no functional improvement after total knee arthroplasty show different kinematics. *Int Orthop.* 2012;36(9):1841–1847.

44. Banks SA, Hodge WA. Implant design affects knee arthroplasty kinematics during stair-stepping. *Clin Orthop Relat Res.* 2004;426:187–193.

45. Kanekasu K, Banks SA, Honjo S, Nakata O, Kato H. Fluoroscopic analysis of knee arthroplasty kinematics during deep flexion kneeling. *J Arthroplasty*. 2004;19(8):998–1003.

46. Duffy GP, Crowder AR, Trousdale RR, Berry DJ. Cemented total knee arthroplasty using a modern prosthesis in young patients with osteoarthritis. *J Arthroplasty*. 2007;22(6 Suppl 2):67–70.

47. Hofmann AA, Heithoff SM, Camargo M. Cementless total knee arthroplasty in patients 50 years or younger. *Clin Orthop Relat Res*. 2002;404:102–107.

48. Idusuyi OB, Morrey BF. *Peroneal nerve palsy after total knee arthroplasty. Assessment of predisposing and prognostic factors. J Bone Joint Surg Am*. 1996;78(2): 177–184.

49. Mehta S, Rigney A, Webb K, et al. Characterizing the recovery trajectories of knee range of motion for one year after total knee replacement. *Physiother Theory Pract*. 2020;36(1):176–185.

Modify What's Modifiable: Smoking, Obesity, Opioid Dependence, and Nutritional Deficiencies

Sandeep Munjal, MD, FAAOS, and Ananya Munjal, MS

INTRODUCTION

Total joint arthroplasties are some of the most commonly performed procedures in orthopedic surgery and have high success rates.[1] These surgeries can greatly improve a patient's quality of life.[2]

Even though these procedures generally have positive patient satisfaction rates, the prevalence of several modifiable risk factors can cause increased risk for postoperative complications. The risks associated with smoking, obesity, opioid use, and malnutrition will be discussed in this chapter. With the drastic anticipated increases in rates of arthroplasty in the United States (a 673% predicted increase in primary total knee arthroplasty [TKA] by 2030), knowledge of these risk factors and suggested mitigation practices are essential for identifying potential risks and achieving optimal postoperative results.[3]

SMOKING

Risks

Studies have shown that exposure to nicotine and cigarette smoke decreases cutaneous blood flow.[4] The nicotine and carbon monoxide from cigarettes can also hinder cell proliferation and epithelial regeneration.[5] Prospective human trials have suggested that collagen synthesis in patients who smoke more than a pack of cigarettes a day was lower than the collagen synthesis in matched nonsmoking patients.[6] Collagen is a major determinant of tensile strength in healing wounds and thus is an essential factor to consider in the recovery of postoperative joint replacement patients. Because of that, smoking may lead to higher rates of postoperative wound infections.

Effects of Cotinine

Nicotine has several metabolites. The primary one is cotinine, a breakdown product found in the blood, saliva, and urine of smokers.[7] Cotinine is the most commonly used biomarker to test for tobacco exposure and therefore can be used by healthcare providers to test for tobacco usage before total joint arthroplasty procedures.[8,9] This test can also be used to encourage patients who are smokers to quit by aiding them in monitoring and tracking their smoking consumption.

Cotinine has a half-life of approximately 20 hours and is available as a blood test. Testing cotinine levels before surgical joint procedures can be an effective method to screen for compliance with smoking cessation. Serum cotinine levels of lower than 10 ng/mL should be used as a cutoff consistent with not smoking.[10] However, it is also important to note that these levels vary with race, age, and sex.[11] It is essential to monitor cotinine levels to assess smoking status. It is important to continue to study the relationship between cotinine levels and potential postoperative complications.

Complications

Studies evaluating postoperative outcomes of patients who smoke have demonstrated that smoking can lead to an increase in hospital length of stay, an increase in intensive care unit admissions, greater rates of wound complications, and increased incidence of perioperative joint infections.[12,13] Metaanalysis studies in rheumatology have evaluated the effects of smoking on total joint arthroplasty. This research has suggested that both current and former smokers are at increased risk for development of complications compared with nonsmokers.

These complications include higher rates of reoperation, revision, implant loosening, deep infection, skin necrosis, and mortality (Fig. 2.1).[14]

Cessation

Research has suggested that cessation of smoking before knee arthroplasty surgery can lessen the risk of postoperative infection. Clinical outcome studies have shown that after 4 to 6 weeks of tobacco cessation, metabolic and immune functions begin to recover and normalize.[15] Other studies have suggested that patients who quit tobacco use 4 to 8 weeks before surgery have decreased morbidity and mortality rates compared with current smokers.[16,17] Although some literature suggests that smoking cessation 4 to 6 weeks before joint arthroplasty surgery can lessen the risks posed by nicotine and other byproducts of smoking, current and former smokers are at greater risk for perioperative complications in comparison with patients who have never smoked.[18]

Smoking cessation is essential for proper wound healing and lowering rates of postoperative complications. Despite targeted efforts to aid patients in stopping smoking before surgery, more than 7% of patients are unsuccessful.[7] An additional 55% of patients who do stop smoking before surgery are unsuccessful in maintaining this cessation 8 years after surgery.[8]

For some patients, especially older adults, the anticipation of surgery itself can serve as a motivating factor for risk-reducing behavioral change and can increase the likelihood of smoking cessation.[19] The need for surgery as a life-improving measure may be the first time a patient seriously considers pursuing an avenue for smoking cessation. Furthermore, smoking cessation for surgery can often serve as a start for long-term smoking cessation. In a study on smoking cessation programs before total joint arthroplasty it was found that 35% (13/37) of patients who quit smoking before surgery were still abstinent 1 year postsurgery.[15]

Total joint arthroplasties have the potential to provide smoking patients with goal-oriented motivation to quit smoking and remain abstinent. For this reason, it is crucial for members of the healthcare team to provide resources, both before and after surgical procedures, to patients who smoke to aid them in establishing and

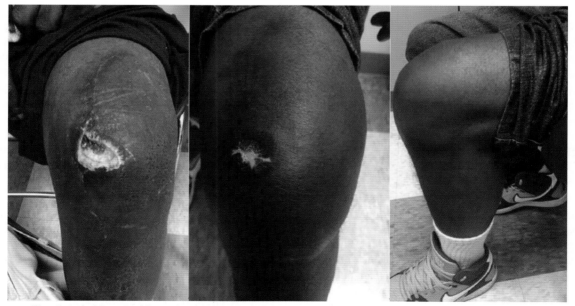

Fig. 2.1 A 62-year-old smoker underwent a primary total knee arthroplasty (TKA) for posttraumatic arthritis. A previous incision was used, and the patient developed skin necrosis on the lateral aspect of the incision. Plastic surgery recommended silver-impregnated dressings. There was no deep tissue necrosis, and infection workup was negative. The patient went on to heal the necrotic area.

maintaining their smoking cessation. These resources include counseling, pharmacotherapy, acupuncture, hypnosis, or a combination of these therapies.[13] Helping all patients achieve these healthy changes has the potential to drastically improve individual patient outcomes and decrease large-scale risks of complications.

OBESITY

The ever-increasing rate of obesity in America today is affecting all sectors of healthcare and poses several risks for detrimental effects for patients pursuing total joint arthroplasty. The Centers for Disease Control and Prevention released a report stating that 54 million obese adults in the United States were affected by osteoarthritis, a common complication of obesity.[20] This number is estimated to rise to approximately 78 million adults by 2040. Preoperative evaluation of surgical risks in total joint arthroplasty patients who are obese is an important period when potential interventions can aid in improving arthroplasty outcomes.[20]

Risks

The risks of having obesity-related complications are greater when combined with joint disease, because this combination can lead to greater pain and increased disability. This presents a specific challenge for orthopedic surgical healthcare teams as positive lifestyle changes and increases in physical activity are difficult to implement when patients are suffering from these negative effects of obesity and osteoarthritis.[20]

It is important to recognize that patients with obesity often have multiple comorbidities, such as coronary artery disease, metabolic syndrome, hypertension, hyperlipidemia, and diabetes mellitus, which increase their risks of postoperative complications and increased lengths of stay.[21] Patients with obesity also have higher rates of postoperative infections and wound complications.[22]

Complications

The mean body mass index (BMI) for patients undergoing arthroplasty in the United States is 33. Patients with obesity (defined as a BMI value ≥30) who pursue TKA have high rates of complications. Patients who are morbidly obese have even greater complications compared with their counterparts who have lower BMI but still have obesity.[23–26] Thus it is suggested that the risk

of complications increases with increased BMI, a trend supported by research demonstrating that increased postoperative complication rates exist at a threshold of BMI >30; these complication rates were even greater in populations with a BMI >40. Predicted causes for these drastically increased complication rates in patients who have BMI >40 are an increase in subcutaneous fat and a greater amount of dead space contributing to seeding of bacteria, which predisposes patients to infection.[22]

Patients with obesity also have unique complications. For example, avulsions of the medial collateral ligament are seen more frequently in this patient population.[27] However, weight and BMI are not the only predictive measures of complications. Distribution of body fat may also be an important factor in determining wound healing and infection risk in knee arthroplasty patients. The prevalence of diabetes, which is an independent risk factor for increased risk of infection postoperatively, is higher in patient populations with obesity.

Prior studies have suggested that the most prevalent complications in patient populations with obesity are venous thromboembolism (VTE) and renal insufficiency.[22] Although there are increased rates of pulmonary embolism in patients with obesity, there is no observed trend of increasing rates with increasing BMI. One hypothesized reason for this correlation is that patients with obesity may be slower to mobilize after surgery, and immobility is a risk factor for VTE. Researchers speculate that rates of renal insufficiency are increased in patients with obesity due to the use of angiotensin II receptor blockers or angiotensin-converting-enzyme inhibitors, drugs that are commonly used in the treatment of hypertension and, if used chronically, can lead to acute kidney injury.[28]

In comparing patient populations with obesity with patients who do not have obesity patients with obesity were suggested to have increased rates of infection, VTE, renal injury, and subsequent unplanned returns to the operating room.[22] In stratifying populations with obesity further, it was noted that patient populations who were morbidly obese had markedly increased risks of postoperative complications compared with other groups with obesity.[22] In considering total joint arthroplasty for patients with obesity morbid obesity should be addressed preoperatively. Several studies have researched the utility of bariatric surgery to decrease a patient's BMI and its effects on outcomes, but this is a risky and controversial approach and the definitive results about the reduction in complications remain uncertain.[29-31]

Patients who have a BMI >30 have been found to have higher wound complication rates and higher hospital readmission and revision surgery rates than patients with BMI <30.[32] Additionally, a retrospective study suggested that a BMI of >40 was a risk factor for developing periprosthetic joint infection after total hip arthroplasty (THA). This finding was supported by a metaanalysis showing that patients with obesity have higher infection rates and significantly higher rates of revision surgery than patients who are not obese. Furthermore, hospital readmission rates for patients with BMI >40 are almost double those of patients who are not obese.[20]

Metabolic Syndrome

When considering patients with obesity, it is imperative to remember that not all patients are the same. Patients who have obesity can sometimes also meet the criteria for metabolic syndrome, which is defined as having a BMI that meets the criteria for obesity (BMI $\geq 30 \, kg/m^2$) and two of the following conditions: hyperlipidemia, hypertriglyceridemia, hypertension, or diabetes.[33] Metabolic syndrome arises from insulin resistance and can lead to many postsurgical complications. Fig. 2.2 shows metabolic syndrome components versus total complication rates and suggests that a diagnosis of metabolic syndrome greatly increases chances for postsurgical complications.[33]

Obesity Reduction Approach

In looking at the drastically increased rates of complications in patient populations with obesity, it is imperative for healthcare teams to encourage these patients to lose weight before surgery. However, several studies have suggested that it is difficult for patients with obesity to lose weight before surgery. Overall, very few patients with obesity can maintain weight loss, even after undergoing total joint arthroplasty. To lessen the risks of postoperative complications, healthcare teams should provide patients with resources for weight loss, counsel them appropriately before surgery, and aid them in the creation of a weight reduction plan preoperatively.[13]

OPIOIDS

The opioid epidemic in the United States is linked with injuries and deaths from medications.[34] To decrease rates of postoperative opioid drug abuse, improved patient and provider education is essential. Multidepartmental research suggests that from 67% to 86% of postoperative patients have access to excessive narcotics from initial prescription, and 92% to 96% of these patients report a lack of information or instruction on how to dispose of unused narcotics.[35] Closing this communication gap between providers and patients and better explaining narcotic disposal options can aid in decreasing the prevalence of narcotic abuse.

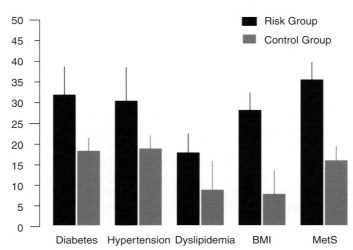

Fig. 2.2 Metabolic syndrome components versus total complication rates. It is important to carefully consider obesity cutoffs for individual patients and keep in mind the risks of metabolic syndrome during preoperative conversations.

Preoperative Testing

Preoperative pain threshold testing has proven to be an objective, simple, reliable, and safe method to help anticipate outpatient narcotic needs in surgical patients.[36] The results of this preoperative sensory test can aid physicians in creating a postoperative medication plan and can aid patients in discontinuing their opioid use postoperatively.[37] A prospective study suggested a significant negative correlation between the results of preoperative pain threshold testing and outpatient narcotic consumption, demonstrating that the higher a patient's measured pain tolerance, the less need there is for narcotic use postoperatively. This information can aid healthcare teams in developing postoperative plans that are tailored specifically for individual patients, thus reducing overprescribing and lessening the potential for abuse, diversion, addiction, or overdose.[36]

Preoperative Opioid Management

Increased rates of opioid use because of increased prescribing have made it very common for patients who have chronic pain to use opioids. This has created a large population of people who consume opioids daily. A large population of patients undergoing surgical procedures are prior chronic prescription opioid users, and these patients require high opioid dose increases after surgery that can persist long into their postoperative care.[38]

To improve patient outcomes, it is recommended that opioid-using patient populations be identified and counseled. Prior studies have suggested that minimizing use of preoperative opioids decreases postoperative risks.[39] Therefore it is imperative for healthcare teams to have discussions regarding opioid dose tapering or cessation before joint surgeries, a practice that is not commonplace. Patients should be educated regarding techniques other than opioid use that can maintain adequate pain control. This practice is especially important in chronic pain patient populations, as prior research suggests that preoperative opioid reduction is protective against adverse postoperative outcomes. The recommendation for care of opioid-using patients is a combination of psychological and opioid screening through a multidisciplinary approach that includes tapering opioid use preoperatively and closely monitoring opioid use postoperatively. It is essential for healthcare teams to establish a pain management system with nonopioid protocols for pain control in these patients.[40]

NUTRITION

Effects of Malnutrition

Studies have suggested that rates of malnutrition in arthroplasty patients can be as high as 26%, and these high rates of malnutrition can lead to decreased immune system function.[41] In a review of patients who had THAs the preoperative presence of malnutrition contributed to joint infection.[42]

Malnutrition in various studies has been defined as serum albumin levels <3.5 or an absolute lymphocyte count <1500, whereas other studies have used other markers such as transferrin or prealbumin. However, these values have been questioned in several studies.[43,44] In a consensus agreement reached through a series of meetings held at the American Society for Enteral and Parenteral Nutrition and European Society for Parenteral and Enteral Nutrition congresses, malnutrition was classified into three groups: starvation-related, chronic disease–related, and acute injury– or disease state–related groups. The classification of malnutrition based on etiology simplifies the issue and also helps determine appropriate management strategies.[45]

Nutritional factors play a crucial role in regulating metabolic pathways and immune system functions. Various nutritional factors that have been identified as playing a role in patients undergoing arthroplasty include serum albumin, serum iron/transferrin, vitamin D, serum zinc, and adiposity.[45]

Role of Vitamins

Vitamin D insufficiency in surgical patients has been associated with increased postoperative pain and increased risk of periprosthetic infections.[46,47] Prior research has suggested that the prevalence of patients who have levels of vitamin D lower than 20 ng/mL is 41%.[48] In patients who had undergone elective joint arthroplasty procedures prevalence of vitamin D deficiency in patients who had periprosthetic fractures was about 66%. The prevalence of vitamin D–deficient patients who had arthroplasties was approximately 54%. Studies on patients who had hip arthroplasties for osteoarthritis have suggested that increased levels of 25-hydroxy-vitamin D in male patients were associated with a 25% increase in need for arthroplasty. Screening and correcting for low vitamin D levels can prove to be instrumental in lessening pain and infection risks associated with joint arthroplasty procedures.

Although vitamin D has a well-recognized role in bone health, it also plays an important role in innate immunity. The immunomodulatory actions of vitamin D are well recognized and are a key factor in innate and adaptive immunity and immunity modulation. Vitamin D may improve outcomes by reducing local and systemic inflammatory responses as a result of modulating cytokine responses and reducing toll-like receptor activation. It also stimulates expression of potent antimicrobial peptides, such as cathelicidin and beta-defensin 2.

Similarly, vitamin C has been identified as an important nutritional variable. Vitamin C has well-recognized antioxidant properties and has been used in arthroplasty to prevent systemic inflammatory response syndrome. It is also known to have immunostimulant, antibacterial, and antiviral properties and has been advocated for the reduction of regional pain syndrome.[45,49–52]

Role of Zinc and Lymphocytes

A prospective research study suggested that the presence of low zinc levels in preoperative arthroplasty patients was correlated with delayed and poor wound healing.[53] This study also suggested a significant correlation between lymphocyte counts <1500 and delayed wound healing in THA patients. Patients should be screened for zinc levels before surgery, and healthcare teams should use a cutoff value of <95 mg/dL to determine which patients should have supplemental zinc before surgery.

Role of Albumin

Protein deficiency causes atrophy of lymphoid organs. This atrophy affects several immune functions such as lymphocyte proliferation, antibody responses, interleukin-2 (IL-2), interferon-gamma, and delayed-type hypersensitivity reactions.[54] In a later study 49,603 primary THA or TKA patients were retrospectively reviewed using the American College of Surgeons National Surgical Quality Improvement Project database. Hypoalbuminemia was identified in 4.0% of cases and was associated with a 2-fold increase in the rate of surgical site infection. This study also demonstrated independent associations between hypoalbuminemia and increased risk of pneumonia, prolonged hospital length of stay, and readmission.[55]

Identification of At-Risk Patients

Obesity, low BMI, prior gastric bypass, malabsorption states, and hypermetabolic states can increase risks.

Referral to a bariatric center for counseling and potential surgical management of obesity may be appropriate in certain cases. However, some forms of bariatric surgery may lead to malabsorption, and monitoring and supplementation are important in these patients.[45] Routine preoperative laboratory studies should include a complete blood count with differential to identify anemia and quantify absolute lymphocyte count. A reticulocyte count is also helpful to determine marrow response to anemia. Serum albumin and transferrin levels and a hemoglobin A1C should be obtained. Optimization of anemia can include iron, vitamin C, and folate supplementation. Patients who have a preoperative hemoglobin <11 g/dL should have additional tests to determine the etiology. Screening for vitamin D deficiency may also be useful.[45]

Preoperative Malnutrition Screenings and Recommendations

For patients undergoing surgical procedures, various malnutrition screening tools are available. The most common serological markers are serum albumin levels <35 mg/dL, lymphocyte counts <1500, and transferrin levels <200. Anthropometric measures and nutritional screening tools have also been described in orthopedic literature as tools for screening. Although anthropometric measures have been useful for nutritional screening, there are no established cutoff values, and their usefulness has been limited.

Correction of Malnutrition in Elective Arthroplasty Patients

Protein supplementation for patients who have protein deficiency can be accomplished with nutritional shakes, with a target intake of 1 g/kg daily. Oral nutritional supplements should be enriched with immune-modulating substances, including arginine, omega-3 fatty acids, and nucleotides.[45]

Simple interventions can include iron supplementation (324 mg per oral three times daily for 3 to 4 weeks) and vitamin C (500 mg per oral daily) to aid iron absorption and collagen cross-linking, which aids wound healing. Zinc (11 mg per oral daily) can also aid in wound healing. Additionally, vitamin D supplementation of 25 mcg daily is recommended for routine maintenance. Patients with vitamin D levels <20 ng/mL should be given greater supplementation with 1250 mcg weekly for 8 weeks followed by maintenance doses of 37.5 to 50 mcg daily with yearly vitamin D level monitoring.

Levels between 20 and 30 ng/dL should be treated with daily vitamin D supplementation of 125 mcg for 3 to 6 months followed by retesting.

CONCLUSION

In approaching joint arthroplasty procedures, evaluation of risk factors is just as important, if not more important, than the quality of the surgery itself. Good surgical outcomes start with good patient selection. The risks and benefits of joint arthroplasty should be carefully weighed in high-risk patients, and surgery should be delayed until appropriate medical optimization has been achieved. Following the famous saying, "Good surgeons know how to operate, better surgeons know when to operate, and the best surgeons know when not to operate," the need for an objective assessment of the likelihood of adverse patient outcomes caused by patient risk factors cannot be overemphasized.

It is essential for healthcare teams to prescreen patients for the four major modifiable risk factors discussed in this chapter: smoking, obesity, opioid abuse, and malnutrition. Teams should have discussions with patients and their families regarding how lifestyle changes, that can be made preoperatively, can lead to better outcomes, more effective healing, and lower complication rates.

Curbing patient expectations is another crucial component of surgery, as patients seeking joint arthroplasties today are younger, better educated, living longer, and have higher expectations. Unrealistic expectations can have a profound effect on surgical outcomes, leading to frustration, dissatisfaction, and unnecessary resource utilization. Communication and transparency, outlining clear and achievable goals, are necessary for correcting unrealistic expectations before surgery. Today, more than ever, we are challenged to provide efficient, high-quality, patient-centered care. Ensuring good outcomes should be a top priority, not just from a financial standpoint but also as a moral obligation. We should strive to be leaders in the face of challenges, using innovation and integrity to produce the best results and advance our profession.[56]

REFERENCES

1. Learmonth ID, Young C. Rorabeck C. The operation of the century: total hip replacement. *Lancet.* 2007;370:1508–1519. https://doi.org/10.1016/S0140-6736(07)60457-7.

2. Hawker G, Wright J, Coyte P, Paul J, Dittus R, Croxford R, et al. Health-related quality of life after knee replacement. *J Bone Jt Surg Am.* 1998;80:163–173. https://doi.org/10.2106/00004623-199802000-00003.

3. Kurtz S, Ong K, Lau E, Mowat F, Halpern M. Projections of primary and revision hip and knee arthroplasty in the United States from 2005 to 2030. *J Bone Jt Surg Am.* 2007;89:780. https://doi.org/10.2106/JBJS.F.00222.

4. Porter SE, Hanley EN. The musculoskeletal effects of smoking. *J Am Acad Orthop Surg.* 2001;9:9–17. https://doi.org/10.5435/00124635-200101000-00002.

5. Sherwin MA, Gastwirth CM. Detrimental effects of cigarette smoking on lower extremity wound healing. *J Foot Surg.* 1990;29:84–87.

6. Jørgensen CC, Kehlet H. Outcomes in smokers and alcohol users after fast-track hip and knee arthroplasty. *Acta Anaesthesiol Scand.* 2013;57:631–638. https://doi.org/10.1111/aas.12086.

7. Hart A, Rainer WG, Taunton MJ, Mabry TM, Berry DJ, Abdel MP. Cotinine testing improves smoking cessation before total joint arthroplasty. *J Arthroplasty.* 2019;34:S148–S151. https://doi.org/10.1016/j.arth.2018.11.039.

8. Kim S. Overview of cotinine cutoff values for smoking status classification. *Int J Environ Res Public Health.* 2016;13:1236. https://doi.org/10.3390/ijerph13121236.

9. Benowitz NL. Biomarkers of environmental tobacco smoke exposure. *Environ Health Perspect.* 1999;107(Suppl 2):349–355. https://doi.org/10.1289/ehp.99107s2349.

10. Hammond SK, Leaderer BP. A diffusion monitor to measure exposure to passive smoking. *Environ Sci Technol.* 1987;21:494–497. https://doi.org/10.1021/es00159a012.

11. Moyer TP, Charlson JR, Enger RJ, Dale LC, Ebbert JO, Schroeder DR, et al. Simultaneous analysis of nicotine, nicotine metabolites, and tobacco alkaloids in serum or urine by tandem mass spectrometry, with clinically relevant metabolic profiles. *Clin Chem.* 2002;48:1460–1471. https://doi.org/10.1093/clinchem/48.9.1460.

12. Singh JA, Houston TK, Ponce BA, Maddox G, Bishop MJ, Richman J, et al. Smoking as a risk factor for short-term outcomes following primary total hip and total knee replacement in veterans. *Arthritis Care Res (Hoboken).* 2011;63:1365–1374. https://doi.org/10.1002/acr.20555.

13. Springer BD. Modifying risk factors for total joint arthroplasty: Strategies that work nicotine. *J Arthroplasty.* 2016;31:1628–1630. https://doi.org/10.1016/j.arth.2016.01.071.

14. Singh JA. Smoking and outcomes after knee and hip arthroplasty: A systematic review. *J Rheumatol.* 2011;38:1824–1834. https://doi.org/10.3899/jrheum.101221.

15. Villebro NM, Pedersen T, Møller AM, Tønnesen H. Long-term effects of a preoperative smoking cessation programme. *Clin Respir J*. 2008;2:175–182. https://doi.org/10.1111/j.1752-699X.2008.00058.x.

16. Møller AM, Kjellberg J, Pedersen T. Health economic analysis of smoking cessation prior to surgery—based on a randomized study. *Ugeskr Laeger*. 2006;168:1026–1030.

17. Lindström D, Azodi OS, Wladis A, Tønnesen H, Linder S, Nåsell H, et al. Effects of a perioperative smoking cessation intervention on postoperative complications: A randomized trial. *Ann Surg*. 2008;248:739–745. https://doi.org/10.1097/SLA.0b013e3181889d0d.

18. Duchman KR, Gao Y, Pugely AJ, Martin CT, Noiseux NO, Callaghan JJ. The effect of smoking on short-term complications following total hip and knee arthroplasty. *J Bone Jt Surg Am*. 2015;97:1049–1058. https://doi.org/10.2106/JBJS.N.01016.

19. McBride CM, Emmons KM, Lipkus IM. Understanding the potential of teachable moments: The case of smoking cessation. *Health Educ Res*. 2003;18:156–170. https://doi.org/10.1093/her/18.2.156.

20. Fournier MN, Hallock J, Mihalko WM. Preoperative optimization of total joint arthroplasty surgical risk: Obesity. *J Arthroplasty*. 2016;31:1620–1624. https://doi.org/10.1016/j.arth.2016.02.085.

21. Allen SR. Total knee and hip arthroplasty across BMI categories: A feasible option for the morbidly obese patient. *J Surg Res*. 2012;175:215–217. https://doi.org/10.1016/j.jss.2011.07.033.

22. Zusmanovich M, Kester BS, Schwarzkopf R. Postoperative complications of total joint arthroplasty in obese patients stratified by BMI. *J Arthroplasty*. 2018;33:856–864. https://doi.org/10.1016/j.arth.2017.09.067.

23. Friedman RJ, Hess S, Berkowitz SD, Homering M. Complication rates after hip or knee arthroplasty in morbidly obese patients. *Clin Orthop Relat Res*. 2013;471:3358–3366. https://doi.org/10.1007/s11999-013-3049-9.

24. Kerkhoffs GMMJ, Servien E, Dunn W, Dahm D, Bramer JAM, Haverkamp D. The influence of obesity on the complication rate and outcome of total knee arthroplasty: A meta-analysis and systematic literature review. *J Bone Jt Surg Am*. 2012;94:1939–1844. https://doi.org/10.2106/JBJS.K.00820.

25. Martin JR, Jennings JM, Dennis DA. Morbid obesity and total knee arthroplasty: A growing problem. *J Am Acad Orthop Surg*. 2017;25:188–194. https://doi.org/10.5435/JAAOS-D-15-00684.

26. Dowsey MM, Choong PFM. Obese diabetic patients are at substantial risk for deep infection after primary TKA. *Clin Orthop Relat Res*. 2009;467:1577–1581. https://doi.org/10.1007/s11999-008-0551-6.

27. Winiarsky R, Earth P, Lotke P. Total knee arthroplasty in morbidly obese patients. *J Bone Jt Surg Am*. 1998;80:1770–1774. https://doi.org/10.2106/00004623-199812000-00006.

28. Kimmel LA, Wilson S, Janardan JD, Liew SM, Walker RG. Incidence of acute kidney injury following total joint arthroplasty: A retrospective review by RIFLE criteria. *Clin Kidney J*. 2014;7:546–551. https://doi.org/10.1093/ckj/sfu108.

29. Severson EP, Singh JA, Browne JA, Trousdale RT, Sarr MG, Lewallen DG. Total knee arthroplasty in morbidly obese patients treated with bariatric surgery. A comparative study. *J Arthroplasty*. 2012;27:1696–1700. https://doi.org/10.1016/j.arth.2012.03.005.

30. Parvizi J, Trousdale RT, Sarr MG. Total joint arthroplasty in patients surgically treated for morbid obesity. *J Arthroplasty*. 2000;15:1003–1008. https://doi.org/10.1054/arth.2000.9054.

31. Inacio MCS, Paxton EW, Fisher D, Li RA, Barber TC, Singh JA. Bariatric surgery prior to total joint arthroplasty may not provide dramatic improvements in post-arthroplasty surgical outcomes. *J Arthroplasty*. 2014;29:1359–1364. https://doi.org/10.1016/j.arth.2014.02.021.

32. Jameson SS, Mason JM, Baker PN, Elson DW, Deehan DJ, Reed MR. The impact of body mass index on patient reported outcome measures (proms) and complications following primary hip arthroplasty. *J Arthroplasty*. 2014;29:1889–1898. https://doi.org/10.1016/j.arth.2014.05.019.

33. Gage MJ, Schwarzkopf R, Abrouk M, Slover JD. Impact of metabolic syndrome on perioperative complication rates after total joint arthroplasty surgery. *J Arthroplasty*. 2014;29:1842–1845. https://doi.org/10.1016/j.arth.2014.04.009.

34. Lucas CE, Vlahos AL, Ledgerwood AM. Kindness kills: The negative impact of pain as the fifth vital sign. *J Am Coll Surg*. 2007;205:101–107. https://doi.org/10.1016/j.jamcollsurg.2007.01.062.

35. Bates C, Laciak R, Southwick A, Bishoff J. Overprescription of postoperative narcotics: A look at postoperative pain medication delivery, consumption and disposal in urological practice. *J Urol*. 2011;185:551–555. https://doi.org/10.1016/j.juro.2010.09.088.

36. Nickel BT, Klement MR, Byrd WA, Attarian DE, Seyler TM, Wellman SS. The James A. Rand Young Investigator's Award: Battling the opioid epidemic with prospective pain threshold measurement. *J Arthroplasty*. 2018;33:S3–S7. https://doi.org/10.1016/j.arth.2018.02.060.

37. Zarling BJ, Yokhana SS, Herzog DT, Markel DC. Preoperative and postoperative opiate use by the arthroplasty patient. *J Arthroplasty*. 2016;31:2081–2084. https://doi.org/10.1016/j.arth.2016.03.061.

38. Gulur P, Nelli AH. The opioid-tolerant patient: Opioid optimization. *J Arthroplasty.* 2020;35:S50–S52. https://doi.org/10.1016/j.arth.2020.01.001.

39. Zywiel MG, Stroh DA, Lee SY, Bonutti PM, Mont MA. Chronic opioid use prior to total knee arthroplasty. *J Bone Jt Surg Am.* 2011;93:1988–1993. https://doi.org/10.2106/JBJS.J.01473.

40. Nguyen LCL, Sing DC, Bozic KJ. Preoperative reduction of opioid use before total joint arthroplasty. *J Arthroplasty.* 2016;31(Suppl 9):282–287. https://doi.org/10.1016/j.arth.2016.01.068.

41. Rai J, Gill SS, Satish Kumar BRJ. The influence of preoperative nutritional status in wound healing after replacement arthroplasty. *Orthopedics.* 2002;25:417–421. https://doi.org/10.3928/0147-7447-20020401-17.

42. Bohl DD, Shen MR, Kayupov E, Cvetanovich GL, Della Valle CJ. Is hypoalbuminemia associated with septic failure and acute infection after revision total joint arthroplasty? A study of 4517 patients from the National Surgical Quality Improvement Program. *J Arthroplasty.* 2016;31:963–967. https://doi.org/10.1016/j.arth.2015.11.025.

43. Gherini S, Vaughn BK, Lombardi AV, Mallory TH. Delayed wound healing and nutritional deficiencies after total hip arthroplasty. *Clin Orthop Relat Res.* 1993;293:188–195. https://doi.org/10.1097/00003086-199308000-00023.

44. Kuzuya M, Kanda S, Koike T, Suzuki Y, Iguchi A. Lack of correlation between total lymphocyte count and nutritional status in the elderly. *Clin Nutr.* 2005;24:427–432. https://doi.org/10.1016/j.clnu.2005.01.003.

45. Golladay GJ, Satpathy J, Jiranek WA. Patient optimization—Strategies that work: Malnutrition. *J Arthroplasty.* 2016;31:1631–1634. https://doi.org/10.1016/j.arth.2016.03.027.

46. Maier GS, Horas K, Seeger JB, Roth KE, Kurth AA, Maus U. Is there an association between periprosthetic joint infection and low vitamin D levels? *Int Orthop.* 2014;38:1499–1504. https://doi.org/10.1007/s00264-014-2338-6.

47. Lavernia CJ, Sierra RJ, Baerga L. Nutritional parameters and short term outcome in arthroplasty. *J Am Coll Nutr.* 1999;18:274–278. https://doi.org/10.1080/07315724.1999.10718863.

48. Forrest KYZ, Stuhldreher WL. Prevalence and correlates of vitamin D deficiency in US adults. *Nutr Res.* 2011;31:48–54. https://doi.org/10.1016/j.nutres.2010.12.001.

49. Chesney RW. Vitamin D and the magic mountain: The anti-infectious role of the vitamin. *J Pediatr.* 2010;156:698–703. https://doi.org/10.1016/j.jpeds.2010.02.002.

50. Hewison M. Vitamin D and immune function: An overview. *Proc Nutr Soc.* 2012;71:50–61. https://doi.org/10.1017/S0029665111001650.

51. Veldman CM, Cantorna MT, DeLuca HF. Expression of 1, 25-dihydroxyvitamin D3 receptor in the immune system. *Arch Biochem Biophys.* 2000;374:334–338. https://doi.org/10.1006/abbi.1999.1605.

52. Conway FJS, Talwar D, McMillan DC. The relationship between acute changes in the systemic inflammatory response and plasma ascorbic acid, alpha-tocopherol and lipid peroxidation after elective hip arthroplasty. *Clin Nutr.* 2015;34:642–646. https://doi.org/10.1016/j.clnu.2014.07.004.

53. Zorrilla P, Gómez LA, Salido JA, Silva A, López-Alonso A. Low serum zinc level as a predictive factor of delayed wound healing in total hip replacement. *Wound Repair Regen.* 2006;14:119–122. https://doi.org/10.1111/j.1743-6109.2006.00100.x.

54. Calder PC. Feeding the immune system. *Proc Nutr Soc.* 2013;72:299–309. https://doi.org/10.1017/S0029665113001286.

55. Bohl DD, Shen MR, Kayupov E, Della Valle CJ. Hypoalbuminemia independently predicts surgical site infection, pneumonia, length of stay, and readmission after total joint arthroplasty. *J Arthroplasty.* 2016;31:15–21. https://doi.org/10.1016/j.arth.2015.08.028.

56. Halawi MJ, Greene K, Barsoum WK. Optimizing outcomes of total joint arthroplasty under the comprehensive care for joint replacement model. *Am J Orthop (Belle Mead NJ).* 2016;45:E112–E113.

3

Optimizing Important Comorbidities: Diabetes, Rheumatoid Arthritis, Peripheral Vascular Disease, and Cardiac Disease

Jesus Fajardo, MD, and Sridhar R. Rachala, MD

The decision to recommend any surgery hinges on the severity of pathology and on the various risk factors the patient has while undergoing surgery. The risk–benefit analysis is an integral part of any surgeon's thought process when offering surgery. Any surgical procedure can be classified into four categories (Fig. 3.1) based on anticipated risk and benefit. In general, surgery is not recommended when the anticipated benefit is low. The ideal scenario is low risk and high benefit, thereby maximizing the success of any surgery. Sometimes it may be necessary to face a scenario where the risk is high but the potential benefit is also high (high risk, high benefit). In this case it is prudent to ask a few questions:

1. Is the risk modifiable? If so, what are the strategies, and how effective are those?
2. If it is a nonmodifiable risk factor, how can the patient be adequately optimized before the surgery?
3. Is the potential benefit worth the risk of going through the surgery?

The surgeon should have an honest discussion with the patient about the risks and benefits and involve them in the decision-making process to maximize the effect of any risk modification. Also, the patients should be given reasonable achievable goals and be directed to appropriate resources to help them accomplish those goals using a team approach that is coordinated by the primary physician.

This chapter deals with optimizing diabetes, rheumatoid arthritis, peripheral vascular disease, and cardiac disease before a total knee arthroplasty (TKA).

DIABETES MELLITUS

Diabetes mellitus is a chronic disease in which the body's ability to properly regulate glucose metabolism is impaired, resulting in high blood glucose levels. Diabetes can occur when the pancreas makes little or no insulin (type 1 diabetes) or when insulin resistance develops and the body fails to respond to endogenous insulin appropriately (type 2 diabetes). Patients who have type 1 diabetes are dependent on insulin for blood glucose control, whereas patients who have type 2 diabetes may receive treatment with a variety of oral and injectable medications, including exogenous insulin. Glycemic control is important, as poorly controlled diabetes can contribute to the development of microvascular and macrovascular complications, including retinopathy, nephropathy, neuropathy, peripheral artery disease, coronary artery disease, and stroke.[1]

Diabetes is a well-documented risk factor for postoperative complications after TKA, especially when it is not well controlled.[2-4] Complications can include superficial infection, deep infection, stroke, deep vein thrombosis, pneumonia, and death.[2,3,5-8] Because TKA is an elective procedure meant to improve patients' quality of life, a marked amount of research has been devoted to determine the best way to assess and optimize diabetes before arthroplasty to reduce the risk of complications.

The American Diabetes Association provides several criteria by which a diagnosis of diabetes can be made, one of which is a hemoglobin A1c (HbA1c)

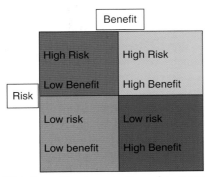

Fig. 3.1 Risk–benefit categorization of surgery.

BOX 3.1 Criteria for the Diagnosis of Diabetes

Fasting plasma glucose $\geq$126 mg/dL. Fasting is defined as no caloric intake for at least 8 hours.
Two-hour plasma glucose $\geq$200 mg/dL during oral glucose tolerance test (glucose load of 75 g glucose in water)
Hemoglobin A1c $\geq$6.5%
In a patient with classic symptoms of hyperglycemia or hyperglycemic crisis a random plasma glucose $\geq$200 mg/dL

Adapted from American Diabetes Association. Classification and diagnosis of diabetes: *Standards of medical care in diabetes–2020. Diabetes Care.* 2020;43(suppl 1):S14–S31.

>6.5% (Box 3.1).[9] The HbA1c test measures glycated hemoglobin and reflects the previous 2 to 3 months of glycemic control in the setting of the usual red blood cell life span of 120 days.[10] HbA1c is used in diagnosing diabetes and monitoring response to antihyperglycemic treatment, so the association between HbA1c and postoperative complications in TKA has been a topic of interest. One study found an increased rate of superficial surgical site infection after TKA in patients who had a preoperative HbA1c $\geq$8% and/or fasting blood glucose $\geq$200 mg/dL[11] Another multicenter, retrospective study found that high HbA1c levels were associated with an increased risk of prosthetic joint infection after total joint arthroplasty, and it identified a threshold HbA1c of 7.7%.[12] Other studies, however, have shown a weak[13] or no[14,15] significant association between HbA1c and the risk of prosthetic knee infection. One study found that even though diabetic patients had a significantly higher risk for infection after TKA compared with nondiabetic patients, HbA1c was not a reliable

predictor of infection.[16] Furthermore, many diabetic patients might not be able to achieve a HbA1c $\leq$7.0%[17] Considering all this, some institutions have adopted a HbA1c target of less than 8%.[18]

Perioperative hyperglycemia has been evaluated in patients undergoing TKA as a predictor of infection and other adverse outcomes. One study found that although HbA1c did not perfectly correlate with the risk of prosthetic joint infection, perioperative hyperglycemia did; patients with a blood glucose level $\geq$194 mg/dL within the 7 days before surgery were at increased risk of developing a prosthetic joint infection.[19] Although the study did not find HbA1c to be a good predictor for prosthetic joint infection, researchers did observe a significantly higher 2-year mortality in patients with HbA1c >7%. In addition to an increased risk for prosthetic joint infection, preoperative hyperglycemia has also been implicated in increasing the risk of revision for aseptic loosening.[20] The effect of postoperative hyperglycemia has been investigated. One study found a linear relationship between postoperative blood glucose levels and periprosthetic joint infection,[21] further highlighting the importance of blood glucose control not only over the previous 3 months, as reflected in the HbA1c, but also during the perioperative period.

The association between the glycemic marker fructosamine and postoperative complications after total joint arthroplasty has been studied. Fructosamines are molecules formed through the glycation of proteins, and the fructosamine test measures the level of glycated proteins in the serum (mainly albumin).[22] In patients who have diabetes mellitus the level of fructosamine molecules in the serum is elevated due the increased blood glucose levels. Because of the relatively short half-life of serum proteins, fructosamine reflects glycemic control over the previous 2 to 3 weeks.[22] A 2017 study found that patients who had preoperative fructosamine levels of $\geq$292 mmol/L had a significantly higher risk of developing adverse outcomes, including prosthetic joint infection, readmission, and reoperation.[23] Although the rate of prosthetic joint infection was 3.3-times higher in patients with HbA1c levels of $\geq$7%, it did not reach statistical significance. A follow-up multicenter prospective study validated fructosamine as a predictor of adverse complications, with a fructosamine level of 293 mmol/L identified as the optimal cutoff associated with adverse outcomes.[24] Patients with elevated fructosamine levels had a 11.2-times higher rate of prosthetic joint infection, 4.2-times higher rate of readmission, and 4.5-times higher rate of reoperation compared with patients who did not have elevated fructosamine levels. HbA1c thresholds of 7% and 7.5%, however, failed to show a significant association with complications. A subset of patients who had elevated fructosamine levels, but a normal HbA1c, were found to have a higher risk of prosthetic joint infection compared with patients with low fructosamine levels and an elevated HbA1c. Because HbA1c reflects the mean blood glucose over the previous 2 to 3 months, spikes in blood glucose levels can be masked if the blood glucose levels are controlled the majority of the time. Because fructosamine reflects the mean blood glucose levels over the previous 2 to 3 weeks, spikes in blood glucose levels are not as easily diluted. Spikes in perioperative blood glucose levels, as some studies have shown, can be a strong predictor of postoperative complications.[14,19–21,25]

In 2018 the International Consensus meeting evaluated the data available at the time and recommended that routine screening for diabetes and glycemic control has the potential to reduce postoperative infections.[26] A study evaluating routine preoperative HbA1c screening in total joint arthroplasty patients found that 33.6% of patients had undiagnosed dysglycemia and 2.6% were undiagnosed diabetics.[27] Similarly, in another study 2.5% of screened patients were found to have undiagnosed diabetes based on HbA1c $\geq 6.5\%$.[23] Therefore consideration should be given to screening all patients being considered for TKA. The optimal glycemic marker for preoperative screening continues to be an active area of research, but an HbA1c threshold of 7.5% to 8.0% is a reasonable cutoff based on the data available at this time. Optimization of glycemic control should be multimodal and should be coordinated with the patient's primary physician or endocrinologist, and it can include pharmacological treatment and dietary modification.

When evaluating a patient who has diabetes mellitus for TKA, it is important to remember the associated comorbidities that are frequently present with diabetes. Patients who have type 2 diabetes are frequently overweight or obese.[28] Obesity has also been identified as a risk factor for postoperative complications after TKA.[29–31] Weight loss can address obesity and improve glycemic control.[32,33] The weight loss strategy can include referral to a weight management program, self-directed exercise, and dietary modifications in consultation with a dietician. Bariatric surgery can also be considered, although the utility of bariatric surgery in reducing perioperative complications remains controversial.[34–37]

Diabetes can result in long-term complications, including peripheral vascular disease and renal insufficiency.[1] The lower extremities should be carefully evaluated preoperatively, with special attention to the peripheral pulses. The presence of decreased or absent pulses, skin changes, hairlessness, or chronic wounds should prompt further evaluation. This can include ankle-brachial indices (ABIs) and referral to a vascular surgeon. With regard to renal insufficiency, modifications might need to be made with regard to perioperative medication dosages to avoid further renal injury.

RHEUMATOID ARTHRITIS

Rheumatoid arthritis is a chronic autoimmune disease that results in systemic inflammation and manifestations in various organ systems, including the musculoskeletal system, cardiovascular system, pulmonary system, hematological system, and renal system. In the musculoskeletal system rheumatoid arthritis is characterized by the presence of synovitis in multiple joints that causes pain, swelling, stiffness, deformity, destruction, and eventual loss of function. Rheumatoid arthritis predominantly affects the small joints of the hands and feet, but it can also affect larger joints such as the hips and knees. Approximately 25% of patients who have rheumatoid arthritis eventually undergo major joint arthroplasty to improve pain and function.[38,39] With advances in the medical management of rheumatoid arthritis with disease-modifying antirheumatic drugs (DMARDs), a decrease in the incidence of total joint arthroplasty in patients with rheumatoid arthritis has been observed.[40–42] It is estimated that approximately 3% of patients undergoing total hip arthroplasty (THA) and TKA have rheumatoid arthritis,[41] and this subset of patients deserves special attention because of the increased risk for associated comorbidities that must be considered preoperatively and the increased risk of postoperative complications.

Rheumatoid arthritis can involve the cervical spine and, through bony erosion and increased ligamentous laxity, cause instability and subluxation. Anterior atlantoaxial subluxation is the most frequently occurring deformity, although other conditions such as cranial settling and subaxial subluxation can also occur.[43] Historically, 30% to 50% of patients who had rheumatoid arthritis also had cervical spine involvement,[44,45] although the use of DMARDs[46,47] has decreased the incidence and progression of cervical spine involvement. Cervical spine instability, when present, can cause cord compression that results in myelopathy and even sudden death.[48] Because of the manipulation of the head and cervical spine involved in direct laryngoscopy and intubation, routine preoperative evaluation of the cervical spine with dynamic flexion and extension lateral radiographs in patients who have rheumatoid arthritis has been recommeneded.[43] Consultation with a spine surgeon should be considered in patients who have abnormal radiographic findings and in patients who have signs and symptoms of myelopathy. Anesthesiologist should also be consulted for consideration of alternative intubation techniques such as fiber optic intubation.

It has been documented that patients who have rheumatoid arthritis are at increased risk of cardiac disease and cardiac events compared with the general population.[48,49] Some studies have even shown that rheumatoid arthritis is comparable with diabetes mellitus as a risk factor for cardiovascular disease and myocardial infarction.[50,51] In addition to coronary artery disease, cardiac manifestations of rheumatoid arthritis can include pericardial effusion and valvular disease.[52] Because of the prevalence of heart disease in the general population and especially in patients who have rheumatoid arthritis, routine preoperative evaluation should include an electrocardiogram. If abnormalities are identified, there should be a low threshold for evaluation with an echocardiogram and consultation with a cardiologist.

Pulmonary manifestations as a result of the disease or the use methotrexate using in treating the disease can occur in patients who have rheumatoid arthritis.[53,54] Interstitial lung disease is the most common type of lung involvement in rheumatoid arthritis, with less common manifestations including interstitial pneumonia, organizing pneumonia, bronchiolitis, bronchiectasis, rheumatoid nodules, and pleural effusion.[55] In severe cases respiratory function may be compromised. Evaluation with pulmonary function tests and arterial blood gas should be considered in severe cases with evidence of dyspnea.

Rheumatoid arthritis can result in anemia of chronic disease and renal insufficiency. The prevalence of anemia in patients who have rheumatoid arthritis is estimated to range between 33% and 60%, with a higher frequency in patients who have severe disease.[56] Correctable iron deficiencies should be addressed to maximize the patient's preoperative hemoglobin. The utility of erythropoietin-stimulating agents to increase hemoglobin is unclear at this time.[57] In patients who have a low hemoglobin level or in whom much blood loss is expected preoperative autologous blood donation and the use of intraoperative autologous blood recovery systems ("cell savers") are options that can be considered. In patients who have renal insufficiency the level of renal function should be taken into account when determining medications and dosages for antibiotics and postoperative pain control.

One of the biggest challenges for the orthopedic surgeon in the management of patients who have rheumatoid arthritis and are undergoing TKA is the perioperative management of DMARDs. Patients who have rheumatoid arthritis are at increased risk of developing deep postoperative infections after TKA,[58] with some studies showing increased risk of infection in patients taking biological DMARDs[59] and other studies showing that continuation of methotrexate treatment does not increase the risk of complications.[60] Because of the wide variety of DMARDs available and the sparse direct evidence on their perioperative management, in 2017 the American College of Rheumatology and American Association of Hip and Knee Surgeons published a joint guideline for the perioperative management of antirheumatic medication in patients with rheumatic diseases undergoing elective THA or TKA.[61] Fig. 3.2 is a summary of their recommendations. They recommend continuation of the nonbiological DMARDs methotrexate, sulfasalazine, hydroxychloroquine, leflunomide, and doxycycline throughout the perioperative period. Biological drugs, however, should be stopped preoperatively, and surgery should be scheduled for the week after the next dose would have been administered. Tofacitinib, despite having a short half-life, is recommended to be withheld for 7 days before surgery because the duration of immunosuppression after it is stopped has yet to be determined. Biological agents may then be restarted a minimum of 14 days after the surgery as long as there is no concern for wound healing problems, surgical site infection, or systemic infection. These recommendation are conditional and may not be universally applicable, so coordination with the patient's rheumatologist is advisable.

Patients who have rheumatoid arthritis may present with specific intraarticular and extraarticular manifestations of disease. Extraarticular manifestations include cardiac disease, pulmonary disease, cervical spine instability, anemia, and renal insufficiency. Evaluation and

DMARDs: CONTINUE these medications through surgery.	Dosing Interval	Continue/Withhold
Methotrexate	Weekly	Continue
Sulfasalazine	Once or twice daily	Continue
Hydroxychloroquine	Once or twice daily	Continue
Leflunomide (Arava)	Daily	Continue
Doxycycline	Daily	Continue
BIOLOGIC AGENTS: STOP these medications prior to surgery and schedule surgery at the end of the dosing cycle. RESUME medications at minimum 14 days after surgery in the absence of wound healing problems, surgical site infection, or systemic infection.	Dosing Interval	Schedule Surgery (relative to last biologic agent dose administered) during
Adalimumab (Humira)	Weekly or every 2 weeks	Week 2 or 3
Etanercept (Enbrel)	Weekly or twice weekly	Week 2
Golimumab (Simponi)	Every 4 weeks (SQ) or every 8 weeks (IV)	Week 5 Week 9
Infliximab (Remicade)	Every 4, 6, or 8 weeks	Week 5, 7, or 9
Abatacept (Orencia)	Monthly (IV) or weekly (SQ)	Week 5 Week 2
Certolizumab (Cimzia)	Every 2 or 4 weeks	Week 3 or 5
Rituximab (Rituxan)	2 doses 2 weeks apart every 4–6 months	Month 7
Tocilizumab (Actemra)	Every week (SQ) or every 4 weeks (IV)	Week 2 Week 5
Anakinra (Kineret)	Daily	Day 2
Secukinumab (Cosentyx)	Every 4 weeks	Week 5
Ustekinumab (Stelara)	Every 12 weeks	Week 13
Belimumab (Benlysta)	Every 4 weeks	Week 5
Tofacitinib (Xeljanz): STOP this medication 7 days prior to surgery.	Daily or twice daily	7 days after last dose
SEVERE SLE-SPECIFIC MEDICATIONS: CONTINUE these medications in the perioperative period.	Dosing Interval	Continue/Withhold
Mycophenolate mofetil	Twice daily	Continue
Azathioprine	Daily or twice daily	Continue
Cyclosporine	Twice daily	Continue
Tacrolimus	Twice daily (IV and PO)	Continue
NOT-SEVERE SLE: DISCONTINUE these medications 1 week prior to surgery	Dosing Interval	Continue/Withhold
Mycophenolate mofetil	Twice daily	Withhold
Azathioprine	Daily or twice daily	Withhold
Cyclosporine	Twice daily	Withhold
Tacrolimus	Twice daily (IV and PO)	Withhold

Fig. 3.2 Recommendations for perioperative anti rheumatic medications for patients undergoing electivetotal joint arthroplasty. *DMARDs,* Disease-modifying antirheumatic drugs; *IV,* intravenous; *PO,* oral; *SLE,* systemic lupus erythematosus. (Adapted from Goodman SM, Springer B, Guyatt G, et al. 2017 American College of Rheumatology/American Association of Hip and Knee Surgeons guideline for the perioperative management of antirheumatic medication in patients with rheumatic diseases undergoing elective total hip or total knee arthroplasty. *J Arthroplasty.* 2017;32:2628–2638.)

optimization of these associated conditions is key to minimizing the risks and optimizing the outcomes for this population when undergoing TKA.

PERIPHERAL VASCULAR DISEASE

Peripheral vascular disease is a progressive condition in which narrowing and blockage of the circulatory system results in reduced blood flow to the extremities. Peripheral vascular disease can markedly affect outcomes after TKA. Peripheral vascular disease has been associated with an increased risk of vascular injury[62] and an increased risk of 90-day mortality.[63] Furthermore, decreased blood flow can result in poor wound healing, and some studies have found peripheral vascular disease to be a significant risk factor for prosthetic joint infection.[63-65] In a study by DeLaurentis et al. peripheral vascular disease was present in 24 out of 1182 (2%) of the TKA patients in their cohort.[66] There were ischemic complications in six patients, all of whom had preexisting peripheral vascular disease, highlighting the importance of preoperative assessment and optimization of peripheral vascular disease in patients undergoing TKA.

Preoperative assessment for peripheral vascular disease begins with the patient history. A medical history of diabetes should raise concern for the presence of peripheral vascular disease because these two conditions are associated.[67,68] A history of prior vascular intervention such as abdominal aortic aneurysm repair, carotid endarterectomy, or coronary artery bypass graft (CABG) is indicative of atherosclerotic disease and should raise concern about the presence of peripheral vascular disease in the lower extremities. These patients should be queried for the presence of intermittent claudication, ischemic rest pain, and poor wound healing, which are indicative of critical limb ischemia. The presence of arterial calcifications on knee radiographs should also raise concern for peripheral vascular disease. In patients who have a history of vascular intervention in the operative extremity such as femoral popliteal bypass or stent placement consultation with a vascular surgeon should be obtained to assess graft function and patency because thrombosis and occlusion of the graft after TKA can have devastating consequences.[69]

A careful preoperative physical examination should be performed on all patients undergoing TKA. On inspection, findings concerning for peripheral vascular disease include the absence of hair and the presence of skin discoloration, dystrophic nails, or chronic wounds. Popliteal and pedal pulses should be palpated. Atherosclerosis of the popliteal artery can result in popliteal aneurysm, thrombosis of which can result in critical limb ischemia and the need for amputation.[70] The popliteal fossa should be evaluated for the presence of a pulsating mass; the majority of popliteal aneurysms can be detected by palpation.[70] Pedal pulses, including posterior tibial artery and dorsalis pedis pulses, should be assessed and documented. Diminished, absent, or asymmetrical pulses are concerning for peripheral vascular disease and warrant further investigation.

If the history and physical examination are concerning for peripheral vascular disease, an ABI study can be obtained for further evaluation. An ABI <0.9 is considered abnormal, and consultation with a vascular surgeon should be considered.[71] It has been shown that patients with an ABI <0.7 are at increased risk for failure and reoperation after TKA.[72] An ABI <0.5 is indicative of severe ischemia, and revascularization may be needed before TKA.[71]

Preoperative consultation with a vascular surgeon should be obtained in patients who have symptoms of critical limb ischemia, patients who have physical examination findings concerning for popliteal aneurysm or peripheral vascular disease, and patients who have abnormal ABI results to determine the need and timing of vascular surgical intervention. Intraoperatively, consideration should be given to performing TKA without a tourniquet in these patients.[73-76] Furthermore, care should be taken when manipulating the extremity intraoperatively[77] to avoid vascular injury, especially from hyperextension of the knee. In patients who have a femoral popliteal bypass graft, tourniquet use should be avoided.[71] As with all patients, an immediate postoperative physical examination should be performed to assess for changes in sensation, motor function, or pedal pulses compared with the preoperative examination. A change in pedal pulses, especially in patients who have peripheral vascular disease, would be concerning for vascular injury and should warrant further workup.

CARDIAC DISEASE

A history of cardiac disease has been shown to be a strong predictor of complications after total joint arthroplasty. Complications can include mortality, cardiovascular complications, and increased lengths of stay.[78,79] Furthermore, postoperative atrial fibrillation and myocardial infarction have been shown to be associated with increased risk of developing periprosthetic joint infections.[81] Therefore identifying and optimizing patients who have cardiac disease and cardiac risk factors is essential to decrease the risk of perioperative adverse events.

In addition to a history of cardiac disease, other factors have been identified that increase the risk of perioperative cardiac complications, including age over 80 years and hypertension requiring the use of antihypertensive medications. Several risk calculators have also been developed to help assess the risk of perioperative cardiac complications, including the Revised Cardiac Risk Index (RCRI), the American College of Surgeons National Surgical Quality Improvement Program (ACS NSQIP) Surgical Risk Calculator, and the Gupta Perioperative Risk for Myocardial Infarction or Cardiac Arrest. Depending on the risk calculator used, several variables are taken into account, including patient age, sex, American Society of Anesthesiologist class, patient functional status, history of cardiovascular disease, presence of diabetes, presence of hypertension, presence of renal disease, presence of chronic obstructive pulmonary disease, history of corticosteroid use, history of smoking, body mass index, and the type of surgical procedure being performed. Using the results from a risk calculator, patients can be risk stratified for surgery, and those requiring further preoperative intervention can be identified.

In 2014 the American College of Cardiology (ACC) and American Heart Association (AHA), in collaboration with the ACS and American Society of Anesthesiologists among others, published the 2014 ACC/AHA Guideline on Perioperative Cardiovascular Evaluation and Management of Patients Undergoing Noncardiac Surgery.[93] They made detailed recommendations on the perioperative evaluation and management of various cardiovascular conditions, including coronary artery disease, heart failure, valvular heart disease, and arrhythmias. Their recommended stepwise approach to perioperative cardiac assessment for coronary artery disease is demonstrated in Fig. 3.3. Because of the age of the patients undergoing TKA, medical comorbidities are often present, including hypertension, hyperlipidemia, and diabetes, which are also risk factors for coronary artery disease. In the

guidelines an emergency procedure is defined as one in which life or limb is threatened if the patient is not in the operating room within 6 hours and if there is time for no or very limited or minimal clinical evaluation. Elective TKA is usually not considered an emergency, and therefore the perioperative risk of major adverse cardiac event is calculated using the ACS NSQIP, RCRI, or other perioperative risk calculator. Based on the risk stratification, further preoperative evaluation may be recommended.

With regard to patients who have prior percutaneous intervention (PCI), the recommended time between PCI and elective noncardiac surgery, such as elective THA, continues to be an area of debate. In 2014 the ACC and AHA published their recommendations, which are shown in Fig. 3.4. Other publications, however, have challenged the recommended interval between PCI and noncardiac elective surgery, especially in patients who have drug-eluting stents.[80,82] Considering the evolving literature and uniqueness of each patient, it is imperative that the optimal timing for THA be determined in conjunction with the patient's primary physician and cardiologist.

Several pharmacotherapies have been investigated for their potential role in preoperative optimization. These include beta blockers, aspirin, lipid-lowering therapies such as statins, and angiotensin-converting enzyme (ACE) inhibitors. The continuation of these medications during the perioperative period and the possible protective effects of the initiation of these therapies in the perioperative period have been researched.

Beta blockers are helpful in the perioperative period by combating the catecholamine surge experienced from surgery. The surge can increase myocardial oxygen demand and result in supply-demand mismatch if coronary artery disease is present, resulting in demand ischemia. Therefore the 2014 ACC/AHA guidelines recommend that beta blockers be continued in patients who have been on beta blockers chronically. Initiation of beta blockers may be reasonable in select patients, and this should be done in consultation with the patient's primary healthcare physician or cardiologist. The generalized use of perioperative beta blockers, especially starting the day of surgery, is not recommended, as one study has shown that perioperative treatment with beta blockers is not a completely harmless therapy.[83]

Likewise, it is considered reasonable to continue aspirin therapy in patients who have prior stents or who do not have prior stents if the risk of cardiac events

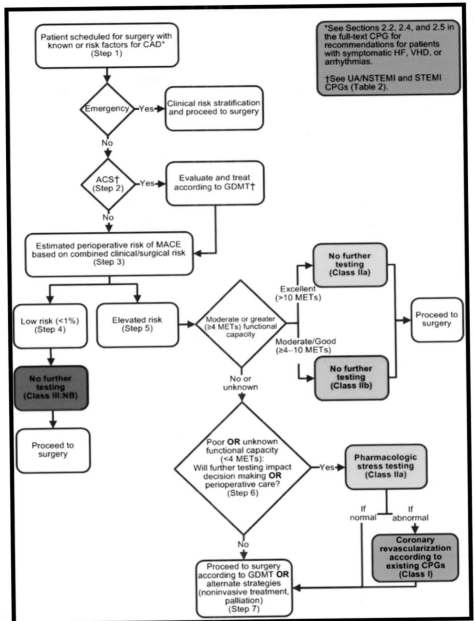

Fig. 3.3 Stepwise approach to perioperative cardiac assessment for coronary artery disease (CAD). *ACS*, Acute coronary syndrome; *CPG*, clinical practice guideline; *GDMT*, guideline-directed medical therapy; *HF*, heart failure; *MACE*, major adverse cardiac event; *MET*, metabolic equivalent; *STEMI*, ST-elevation myocardial infarction; *UA/NSTEMI*, unstable angina/non–ST-elevation myocardial infarction; *VHD*, valvular heart disease. (Fleisher LA, Fleischmann KE, Auerbach AD, Barnason SA, Beckman JA, Bozkurt B, Davila-Roman VG, Gerhard-Herman MD, Holly TA, Kane GC, Marine JE, Nelson MT, Spencer CC, Thompson A, Ting HH, Uretsky BF, Wijeysundera DN. 2014 ACC/AHA guideline on perioperative cardiovascular evaluation and management of patients undergoing noncardiac surgery: a report of the American College of Cardiology/American Heart Association Task Force on Practice Guidelines. Circulation. 2014 Dec 9;130(24):e278-333. doi: 10.1161/CIR.0000000000000106. Epub 2014 Aug 1. PMID: 25085961.)

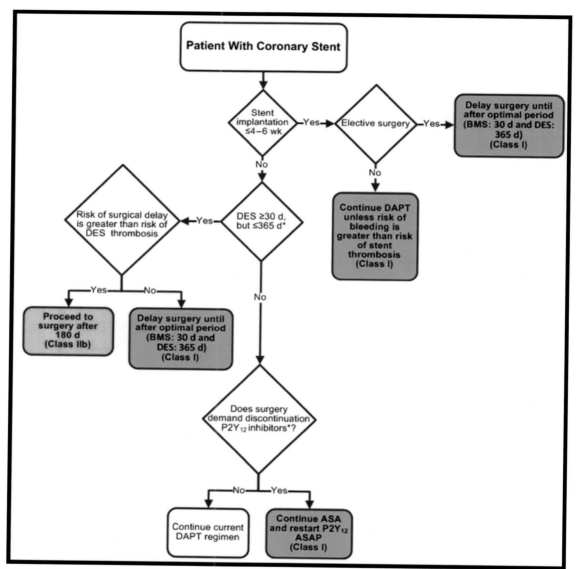

Fig. 3.4 Algorithm for antiplatelet management in patients with percutaneous coronary intervention (*PCI*) and noncardiac surgery. Colors correspond to the classes of recommendations. *Assuming patient is currently on dual antiplatelet therapy (*DAPT*). *ASA*, Acetylsalicylic acid (aspirin); *ASAP*, as soon as possible; *BMS*, bare metal stent; *d*, day; *DES*, drug-eluting stent; *wk*, week. (Fleisher LA, Fleischmann KE, Auerbach AD, Barnason SA, Beckman JA, Bozkurt B, Davila-Roman VG, Gerhard-Herman MD, Holly TA, Kane GC, Marine JE, Nelson MT, Spencer CC, Thompson A, Ting HH, Uretsky BF, Wijeysundera DN. 2014 ACC/AHA guideline on perioperative cardiovascular evaluation and management of patients undergoing noncardiac surgery: a report of the American College of Cardiology/American Heart Association Task Force on Practice Guidelines. Circulation. 2014 Dec 9;130(24):e278–333. doi: 10.1161/CIR.0000000000000106. Epub 2014 Aug 1. PMID: 25085961.)

outweighs the risk of increased bleeding. Generalized initiation of aspirin in the perioperative period in patients who do not have prior stenting is not helpful and is not recommended; it may result in increased risk of bleeding without providing benefit.[84]

Statins for the prevention of perioperative complications have been investigated; some studies showed significant reductions in perioperative mortality,[85-87] and other studies found no evidence to support the routine use of perioperative statins.[88] The 2014 ACC/AHA guidelines recommend continuing statins in patients who are taking statins and are scheduled for noncardiac surgery, and they state that perioperative initiation of statin use may be reasonable in patients undergoing vascular surgery.

The use of ACE inhibitors in the perioperative period has also been investigated, with some studies showing increased rates of intraoperative hypotension with continuation of ACE inhibitor therapy compared with preoperative discontinuation of ACE inhibitor therapy but no difference in important cardiovascular outcomes such as myocardial infarction, stroke, or death.[89-92] Taking the limited data into consideration, the 2014 ACC/AHA recommendations state that continuation of ACE inhibitors or angiotensin-receptor blockers perioperatively is reasonable. If these agents are discontinued preoperatively, they may be resumed postoperatively as soon as clinically feasible.

Cardiac disease has been shown to be a risk factor for postoperative complications after TKA, and preoperative optimization is important in minimizing adverse events and maximizing outcomes. Because of the wide spectrum of cardiac disease, the evolving literature in the field, and the uniqueness of each patient, it is important to have a collaborative relationship with the patient's primary physician and cardiologist determine the best optimization strategy.

REFERENCES

1. Beckman JA, Creager MA. Vascular complications of diabetes. *Circ Res.* 2016;118(11):1771–1785.
2. Iorio R, Williams KM, Marcantonio AJ, Specht LM, Tilzey JF, Healy WL. Diabetes mellitus, hemoglobin A1C, and the incidence of total joint arthroplasty infection. *J Arthroplasty.* 2012;27(5):726–729. e1.
3. Marchant Jr MH, Viens NA, Cook C, Vail TP, Bolognesi MP. The impact of glycemic control and diabetes mellitus on perioperative outcomes after total joint arthroplasty. *J Bone Joint Surg Am.* 2009;91(7):1621–1629. https://doi.org/10.2106/JBJS.H.00116.
4. Jämsen E, Nevalainen P, Eskelinen A, Huotari K, Kalliovalkama J, Moilanen T. Obesity, diabetes, and preoperative hyperglycemia as predictors of periprosthetic joint infection: A single-center analysis of 7181 primary hip and knee replacements for osteoarthritis. *J Bone Joint Surg Am.* 2012;94(14):e101.
5. Zhao Z, Wang S, Ma W, et al. Diabetes mellitus increases the incidence of deep vein thrombosis after total knee arthroplasty. *Arch Orthop Trauma Surg.* 2014;134(1):79–83.
6. Martínez-Huedo MA, Jiménez-García R, Jiménez-Trujillo I, Hernández-Barrera V, Del Rio Lopez B, López-de-Andrés A. Effect of type 2 diabetes on in-hospital postoperative complications and mortality after primary total hip and knee arthroplasty. *J Arthroplasty.* 2017;32(12):3729–3734. e2.
7. Belmont Jr PJ, Goodman GP, Waterman BR, Bader JO, Schoenfeld AJ. Thirty-day postoperative complications and mortality following total knee arthroplasty: Incidence and risk factors among a national sample of 15,321 patients. *J Bone Joint Surg Am.* 2014;96(1):20–26.
8. Bolognesi MP, Marchant Jr MH, Viens NA, Cook C, Pietrobon R, Vail TP. The impact of diabetes on perioperative patient outcomes after total hip and total knee arthroplasty in the United States. *J Arthroplasty.* 2008;23(6 Suppl 1):92–98.
9. American Diabetes Association. Classification and diagnosis of diabetes: Standards of medical care in diabetes—2020. *Diabetes Care.* 2020;43(Suppl 1):S14–S31.
10. American Diabetes Association. Tests of glycemia in diabetes. *Diabetes Care.* 2004;27(suppl 1):S91–S93.
11. Hwang JS, Kim SJ, Bamne AB, Na YG, Kim TK. Do glycemic markers predict occurrence of complications after total knee arthroplasty in patients with diabetes? *Clin Orthop Relat Res.* 2015;473(5):1726–1731.
12. Tarabichi M, Shohat N, Kheir MM, et al. Determining the threshold for HbA1c as a predictor for adverse outcomes after total joint arthroplasty: A multicenter, retrospective study. *J Arthroplasty.* 2017;32(9S):S263–S267. e1.
13. Cancienne JM, Werner BC, Browne JA. Is there an association between hemoglobin A1C and deep postoperative infection after TKA? *Clin Orthop Relat Res.* 2017;475(6):1642–1649.
14. Maradit Kremers H, Lewallen LW, Mabry TM, Berry DJ, Berbari EF, Osmon DR. Diabetes mellitus, hyperglycemia, hemoglobin A1C and the risk of prosthetic joint infections in total hip and knee arthroplasty. *J Arthroplasty.* 2015;30(3):439–443.
15. Adams AL, Paxton EW, Wang JQ, et al. Surgical outcomes of total knee replacement according to diabetes status

and glycemic control, 2001 to 2009. *J Bone Joint Surg Am.* 2013;95(6):481–487.

16. Iorio R, Williams KM, Marcantonio AJ, Specht LM, Tilzey JF, Healy WL. Diabetes mellitus, hemoglobin A1C, and the incidence of total joint arthroplasty infection. *J Arthroplasty.* 2012;27(5):726–729. e1.

17. Giori NJ, Ellerbe LS, Bowe T, Gupta S, Harris AH. Many diabetic total joint arthroplasty candidates are unable to achieve a preoperative hemoglobin A1c goal of 7% or less. *J Bone Joint Surg Am.* 2014;96(6):500–504.

18. Edwards PK, Mears SC, Stambough JB, Foster SE, Barnes CL. Choices, compromises, and controversies in total knee and total hip arthroplasty modifiable risk factors: What you need to know. *J Arthroplasty.* 2018;33(10):3101–3106.

19. Chrastil J, Anderson MB, Stevens V, Anand R, Peters CL, Pelt CE. Is hemoglobin A1c or perioperative hyperglycemia predictive of periprosthetic joint infection or death following primary total joint arthroplasty? *J Arthroplasty.* 2015;30(7):1197–1202.

20. Maradit Kremers H, Schleck CD, Lewallen EA, Larson DR, Van Wijnen AJ, Lewallen DG. Diabetes mellitus and hyperglycemia and the risk of aseptic loosening in total joint arthroplasty. *J Arthroplasty.* 2017;32(9S):S251–S253.

21. Kheir MM, Tan TL, Kheir M, Maltenfort MG, Chen AF. Postoperative blood glucose levels predict infection after total joint arthroplasty. *J Bone Joint Surg Am.* 2018;100(16):1423–1431.

22. Armbruster DA. Fructosamine: Structure, analysis, and clinical usefulness. *Clin Chem.* 1987;33(12):2153–2163.

23. Shohat N, Tarabichi M, Tischler EH, Jabbour S, Parvizi J. Serum fructosamine: A simple and inexpensive test for assessing preoperative glycemic control. *J Bone Joint Surg Am.* 2017;99(22):1900–1907.

24. Shohat N, Tarabichi M, Tan TL, et al. 2019 John Insall Award: Fructosamine is a better glycaemic marker compared with glycated haemoglobin (HbA1C) in predicting adverse outcomes following total knee arthroplasty: A prospective multicentre study. *Bone Joint J.* 2019;101-B(7_Supple_C):3–9.

25. Shohat N, Restrepo C, Allierezaie A, et al. Increased postoperative glucose variability is associated with adverse outcomes following total joint arthroplasty. *J Bone Joint Surg Am.* 2018;100-A:1110–1117.

26. Jiranek W, Kigera JWM, Klatt BA, et al. General Assembly, Prevention, Host Risk Mitigation—General Factors: Proceedings of International Consensus on Orthopedic Infections. *J Arthroplasty.* 2019;34(2S):S43–S48.

27. Capozzi JD, Lepkowsky ER, Callari MM, Jordan ET, Koenig JA, Sirounian GH. The prevalence of diabetes mellitus and routine hemoglobin A1c screening in elective total joint arthroplasty patients. *J Arthroplasty.* 2017;32(1):304–308.

28. Carolyn TB, Clare JL, Kimberly AG. Treatment of obesity in patients with diabetes. *Diabetes Spectr.* 2017;30(4): 237–243.

29. George J, Piuzzi NS, Ng M, Sodhi N, Khlopas AA, Mont MA. Association between body mass index and thirty-day complications after total knee arthroplasty. *J Arthroplasty.* 2018;33(3):865–871.

30. Wagner ER, Kamath AF, Fruth K, Harmsen WS, Berry DJ. Effect of body mass index on reoperation and complications after total knee arthroplasty. *J Bone Joint Surg Am.* 2016;98(24):2052–2060.

31. Zusmanovich M, Kester BS, Schwarzkopf R. Postoperative complications of total joint arthroplasty in obese patients stratified by BMI. *J Arthroplasty.* 2018;33(3):856–864.

32. Goldstein DJ. Beneficial health effects of modest weight loss. *Int J Obes Relat Metab Disord.* 1992;16(6):397–415.

33. Lau DC, Teoh H. Benefits of modest weight loss on the management of type 2 diabetes mellitus. *Can J Diabetes.* 2013;37(2):128–134.

34. Smith TO, Aboelmagd T, Hing CB, MacGregor A. Does bariatric surgery prior to total hip or knee arthroplasty reduce post-operative complications and improve clinical outcomes for obese patients? Systematic review and meta-analysis. *Bone Joint J.* 2016;98-B(9):1160–1166.

35. Lee GC, Ong K, Baykal D, Lau E, Malkani AL. Does prior bariatric surgery affect implant survivorship and complications following primary total hip arthroplasty/ total knee arthroplasty? *J Arthroplasty.* 2018;33(7): 2070–2074. e1.

36. Li S, Luo X, Sun H, Wang K, Zhang K, Sun X. Does prior bariatric surgery improve outcomes following total joint arthroplasty in the morbidly obese? A meta-analysis. *J Arthroplasty.* 2019;34(3):577–585.

37. Gu A, Cohen JS, Malahias MA, Lee D, Sculco PK, McLawhorn AS. The effect of bariatric surgery prior to lower-extremity total joint arthroplasty: A systematic review. *HSS J.* 2019;15(2):190–200.

38. Kapetanovic MC, Lindqvist E, Saxne T, Eberhardt K. Orthopaedic surgery in patients with rheumatoid arthritis over 20 years: Prevalence and predictive factors of large joint replacement. *Ann Rheum Dis.* 2008;67(10):1412–1416.

39. Wolfe F, Zwillich SH. The long-term outcomes of rheumatoid arthritis: A 23-year prospective, longitudinal study of total joint replacement and its predictors in 1,600 patients with rheumatoid arthritis. *Arthritis Rheum.* 1998;41:1072–1082.

40. Young BL, Watson SL, Perez JL, McGwin G, Singh JA, Ponce BA. Trends in joint replacement surgery in patients with rheumatoid arthritis. *J Rheumatol.* 2018;45(2): 158–164.

41. Jain A, Stein BE, Skolasky RL, Jones LC, Hungerford MW. Total joint arthroplasty in patients with rheumatoid

arthritis: A United States experience from 1992 through 2005. *J Arthroplasty*. 2012;27(6):881–888.

42. Hekmat K, Jacobsson L, Nilsson J, et al. Decrease in the incidence of total hip arthroplasties in patients with rheumatoid arthritis—results from a well defined population in south Sweden. *Arthritis Res Ther*. 2011;13:R67.

43. Wasserman BR, Moskovich R, Razi AE. Rheumatoid arthritis of the cervical spine-clinical considerations. *Bull NYU Hosp Jt Dis*. 2011;69(2):136–148.

44. Paimela L, Laasonen L, Kankaanpää E, Leirisalo-Repo M. Progression of cervical spine changes in patients with early rheumatoid arthritis. *J Rheumatol*. 1997;24(7):1280–1284.

45. Wasserman BR, Moskovich R, Razi AE. Rheumatoid arthritis of the cervical spine-clinical considerations. *Bull NYU Hosp Jt Dis*. 2011;69(2):136–148.

46. Sandström T, Rantalaiho V, Yli-Kerttula T, et al. NEO-RACo Study Group. Cervical spine involvement is very rare in patients with rheumatoid arthritis treated actively with treat to target strategy. Ten-year results of the NEORACo Study. *J Rheumatol*. 2020;27:1160–1164.

47. Kauppi MJ, Neva MH, Laiho K, Kautiainen H, Luukkainen R, Karjalainen A, Hannonen PJ, Leirisalo-Repo M, Korpela M, Ilva K, Möttönen T; FIN-RACo Trial Group. Rheumatoid atlantoaxial subluxation can be prevented by intensive use of traditional disease modifying antirheumatic drugs. *J Rheumatol*. 2009 Feb;36(2):273–8. doi: 10.3899/jrheum.080429. PMID: 19132793.

48. Maradit-Kremers H, Crowson CS, Nicola PJ, et al. Increased unrecognized coronary heart disease and sudden deaths in rheumatoid arthritis: A population-based cohort study. *Arthritis Rheum*. 2005;52:402–411.

49. Solomon DH, Goodson NJ, Katz JN, et al. Patterns of cardiovascular risk in rheumatoid arthritis. *Ann Rheum Dis*. 2006;65:1608–1612.

50. Peters MJ, van Halm VP, Voskuyl AE, et al. Does rheumatoid arthritis equal diabetes mellitus as an independent risk factor for cardiovascular disease? A prospective study. *Arthritis Rheum*. 2009;61:1571Y1579.

51. Lindhardsen J, Ahlehoff O, Gislason GH, et al. The risk of myocardial infarction in rheumatoid arthritis and diabetes mellitus: A Danish nationwide cohort study. *Ann Rheum Dis*. 2011;70:929Y934.

52. Corrao S, Messina S, Pistone G, Calvo L, Scaglione R, Licata G. Heart involvement in rheumatoid arthritis: Systematic review and meta-analysis. *Int J Cardiol*. 2013;167(5):2031–2038.

53. Farquhar H, Vassallo R, Edwards AL, Matteson EL. Pulmonary complications of rheumatoid arthritis. *Semin Respir Crit Care Med*. 2019;40(2):194–207. https://doi.org/10.1055/s-0039-1683995. Epub 2019 May 28.

54. Duarte AC, Porter JC, Leandro MJ. The lung in a cohort of rheumatoid arthritis patients-an overview of different types of involvement and treatment. *Rheumatology (Oxford)*. 2019;58(11):2031–2038.

55. Duarte AC, Porter JC, Leandro MJ. The lung in a cohort of rheumatoid arthritis patients-an overview of different types of involvement and treatment. *Rheumatology (Oxford)*. 2019;58(11):2031–2038.

56. Wilson A, Yu HT, Goodnough LT, Nissenson AR. Prevalence and outcomes of anemia in rheumatoid arthritis: A systematic review of the literature. *Am J Med*. 2004;116(Suppl 7A):50–57.

57. Martí-Carvajal AJ, Agreda-Pérez LH, Solà I, Simancas-Racines D. Erythropoiesis-stimulating agents for anemia in rheumatoid arthritis. *Cochrane Database Syst Rev*. 2013;2:CD000332.

58. Jämsen E, Huhtala H, Puolakka T, Moilanen T. Risk factors for infection after knee arthroplasty. A register-based analysis of 43,149 cases. *J Bone Joint Surg Am*. 2009;91(1):38–47.

59. Momohara S, Kawakami K, Iwamoto T, et al. Prosthetic joint infection after total hip or knee arthroplasty in rheumatoid arthritis patients treated with nonbiologic and biologic disease-modifying antirheumatic drugs. *Mod Rheumatol*. 2011;21(5):469–475.

60. Grennan DM, Gray J, Loudon J, Fear S. Methotrexate and early postoperative complications in patients with rheumatoid arthritis undergoing elective orthopaedic surgery. *Ann Rheum Dis*. 2001;60:214e7.

61. Goodman SM, Springer B, Guyatt G, et al. 2017 American College of Rheumatology/American Association of Hip and Knee Surgeons guideline for the perioperative management of antirheumatic medication in patients with rheumatic diseases undergoing elective total hip or total knee arthroplasty. *J Arthroplasty*. 2017;32(9):2628–2638.

62. Ko LJ, DeHart ML, Yoo JU, Huff TW. Popliteal artery injury associated with total knee arthroplasty: Trends, costs and risk factors. *J Arthroplasty*. 2014;29(6):1181–1184.

63. Bozic KJ, Lau E, Kurtz S, Ong K, Berry DJ. Patient-related risk factors for postoperative mortality and periprosthetic joint infection in medicare patients undergoing TKA. *Clin Orthop Relat Res*. 2012;470:130e7.

64. Jiang SL, Schairer WW, Bozic KJ. Increased rates of periprosthetic joint infection in patients with cirrhosis undergoing total joint arthroplasty. *Clin Orthop Relat Res*. 2014;472:2483e91.

65. Lenguerrand E, Whitehouse MR, Beswick AD, et al. National Joint Registry for England, Wales, Northern Ireland and the Isle of Man. Risk factors associated with revision for prosthetic joint infection following knee replacement: An observational cohort study from England and Wales. *Lancet Infect Dis*. 2019;19(6):589–600.

66. DeLaurentis DA, Levitsky KA, Booth RE, et al. Arterial and ischaemia aspects of total knee arthroplasty. *Am J Surg.* 1992;164:237–240.

67. Beckman JA, Creager MA. Vascular complications of diabetes. *Circ Res.* 2016;118(11):1771–1785.

68. Park IH, Lee SC, Park IS, et al. Asymptomatic peripheral vascular disease in total knee arthroplasty: Preoperative prevalence and risk factors. *J Orthop Traumatol.* 2015;16(1):23–26.

69. John TG, Stonebridge PA, Kelman J, Murie JA, Jenkins AM, Ruckley CV. Above-knee femoropopliteal bypass grafts and the consequences of graft failure. *Ann R Coll Surg Engl.* 1993;75:257–260.

70. Downing R, Ashton F, Grimley RP, Slaney G. Problems in diagnosis of popliteal aneurysms. *J R Soc Med.* 1985;78:440.

71. Smith DE, McGraw RW, Taylor DC, Masri BA. Arterial complications and total knee arthroplasty. *J Am Acad Orthop Surg.* 2001;9(4):253–257.

72. Gad BV, Langfitt MK, Robbins CE, Talmo CT, Bono OJ, Bono JV. Factors influencing survivorship in vasculopathic patients. *J Knee Surg.* 2020;33:1004–1009.

73. Rush JH, Vidovich JD, Johnson MA. Arterial complications of total knee replacement: The Australian experience. *J Bone Joint Surg Br.* 1987;69:400–402.

74. Rand JA. Vascular complications of total knee arthroplasty: Report of three cases. *J Arthroplasty.* 1987;2:89–93.

75. Kumar SN, Chapman JA, Rawlins I. Vascular injuries in total knee arthroplasty: A review of the problem with special reference to the possible effects of the tourniquet. *J Arthroplasty.* 1998;13:211–216.

76. Calligaro KD, DeLaurentis DA, Booth RE, Rothman RH, Savarese RP, Dougherty MJ. Acute arterial thrombosis associated with total knee arthroplasty. *J Vasc Surg.* 1994;20:927–932.

77. Holmberg A, Milbrink J, Bergqvist D. Arterial complications after knee arthroplasty: Four cases and a review of the literature. *Acta Orthop Scand.* 1996;67:75–78.

78. Belmont Jr PJ, Goodman GP, Kusnezov NA, et al. Postoperative myocardial infarction and cardiac arrest following primary total knee and hip arthroplasty: Rates, risk factors, and time of occurrence. *J Bone Joint Surg Am.* 2014;96(24):2025.

79. Elsiwy Y, Jovanovic I, Doma K, Hazratwala K, Letson H. Risk factors associated with cardiac complication after total joint arthroplasty of the hip and knee: A systematic review. *J Orthop Surg Res.* 2019;14(1):15.

80. Wijeysundera DN, Wijeysundera HC, Yun L, et al. Risk of elective major noncardiac surgery after coronary stent insertion: A population-based study. *Circulation.* 2012;126(11):1355–1362.

81. Pulido L, Ghanem E, Joshi A, Purtill JJ, Parvizi J. Periprosthetic joint infection: The incidence, timing, and predisposing factors. *Clin Orthop Relat Res.* 2008;466:1710e5.

82. Hawn MT, Graham LA, Richman JS, et al. Risk of major adverse cardiac events following noncardiac surgery in patients with coronary stents. *JAMA.* 2013;310(14):1462–1472.

83. POISE Study Group Devereaux PJ, Yang H, et al. Effects of extended-release metoprolol succinate in patients undergoing non-cardiac surgery (POISE trial): A randomised controlled trial. *Lancet.* 2008;371(9627):1839–1847.

84. Devereaux PJ, Mrkobrada M, Sessler DI, et al. Aspirin in patients undergoing noncardiac surgery. *N Engl J Med.* 2014;370(16):1494–1503.

85. Ma B, Sun J, Diao S, Zheng B, Li H. Effects of perioperative statins on patient outcomes after noncardiac surgery: A meta-analysis. *Ann Med.* 2018;50(5):402–409.

86. Chopra V, Wesorick DH, Sussman JB, et al. Effect of perioperative statins on death, myocardial infarction, atrial fibrillation, and length of stay: A systematic review and meta-analysis. *Arch Surg.* 2012;147(2):181–189.

87. Desai H, Aronow WS, Ahn C, et al. Incidence of perioperative myocardial infarction and of 2-year mortality in 577 elderly patients undergoing noncardiac vascular surgery treated with and without statins. *Arch Gerontol Geriatr.* 2010;51(2):149–151.

88. Kapoor AS, Kanji H, Buckingham J, Devereaux PJ, McAlister FA. Strength of evidence for perioperative use of statins to reduce cardiovascular risk: Systematic review of controlled studies. *BMJ.* 2006;333(7579):1149.

89. Turan A, You J, Shiba A, et al. Angiotensin converting enzyme inhibitors are not associated with respiratory complications or mortality after noncardiac surgery. *Anesth Analg.* 2012;114:552–560.

90. Rosenman DJ, McDonald FS, Ebbert JO, et al. Clinical consequences of withholding versus administering renin-angiotensin-aldosterone system antagonists in the preoperative period. *J Hosp Med.* 2008;3:319–325.

91. Brabant SM, Bertrand M, Eyraud D, et al. The hemodynamic effects of anesthetic induction in vascular surgical patients chronically treated with angiotensin II receptor antagonists. *Anesth Analg.* 1999;89:1388–1392.

92. Bertrand M, Godet G, Meersschaert K, et al. Should the angiotensin II antagonists be discontinued before surgery? *Anesth Analg.* 2001;92:26–30.

93. Fleisher LA, Fleischmann KE, Auerbach AD, Barnason SA, Beckman JA, Bozkurt B, Davila-Roman VG, Gerhard-Herman MD, Holly TA, Kane GC, Marine JE, Nelson MT, Spencer CC, Thompson A, Ting HH, Uretsky BF, Wijeysundera DN. 2014 ACC/AHA guideline on perioperative cardiovascular evaluation and management of patients undergoing noncardiac surgery: a report of the American College of Cardiology/American Heart Association Task Force on Practice Guidelines. *Circulation.* 2014 Dec 9;130(24):e278–333. doi: 10.1161/CIR.0000000000000106. Epub 2014 Aug 1. PMID: 25085961.

4

Assessment of Surgical Difficulty

Curtis Miller, MD

"Plan for what is difficult while it is easy."[1]
Sun Tzu

Although surgery cannot be compared with war, Sun Tzu's philosophies, as written in *The Art of War*, have been used often in other fields, such as business, politics, and sports. Perhaps some of his principles can be applied when approaching surgery in general and total knee arthroplasty (TKA) specifically. None of us ever wants to be in the uncomfortable position of being "knee deep" into a TKA surgery and being faced with a surprise that we had not planned for. Even careful planning will not prevent all intraoperative surprises, but careful assessment of the patient's physical examination, a careful review of their medical and surgical histories, and interpretation of all appropriate laboratory and imaging studies can minimize surprises. The scope of this chapter is not specifically about preoperative planning, but careful preoperative planning can help one to assess the difficulties that might occur at the time of TKA. Dr. Lavernia will go further in depth regarding preoperative planning in Chapter 5.

I learned a critical lesson about assessing a patient in my fellowship year with Kenneth Krackow. In the first few months of my fellowship I was with a first-year orthopedic resident who was on the first day of his total joint rotation. Dr. Krackow had his usual line up of cases that day. Because it was the first day of his rotation, the resident had not seen the patients in the clinic weeks earlier when they had undergone their initial surgical consultations. The resident did not get to examine the patients, and he had not been present at the evaluation of radiographs and testing. Additionally, and most importantly, he did not get to witness the thought process and planning that Dr. Krackow had put into the case at the time the decision was made to proceed with surgery. This was in an era before electronic documentation. Dr. Krackow, as was his habit, had made index cards on every patient, whether

their surgery was routine or otherwise. On those cards, he documented items such as previous surgery with scars, retained hardware, knee stability, range of motion of the knee, deformity, bone loss, and vascularity and whether or not the patient needed any further subspecialty consultation before surgery (i.e., vascular surgery or plastic surgery). A thorough plan was in place weeks before surgery. Dr. Krackow would then review this information with the residents and the fellow on his rotation before the surgery at preoperative rounds to make sure this thorough plan was indeed going to proceed with as few unknowns as possible. This review included verifying instrumentation and specialized prosthetics necessary to treat any instability/deformity or defect present, the need for intraoperative imaging or navigation (in trial at the time), having appropriate consultants available as backup if needed, verifying that bone graft was available if needed, having instrumentation available to remove any hardware that was present that might interfere with the procedure, and having available the ability for advanced soft tissue balancing (i.e., medial collateral ligament advancement; see Chapter 9). He then brought the index cards into the operating room and reviewed them before each case. For at least the third time, he verified that everything that he anticipated needing for that particular patient and surgery was present, whether the surgery was considered routine or not.

On that first day of the junior resident's rotation, we had just finished a very complex valgus, flexion contracture knee arthroplasty case with severe deformity, bone loss, and medial collateral ligament laxity when the young resident and I received a lesson that became entrenched in our memories. The resident had been told before surgery that the TKA would be a difficult surgery. Not surprisingly, with Dr. Krackow's surgical skills and his thorough preoperative planning, the surgery occurred without a hitch. Afterward, the resident, I am assuming to credit Dr. Krackow for a job well done, made the statement: "I am not sure what you guys were talking about, but that was easy!" Dr. Krackow, seeing the opportunity for a teaching moment, immediately corrected the resident: "You have no idea what exactly went into that surgery in the weeks prior to today to make it look so easy. Do not be fooled into thinking you can just show up and perform every total knee that is on the schedule." He did not do this to admonish the resident but to teach him about the need for extensive preoperative planning.

Prolonged surgical time has been associated with increased risk of surgical infection.[2] Therefore one can conclude that anything that makes a surgery more difficult could lead to increased complication rates. Most TKAs are straightforward and, possibly, even routine. Advances in imaging, surgical technique, technology, fixation, augmentation, instrumentation, navigation, tribology, and prosthetics now make most TKAs very manageable. However, the occasional TKA may be anything but routine. If one takes to heart Sun Tzu's principles of planning for war and adapts them to surgery while following the example of Dr. Krackow in planning every detail on even the most apparently routine TKA, rarely will one be surprised with something unexpected during surgery. As Dr. Krackow said, "it is almost impossible to imagine that a total knee arthroplasty performed on a thin patient with good preoperative range of motion, no major deformity, and uniformly good bone quality could be anything other than straightforward from a technical standpoint, especially if one assumes no special problems with local tissues, circulation, or hemostasis" (p. 75).[3]

This chapter will discuss items that can be considered as screening factors for difficulty in the performance of a TKA: surgical exposure and soft tissue factors excluding ligamentous instability, deformity, retained hardware, bone quality and bone loss, and ligamentous instability.

SURGICAL EXPOSURE AND SOFT TISSUE FACTORS EXCLUDING LIGAMENTOUS INSTABILITY

There are data that many comorbidities can affect the outcome of TKA. This chapter only mentions comorbidities as they relate to the potential for adding difficulty to the surgical procedure and not how they might affect the ultimate outcome. Chapters 1 to 3 have covered comorbidities

and their relationships to outcome. Additionally, surgical exposures and techniques are discussed in Chapter 7. This chapter discusses how soft tissue factors can make a TKA more difficult to perform.

Morbid Obesity

Obesity in the United States is reaching epidemic proportions, and it has a major impact on lower-extremity Fig. 4.1 total joint arthroplasty, particularly TKA.[4] Although it has been shown that patients who are morbidly obese (body mass index [BMI] >40) and undergo TKA have a higher 30-day postoperative complication rate[5] and patients who are obese (BMI >35) have a higher risk of infection,[6] have a higher cost of care, have longer hospital stays,[7] have a greater odds ratio of revision from any cause,[8] and have a higher mid- to long-term revision rate[9] compared with patients who are not obese. Some sources conclude that patients who are obese should not be excluded from the benefit of TKA, because their overall improvement may be similar to those of patients who have a lower BMI.[10] As the rate of obesity and morbid obesity rises in the United States, one can extrapolate that TKA in patients who are obese or morbidly obese will become more commonplace. Krackow instructs that "it is sufficient to state, for our present purposes, that obesity makes the entire total knee arthroplasty operation more difficult … one is cautioned not to disregard obesity" (p. 84).[3] The bulky soft tissues of the calf and thigh in the patient who is obese do not allow typical flexion of the joint during surgery, thus making exposure, especially of the tibia, more challenging.[3] The thick soft tissue envelope can also render routine instrumentation and retractors insufficient.[3] The surgical incision must typically be longer owing to the depth of the subcutaneous fat layer.[3] All of these factors can lead to a TKA being more difficult in patients who are obese or morbidly obese. Whiteside[11] has described the formation of a lateral subfascial pocket to hold the patella in the everted position to aid in surgical exposure in the patient who is obese and undergoing TKA.

Previous Surgical Scars

Wound complications are obviously better avoided than treated. However, occasionally patients present with poor skin quality. Patients who have previous surgical scars, trauma, burns, and skin grafts can present for TKA. It has been shown that oxygen tension of the lateral and medial skin flaps on postoperative day one in previously unoperated knees is higher in the standard

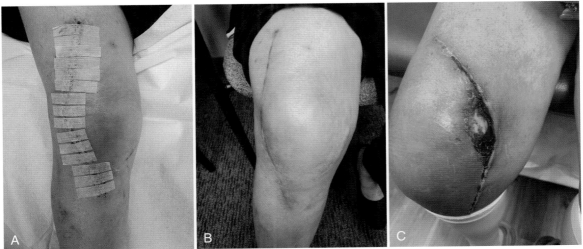

Fig. 4.1 (A) Two-week postoperative photograph of a patient that underwent total knee arthroplasty using a previous open lateral meniscectomy scar and a medial parapatellar approach. The faint blue line medially depicts an old open medial meniscectomy scar. (B) Same patient at 6 weeks postoperatively showing healthy skin flap. The previous medial meniscectomy scar is more readily seen in this photograph. (C) Six-week postoperative photograph of a patient that underwent total knee arthroplasty using a previous open meniscectomy scar. Skin slough and eschar are noted on the junction of the old meniscectomy scar and also where the approach was brought toward the midline for surgical exposure. The surgeon felt that a standard midline incision would leave a narrow skin bridge and be more prone to skin slough. Subsequent excision of eschar and primary wound closure healed well without further complications. (Courtesy Curtis Miller, MD and J. F. Davidson, MD)

anterior midline TKA approach than in the medial parapatellar and curved medial incisions.[12,13] Previous arthroscopy scars seem of little consequence. But, surgical scars from open meniscectomy, ligament reconstruction, previous osteotomy, and trauma, including surgical fixation of fractures, have the potential to be problematic. A standard anterior midline approach cannot always be used. Anything that would place a surgical incision at risk of necrosis is best avoided. Previous surgical incisions could require alteration of the standard anterior midline TKA approach. (Fig. 4.1). According to Sanna et al.,[14] there are some practical rules that can be helpful in choosing the most suitable incision site for TKA when presented with previous surgical incisions:

- In the presence of a single previous incision the scar, providing it is suitable, can be used.
- If it is not possible to incorporate the scar, the distance between the old and the new incisions should be no less than two-thirds of the length of the scar, and there must be a minimum of at least a 5-cm bridge of skin between the two incisions.

- A previous horizontal incision must be crossed perpendicularly.
- In the presence of multiple previous incisions the most lateral one should be used. To avoid excessive prefascial separations, the medial one can be used, but only if the bridge of skin between the two incisions is greater than 5 cm.

The use of a sham incision technique has been described.[14] This technique was used occasionally during my fellowship in the late 1990s. Although this technique is preferable to postoperative wound necrosis and wound complications, its use today, at least in the United States, is limited as a result of insurance requirements and the potential for other complications from a second surgical exposure.

The use of consultants, especially plastic surgery and vascular surgery, can be helpful in extreme situations. Consultation preoperatively can help in the planning of difficult surgical exposures. The benefit of this option is 2-fold. First, the best surgical approach can be planned before the actual surgery. An additional benefit comes from the fact that should a major wound complication occur, the consultant is already familiar with the patient and the situation and is ready to assist with wound care. The consultant's availability postoperatively and possibly intraoperatively can help avoid or treat any important wound complications.

Soft Tissue Contractures and Range of Motion

TKA soft tissue balancing will be discussed in Chapter 9. This section will therefore not go into soft tissue releases and balancing. In Chapter 5 implant selection will be discussed in detail. With extensive soft tissue balancing, occasionally specialized implants with additional constraint and stems should be available for TKA. In a case with either a fixed, severe deformity or limited preoperative range of motion specialized techniques may be required for exposure. The use of a tibial tubercle osteotomy in extension contractures can be useful in gaining intraoperative exposure and flexion (Fig. 4.2). The extreme of extension contractures is seen in the case of converting a previous knee fusion to a TKA. Krackow has advocated the consideration of a tibial tubercle osteotomy for exposure in such cases.[3] The use of additional incisions for osteophyte removal that cannot be

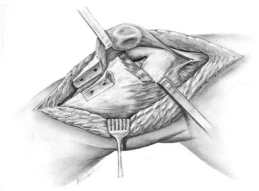

Fig. 4.2 Tibial tubercle osteotomy. (Courtesy Krackow, K. *The Technique of Total Knee Arthroplasty.* Mosby; 1990.)

accomplished with the standard TKA approaches may rarely, but occasionally, be required (Fig. 4.3).[3] One must be prepared to consider those techniques when indicated, and alternative approaches should be in the armamentarium of any TKA surgeon. Krackow has suggested that patients with a severely limited preoperative range of motion should also be informed before TKA

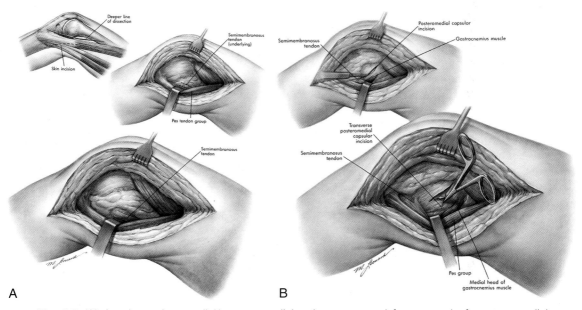

A   B

Fig. 4.3 (A) An alternative medial/posteromedial arthrotomy used for removal of posteromedial osteophytes in the case of limited intraoperative flexion. (B) Deeper dissection in the medial/posteromedial arthrotomy used for removal of posteromedial osteophytes in the case of limited intraoperative flexion. (Courtesy Krackow, K. *The Technique of Total Knee Arthroplasty.* Mosby; 1990.)

that "poor preoperative range of motion correlates to some degree with poorer than average postoperative range of motion." (p. 79)[3]

DEFORMITY

Preoperative deformity can be split into two categories, extraarticular and articular. This section will address articular deformities followed by a brief discussion of extraarticular deformities. These are briefly discussed as they relate to the assessment of surgical difficulty. These topics will be discussed extensively in Chapter 5.

Articular Deformities

TKA balancing techniques will be discussed in detail in Chapter 8 and implant selection and surgical technique will be discussed in Chapter 5. This section will therefore not go into detail regarding these. It stands to reason that larger deformities will be more difficult to balance than smaller deformities and may require more soft tissue balancing and more constrained prostheses. (Fig. 4.4) Therefore it also stands to reason that larger deformity TKAs will be more difficult to perform and may require longer surgical time to correct those deformities. Dr. Krackow cautions us to not "understate the magnitude of the problem at hand" (p. 79).[3] I have also heard the expression during my training that a simple valgus deformity is harder to correct than a difficult varus deformity. Although not always the case, some deformities, perhaps because of their decreased incidence and perhaps because of our limited experience with those deformities, are harder to correct and can make TKA surgery more difficult. It is suggested that one's surgical armamentarium should have ligament advancement techniques for cases in which attenuated soft tissue sleeves are present on the convex side of the deformity.[15]

Extraarticular Deformities

In the case of classical alignment TKA surgery involves placing the femoral component so that the femoral component articular surface lies perpendicular to a line drawn from the center of the hip to the center of the knee in the coronal plane. Additionally it involves placing the tibial component articular surface such that it lies perpendicular to the line drawn from the center of the knee to the center of the ankle in the coronal plane.[3] Soft tissue balancing is then done to equalize and rectangularize the flexion and extension gaps. In this scenario with the

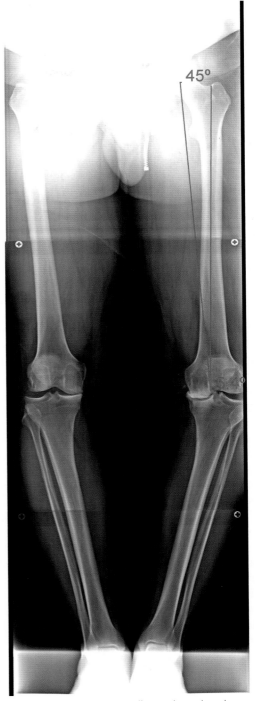

Fig. 4.4 Long standing radiographs showing varus deformity, degenerative arthrosis with medial tibial bone loss, and articular deformity of the left knee. (Courtesy Curtis Miller, MD)

appropriately sized tibial insert thickness, one has a well-aligned, well-balanced, and therefore stable TKA. In cases where there is no extraarticular deformity the principles of soft tissue balancing, as discussed in Chapter 8, will be helpful.

Extraarticular deformities are often the result of previous trauma, but they may be seen in other conditions such as congenital and developmental issues and previous corrective surgery (i.e., osteotomies). An extraarticular deformity may or may not have an important effect on any planned TKA. In general, the smaller the deformity and the further it is away from the knee joint, the less effect it will have on the TKA.[3] Conversely, the larger the deformity and the closer it is to the knee joint, the more effect it will have on the TKA.[3] The goal of any TKA is to end up with a well-aligned, well-balanced TKA. The reason an extraarticular deformity can affect TKA surgery stems from the fact that, according to Krackow, "its special significance derives from ligament attachment points that are, in certain respects, normal, whereas, the orientations of the femur or the femoral or tibial joint line to the overall shaft axis is abnormal."[3] Krackow also states, "Because of the potential impact of a significant shaft deformity relatively close to the knee in terms of altering the distal femoral or proximal tibial cut line in their relationship to the ligament attachments, it may be prudent to plan corrective osteotomy surgery" (p. 100).[3]

According to Krackow,[3] several points should be considered when dealing with extraarticular deformities:

- Extraarticular shaft or metaphyseal deformity can lead to important joint line abnormality, which would make ligament balancing difficult. (Fig. 4.5)
- The amount of such deformity, or its effect on the knee, is nearly proportional to its proximity to the joint.
- If an osteotomy is performed, in addition to a TKA, its timing should be carefully planned so that postoperative requirements of each do not interfere with the other.

Even if corrective osteotomy is not required, the use of standard alignment techniques (intramedullary alignment instrumentation) may be difficult (Fig. 4.6). Newer techniques (discussed in detail in Chapter 10) such as patient-specific cutting blocks and computer navigation may be required to perform the TKA adequately in the setting of extraarticular deformity. (Fig. 4.7)

The case of extraarticular deformity emphasizes the need for adequate imaging preoperatively. Full length,

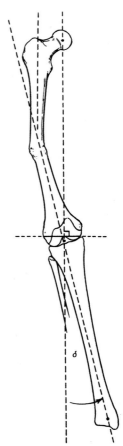

Fig. 4.5 An extraarticular varus deformity of the femur and its effect on joint alignment. *d*, resultant joint deformity from extraarticular deformity of the femur. (Courtesy Krackow, K. *The Technique of Total Knee Arthroplasty.* Mosby; 1990.)

standing, hip-to-ankle films are imperative in this setting, and they are often a minimum radiographic workup in these cases. CT scanning may be indicated to evaluate deformities, especially in the case of previous fracture, and the possibility of nonunion. The use of patient-specific blocks and some computer navigation systems require hip-to-knee three-dimensional imaging for planning purposes as well.

RETAINED HARDWARE

Retained hardware from previous surgery can either be ignored or compensated for during a TKA procedure. However, not infrequently, the retained hardware

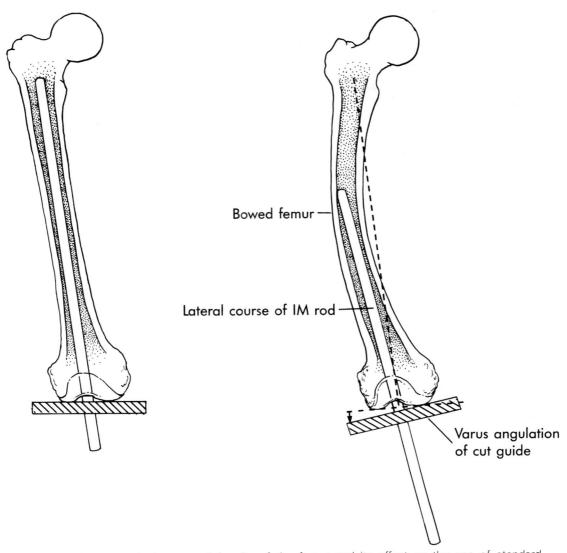

Bowed femur

Lateral course of IM rod

Varus angulation
of cut guide

Fig. 4.6 An extraarticular varus deformity of the femur and its effect on the use of standard intramedullary alignment cutting jigs in total knee arthroplasty. *IM,* intramedullary. (Courtesy Krackow, K. *The Technique of Total Knee Arthroplasty.* Mosby; 1990.)

needs to be addressed (Fig. 4.8). Anything that prolongs TKA surgical time can result in increased perioperative complications, including infection.[2] Therefore removal of retained hardware can be problematic. Additionally, the presence of retained hardware around the knee in patients undergoing TKA may predispose the patient to mechanical complications of the implant after TKA.[16] There is no one right answer for every case; the options

come down to retaining the hardware; removing it, either partially or completely at the time of the TKA; or staging the removal of hardware and the TKA as two separate procedures.

Retention of hardware, if distant from the TKA or if incidental (i.e., retained interference screws or staples from previous ligament reconstruction), may cause little, if any, change in surgical technique. Retained hardware

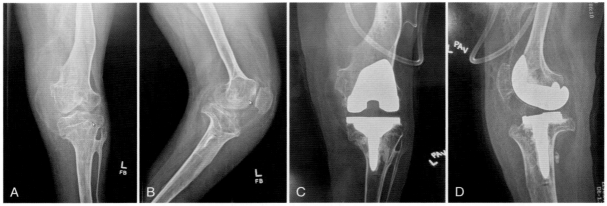

Fig. 4.7 (A) The anteroposterior (AP) radiograph of a patient with multiple osteochondromas, degenerative joint disease, and deformities of the tibia and femur. (B) The lateral radiographs of the same patient. These preoperative radiographs show the difficulty a surgeon might have in performing a total knee arthroplasty using standard cutting jigs. (C) Postoperative AP radiograph of the same patient after total knee arthroplasty that was performed using computer-assisted surgery. Note the residual pin holes that are present from the placement of fixed infrared sensors that were used during the procedure. (D) The lateral postoperative radiograph of the same patient. (Courtesy Chad Hill, MD.)

that prevents intramedullary instrumentation of the femur, more so than the tibia, must be compensated for by the use of either preoperative planning with patient-specific cutting blocks (which can be obtained through many implant companies) or with the use of intraoperative computer navigation (which also can be obtained from many implant companies). One should also be aware of the standard peg length and box depth when using a cruciate substituting femoral component, the keel length on the tibial components, and any additional stem and/or augmentation requirements of the individual implants used when retaining hardware.

Removal of hardware, either partial or complete at the time of TKA, saves one surgical procedure, but it should not cause undo lengthening of the surgical time over what is acceptable. Additionally, this option requires having the appropriate equipment on hand to remove the hardware (e.g., system-specific instrumentation, universal hardware removal instrumentation, and possibly broken screw removal instrumentation along with any high-speed cutting devices as needed). Previous operative reports and implant records are helpful in ensuring that appropriate instrumentation is

available. Bone grafting of defects and the use of stems to bypass defects can be considered as needed. The use of stems to bypass defects and stress risers can also render a standard TKA more difficult and more costly.

The use of staging procedures with removal of hardware as a separate surgery followed by delayed TKA can be considered. The optimal timing between stages is not known, and further study has been recommended.[16] Additionally, it is recommended that the patient should be informed about the potential increased risks of TKA with previous hardware.[16] Staging has been recommended in cases of suspected bacterial colonization or of known previous infection from retained hardware,[16] with appropriate workup and treatment as indicated before consideration for TKA.

One last consideration of retained hardware in conjunction with TKA is the battery effect that may be present with differing metals. Obviously, the potential for a galvanic response to two different metals in a solution is a possibility when those metals come into contact or are in very close proximity to each other. This could require the removal of hardware that is of a dissimilar metal from a TKA implant that might otherwise not require removal.

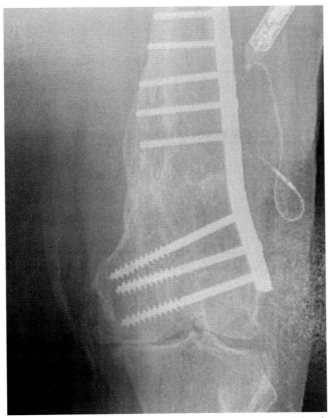

Fig. 4.8 Retained hardware from the previous fixation of a supracondylar femur fracture in a patient with degenerative arthrosis of the knee. This shows the potential difficulty of using standard total knee arthroplasty alignment techniques such as intramedullary alignment jigs. Hardware removal, either partial or complete and either staged or performed during the arthroplasty, or use of computer-assisted surgery or patient-specific cutting blocks must be considered. (Courtesy Curtis Miller, MD)

BONE QUALITY AND BONE LOSS

When implanting a TKA, the goal is to end up with a bond between the host bone and the prosthesis. This can be achieved almost instantly with methylmethacrylate or over time with porous ingrowth prostheses. Both methods are dependent on the quality of the host bone and the quantity (surface area) of host bone available for either methylmethacrylate interdigitation or bony ingrowth.[3] These techniques are briefly mentioned as they relate to the assessment of difficulty in TKA. Chapter 5 will go into detail regarding these topics.

Bone Quality

Osteoarthritis (OA) of the knee accounts for more than 90% of all TKAs.[17] It has been reported that OA and osteoporosis do not normally occur together and that most patients who suffer from OA have a bone density that is greater than normal for their age.[18] Bone reacts to stress; it becomes stronger mechanically by remodeling and becomes denser with the stresses induced with weight bearing. In the case of OA especially associated with deformity, increased stress can lead to increased density of bone. For instance, in a varus knee the bone is denser and harder to cut on the medial side of the femur and tibia than on the lateral side of each. The reverse is true with a valgus knee. The mechanical axis shifts medially in a varus knee and laterally in a valgus knee. The greater the deformity, the greater the shift of the mechanical axis. The greater the shift of the mechanical axis from the center of the knee, the more stress is imparted upon that bone on the concave side of the deformity especially compared with the bone on the convex side of the deformity. This leads to typically denser bone on the concave side of the deformity than the bone on the convex side of the deformity. Dr. Krackow liked to describe this phenomenon seen intraoperatively as the "differential density" of deformity.[3] It might be counterintuitive, but dense bone can cause difficulties in TKA surgery. "Unusually dense or sclerotic bone may pose problems of difficulty in effective use of a bone saw, because such bone is simply difficult to cut. Hard bone also can create problems related to fixation aspects in both cemented and uncemented arthroplasties. Areas of dense sclerotic bone do not permit good cement intrusion and may require extra drilling or preparation of 'keying' fixation holes. In the case of uncemented arthroplasties, dense, sclerotic bone surfaces are notoriously unyielding with regard to prosthetic component fit… the slightest imperfection of cut can lead to persistence of undesirable gaps" (p. 81).[3] In the case of uncemented TKA it is obvious that the greatest contact area between the host bone and the porous-coated prosthesis is most desirable to obtain maximum ingrowth and fixation.

However, if 90% of TKAs are performed in patients who have OA, then that implies that 10% are performed in patients who have other etiologies of arthrosis including inflammatory arthropathies. Rheumatoid arthritis (RA) patients routinely have osteopenic bone secondary to many mechanisms (e.g., disuse, medications used to treat RA). It has been estimated that fully one-quarter of all total joint patients meet the criteria to receive osteoporosis medications, but only 5% receive therapy preoperatively or postoperatively.[19] That implies that not all patients with OA have denser bone associated with deformity. The effect of TKA on host bone is to lower the bone mineral density (BMD) of the host bone after surgery.[20] Krackow states that "in many respects, soft bone may pose more significant problems (in TKA) than hard bone. A point relevant to both cemented and uncemented arthroplasties is that in the presence of osteoporotic bone, one has to be especially careful not to damage the bone as the knee is handled and as instruments are brought to and taken away from cut surfaces" (p. 81).[3] Damage has been

caused by retractors, lamina spreaders, and gap balancing blocks when operating on osteoporotic bone.

Krackow goes on to say that although "relatively osteoporotic bone provides large spaces for good cement intrusion, in the case of uncemented arthroplasty, the presence of *grossly* osteoporotic bone should raise serious questions about the practicality of carrying out uncemented fixation."[3] The choice of implants will be discussed in Chapter 5 and cement technique in Chapter 11. Therefore this chapter is not the place for the "to cement or not cement" debate. Additionally, current ingrowth prostheses may be better suited than previous designs for bony ingrowth. There may not be a platform of support for uncemented TKA in the severely osteoporotic host. These considerations could make the seemingly routine TKA more difficult.

Bone Loss

Bone loss is more frequently seen in revision arthroplasty than in primary TKA. However, bone loss because of wear, osteonecrosis with collapse, insufficiency fractures, and trauma can occur and be present during primary TKA (Fig. 4.9). These topics will be extensively discussed in Chapter 5. They are briefly discussed here in the context of assessing surgical difficulty.

Bone defects on the tibia and femur can be classified as contained or enclosed and uncontained or peripheral. The treatment of bone loss can include further resection of bone to minimize the defect (i.e., more

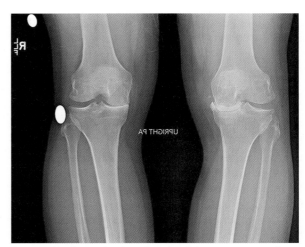

Fig. 4.9 Radiograph showing medial compartment bone loss in a patient with a moderate varus deformity considering total knee arthroplasty. (Courtesy Curtis Miller, MD)

commonly done on the tibia because further resection of the tibia affects both the flexion and extension gaps) within reason so as not to overresect bone. Doing so could compromise ligamentous attachments and markedly affect the size of the tibial component. Some prosthetic designs limit the amount of mismatching of sizes between the tibial and femoral components. Cement and bone graft to fill defects or specialized prosthetics to treat defects (e.g., sleeves/cones for large contained or central defects and use of augments for uncontained or peripheral defects) can be used (Fig. 4.10). Obviously, the larger the defect, the more likely some treatment in addition to routine TKA will be required. Assessing this preoperatively with appropriate imaging (e.g., routine radiographs, CT scanning for assessment of large bone defects, and MRI to assess the effect a large defect may have upon ligament insertion/origin) may be indicated. Defects can increase the difficulty of primary TKA and may require the availability of bone graft, additional hardware (e.g., screw augmentation of cement that fills larger defects, screw and/or staple fixation of bone graft for uncontained or peripheral defects), or specialized prosthetics (e.g., cones/sleeves for contained or central defects, augments for uncontained or peripheral defects,

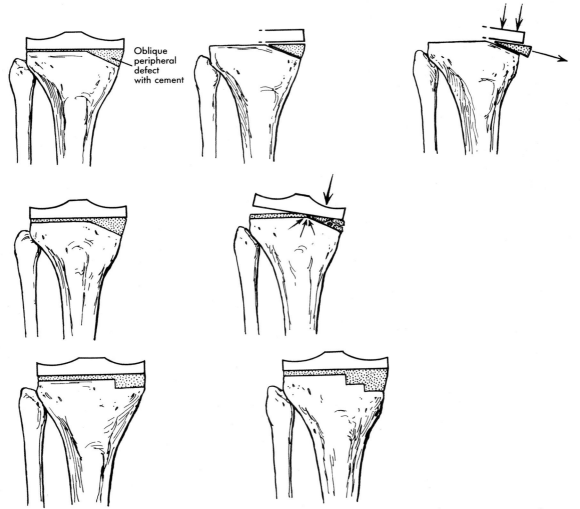

Fig. 4.10 Medial tibial bone loss and surgical techniques using cement or bone to compensate for the defect during total knee arthroplasty. (Courtesy Krackow, K. *The Technique of Total Knee Arthroplasty.* Mosby; 1990.)

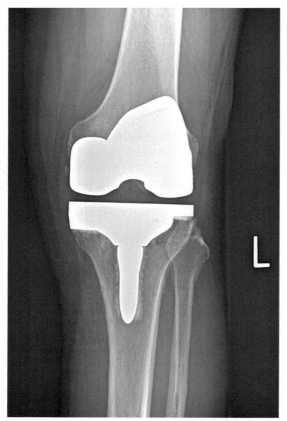

Fig. 4.11 Postoperative radiograph of a patient with medial tibial bone loss that underwent total knee arthroplasty using a medial tibial augment to compensate for the bone loss. (Courtesy Curtis Miller, MD)

and stems to bypass larger defects) that would allow for adequate fixation of the TKA (Fig. 4.11).

LIGAMENT INSTABILITY

The goal of every TKA surgeon is to provide a fixed, well-aligned, well-balanced, and therefore stable TKA. Assessment of the difficulties with alignment and fixation have been discussed previously in this chapter. This section will discuss ligament instability as it relates to the assessment of difficulty in TKA. TKA soft tissue balancing will be discussed extensively in Chapter 8 and specialized implants with additional constraint will be discussed in Chapter 5. However, these issues need to be considered when assessing the difficulty of TKA and will be mentioned here for that purpose only. If adequate ligamentous stability cannot be obtained with routine soft tissue

balancing, one must be prepared to either perform more advanced ligament balancing or ensure that adequate constraint is available in the prosthesis that is used.

For most TKA surgeries with routine deformities, adequate soft tissue balancing can be achieved at the time of TKA to obtain ligamentous stability. Occasionally, with large varus or valgus deformities, the soft tissues on the convex side of the deformity can become lax over years of a progressive deformity. In the case of previous trauma with ligament injury, even if the patient has had previous ligament reconstruction, adequate stability may not be present at the time of TKA to provide the required stability necessary for a good outcome. Techniques for ligament advancement and/or augmentation will be discussed in Chapter 9. However, the problem can be recognized in advance during the initial physical examination and through appropriate imaging, including MRI, to evaluate the soft tissue structures involved. After assessment of the potential need for advanced surgical techniques, one can plan for the appropriate equipment and graft material (i.e., autograft or allograft) necessary to aid in achieving the adequate soft tissue balance. To perform these more technical ligament advancements, augmentations, and reconstructions, one must be comfortable performing the techniques discussed in Chapter 9 or consider referral to a total joint arthroplasty surgeon who is familiar and comfortable performing such procedures. Ligament reconstruction/advancement during TKA has been shown to be a viable option to address ligament instability encountered during TKA.[21]

When adequate ligament balancing cannot be obtained, another consideration to help provide stability would be to use greater constraint in the prosthesis. Chapter 5 discusses the choice of the appropriate implant. For the purposes of this discussion about assessment of difficulty, suffice it to say that most implant companies have multiple levels of constraint available running the full gamut from cruciate retaining to fully constrained hinged prostheses for those with severe instability. The utilization of hinged arthroplasty should typically be reserved for those cases of severe distal femoral bone loss, severe flexion gap instability that cannot be matched by the extension gap, and in the presence of a totally disrupted medial collateral ligament in an elderly patient.[22] Often, multiple levels of constraint can be obtained using the surgeon's preferred implant company. Familiarity with the recommended techniques of the various implant companies when using more constrained prosthetics (i.e., the need for stem fixation when using some total stabilized or hinged prostheses) is necessary when implanting these devices.

The debate about using more advanced ligament reconstruction techniques versus substituting for ligament reconstruction with more implant constraint is not the topic of this chapter. However, one must anticipate the potential need for these options and ensure that the appropriate equipment for performing these advanced ligament techniques or the implant with the appropriate constraint is available before surgery. Additionally, one must recognize that these techniques will add surgical time and difficulty to the procedure.

SUMMARY

Although not every difficult situation can be anticipated before TKA, many, if not most, can be anticipated with careful preoperative planning. As Sun Tzu stated in *The Art of War*, "Every battle is won before it is fought" (p. 13).[23] TKA surgery cannot be exactly compared with battle, but Tzu's philosophy, when applied to TKA surgery, can render even the most difficult TKA manageable.

After spending a year with Dr. Krackow, my biggest takeaways from him were to not underestimate any surgery and that meticulous preparation is not wasted time but rather is time well invested in making even the most difficult TKA seem, as that inexperienced first-year resident once stated, "easy." Krackow states, "It is appropriate to reemphasize the importance of preoperative analyses directed toward predicting intraoperative difficulty. It is difficult, if not impossible, to be prepared adequately when the complexity of a given case goes unrecognized … Careful attention to them (these potential difficulties discussed above) should improve the quality of preoperative planning and result in a much smoother time in the operating room" (p. 85).[3]

REFERENCES

1. Tzu S. *The Art of War*. Shambhala Publications; 2005:6.
2. Ravi, et al. Surgical duration is associated with an increased risk of periprosthetic infection following total knee arthroplasty: a population-based retrospective cohort Study. *EClinical Medicine*. October 22, 2019.
3. Krackow K. *The Technique of Total Knee Arthroplasty*. The C. V. Mosby Company; 1990:75–248.
4. Clark CR. Obesity and total knee arthroplasty. *Clin Summ, J Bone Joint Surg Am*. May 11, 2021.
5. Belmont, et al. Thirty-day postoperative complications and mortality following total knee arthroplasty: incidence and risk factors among a national sample of 15,321 patients. *J Bone Joint Surg Am*. 2014;96(1):20–26.
6. Namba, et al. Obesity and perioperative morbidity in total hip and total knee arthroplasty patients. *J. Arthroplasty*. 2005;20(Suppl 3):46–50.
7. Kremers, et al. The effect of obesity on direct medical costs in total knee arthroplasty. *J Bone Joint Surg Am*. 2014;96(9):718–724.
8. Kerkhoffs, et al. The influence of obesity on the complication rate and outcome of total knee arthroplasty: a meta-analysis and systematic literature review. *J Bone Joint Surg Am*. 2012;94(20):1839–1844.
9. Boyce, et al. The outcomes of total knee arthroplasty in morbidly obese patients: a systematic review of the literature. *Arch Orthop Trauma Surg*. 2019;139(4):553–560.
10. Baker, et al. The association between body mass index and the outcomes of total knee arthroplasy. *J Bone Joint Surg Am*. 2012;94(16):1501–1508.
11. Whiteside L. Surgical exposure in revision total knee arthroplasty. *Instr Course Lect*. 1997;46:221–225.
12. Johnson, et al. Anterior midline or medial parapatellar incision for arthroplasty of the knee. A comparative study. *J Bone Joint Surg Br*. 1986;68(5):812–814.
13. Johnson, et al. Midline or parapatellar incision for knee arthroplasty. A comparative study of wound viability. *J Bone Joint Surg Br*. 1988;70(4):856–858.
14. Sanna, et al. Surgical approaches in total knee arthroplasty. *Joints*. 2013;1(2):33–44.
15. Krackow K. *The Technique of Total Knee Arthroplasty*. The C. V. Mosby Company; 1990:327–370.
16. Manrique, et al. Total knee arthroplasty in patients with retention of prior hardware material: what is the outcome? *Arch Bone Jt Surg*. 2018;6(1):23–26.
17. Lohmander SL. Knee replacement for osteoarthritis: facts, hopes and fears. *Medicographia*. 2013;35(2):181–188.
18. Foss M, Byers P. Bone density, osteoarthosis of the hip, and fracture of the upper end of the femur. *Ann Rheum Dis*. 1972;31:39.
19. Bernatz, et al. Osteoporosis is common and undertreated prior to total joint arthroplasty. *J Arthroplasty*. 2019;34(7):1347–1353.
20. Gundry, et al. A review on bone mineral density loss in total knee replacements leading to increased fracture risk. *Clin Rev Bone Miner Metab*. 2017;15(4):162–174.
21. Jain JK, Agarwal S, Sharma RK. Ligament reconstruction/advancement for management of instability due to ligament insufficiency during total knee arthroplasty: a viable alternative to constrained implant. *J Orthop Sci*. 2014;19:564–569.
22. Indelli, et al. Level of constraint in revision total knee arthroplasty. *Curr Rev Muculoskelet Med*. 2015;8(4):390–397.
23. Tzu S. *The Art of War: Bilingual Edition Complete Chinese and English Text*. Tuttle Publishing; 2012:13.

5

Preoperative Planning From Medical Issues to Implants

Jose C. Alcerro, MD, and Carlos J. Lavernia, MD

There is no straightforward answer as to "when to pull the trigger" and offer surgery to a patient with severe knee disease. Surgeons would require a patient to report chronic knee pain and has functional impairment before they proceed with an arthroplasty. How bad is the pain? Is a patient impaired enough? Are the radiographs bad enough? Is the patient too young or too old? Is the patient too overweight? Is the deformity severe enough? Some of these questions are extremely difficult to answer, and the answers have a large subjective component. Appropriate patient selection is probably one of the most understudied issues in surgery and one of the most frequent causes of suboptimal outcomes. As in all clinical medicine, history taking and physical examination are the cornerstones of making the right diagnosis and recommending the correct treatment. Additional studies such as plain radiographs, CT, and MRI have an important but secondary place in the decision-making process.

PATIENT HISTORY

Although there is currently not a reliable "pain-o-meter," every effort should be made to quantitate and qualify the pain that the patient is having. Details of the type, intensity, and nature of the pain should be noted. The nature of the pain needs to be described in simple terms such as dull, sharp, or electric in nature. Location and radiation of the pain and frequency and time of the day when it affects the patient are key elements. How this pain modifies the patient's function is probably one the most crucial elements in the decision-making process. A detailed history of when the pain appeared and its relationship to spatial events is also very important. Medical legal issues can cloud the patient's description of the problem. For instance, it has been reported that the effect of disability

of patients who are receiving workers compensation can be linked with greater experience of pain and reduced treatment efficacy.[1] Questions to be asked include: When did it begin? Did it appear spontaneously? Was there a traumatic event? Where is the location of the pain; has it gotten any worse since it began? How often is it present? When present, is the intensity the same or does it vary? Does the activity make it worse? Does it require the use of pain medication? How often? Does it wake the patient from sleep? In essence, the amount of detail for the symptom being described and how it affects the patient's life will help identify how this problem is impairing the patient's quality of life. Statements such as "severe pain that does not improve with medication and limits activities of daily living" are not as informative as "severe pain that deprives the patient of sleep, requires daily narcotic intake to slightly reduce its intensity, and exacerbates with minimal activity that can only be performed with the use of assisted devices." Clearly, the latter is a description of a more severe disruption that will probably require surgery.

After all adjectives that better describe the current state of the patient's pain have been outlined, focus needs to be directed toward the pain's effects on function. It is essential to record activities the patient can do or is unable to do as a result of the knee problem. It is important to establish whether the limitations are directly related to the knee problem and not a consequence of other medical conditions (i.e., vascular insufficiency or heart disease). The need for assistive devices, the type of devices, and the patient's dependence on the devices to perform activities of daily living should be clearly identified and documented. As with pain, a comprehensive characterization of the patient's function will aid the surgeon in determining what intervention would be of greater benefit. It is appropriate to include a segment of the patient's socioeconomic background at this time. If the patient is working, it will be important to determine how this condition limits their ability to perform their duties. A conversation on how surgery will affect the patient's ability to work in their current job is important. The time to return to work will be different for someone who is an office clerk rather than a construction worker.

Severity of the functional impairment has been shown to affect outcome.[2,3] Several reports have clearly shown that waiting too long to offer a patient knee replacement arthroplasty will result in a suboptimal outcome.[2-4]

The patient's socioeconomic and medical history will also be very helpful in the decision-making process. It is imperative that all medical events and problems a person has experienced and relevant health-related information be carefully explored and documented.

After establishing the status of the condition, expectations need to be discussed. It has been estimated that one in five primary total knee arthroplasty (TKA) patients is not satisfied with their outcome and that satisfaction (the strongest predictor) is primarily determined by unmet patient expectations.[5,6] What does the patient expect to get out of this procedure? Do the expectations match what the procedure has clinically proven to achieve with regard to pain and function?

Another key aspect is a thorough understanding of the attempts to manage the problem without surgery. A detailed history of the use of antiinflammatory and analgesic drugs has to be obtained. The use of oral pharmacological agents to manage the patient's problem needs to be documented, and in most cases these agents should be tried before offering surgery. The frequency and appropriateness of these oral pharmacological agents needs to be assessed by the surgeon. Intraarticular injections should also be tried before surgical intervention. The type and timing of any intraarticular injection needs to be noted because recent data have demonstrated an increased risk of infection after injections are performed within 3 months of a surgical intervention.[7] Hyaluronic acid and corticosteroids are key modalities in the nonoperative management of severe knee pain. The use of platelet-rich plasma or stem cells remains controversial and has not been shown to be safe and effective in the treatment of arthritis.[8] Additional modalities that need to be considered include physical therapy and bracing, although both of these are temporary solutions; their effectiveness has been questioned particularly in the face of severe radiological changes.[9,10]

The opioid crisis in the United States clearly illustrates the importance of addressing narcotics and their use for any type of chronic pain that has a surgical solution. It has been well established that patients who have been exposed to high opioid doses for a prolonged period of time will display less favorable response to any pain management treatment after surgery.[11,12]

Planning the postdischarge process after knee arthroplasty should be a key portion of the preoperative evaluation. The proper aftercare of patients requires a detailed assessment of the socioeconomic status of the patient. Having a significant other, having social support, and belonging to a faith group have been shown to improve outcomes.[13] Attempts should be made to send the patient straight home after surgery. Several studies have shown that discharge disposition to home results in improved outcomes after TKA compared with discharge to skilled nursing facilities.[14] It is imperative to determine the robustness of the patient's support group. Information about living arrangements, availability of relatives to accompany the patient in the aftercare process, and rehabilitation will aid the discussion on how the patient can prepare in case of undergoing the procedure.

A detailed evaluation of the patient's medical history must be performed. Most of these issues have been addressed in prior chapters. However, the importance of such information will elucidate not only the patient's probabilities of surgical morbidity and mortality but also the potential for complications related to the procedure. Based on this fact (i.e., comorbid conditions), individuals can be classified into one of two groups: (1) medically stable (Figs. 5.1 and 5.2) medically unstable. Patients who are medically unstable will require a multidisciplinary approach. In general, patients will require a preoperative workup that will contain a general medical evaluation including laboratory tests, electrocardiogram, and chest radiography. Drug history of the patient should determine which medication needs to be discontinued, bridged, and/or continued without negative effects. Sources of infection such as dental, dermatological, urinary, or respiratory must be ruled out. Age has not been found to be an absolute contraindication for surgery, however, age-related comorbidities should be considered.[15]

In addition to the aforementioned, it is important to evaluate the patient's nutritional status and vitamin D levels. Lavernia et al.[16] have previously reported that there was a direct correlation between patients

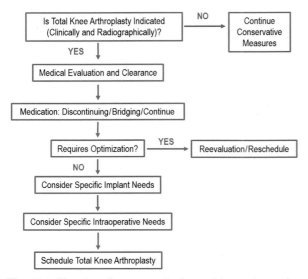

Fig. 5.1 Planning for a medically stable patients (no comorbid conditions).

undergoing joint arthroplasty who presented preoperatively with low levels of total lymphocyte count (TLC: calculated by multiplying the total number of white blood cells by the percentage of lymphocytes) and albumin and increased length of stay, operative time, and resource consumption compared with patients with normal levels. Calcifediol is the serum marker commonly used to determine a patient's vitamin D status. Although there is no consensus on what level defines the low end of the normal range and its associations with pathological conditions, research has shown that suboptimal levels of vitamin D are associated with lower preoperative and postoperative objective scores in total hip arthroplasty.[17] Modification of most risk factors or personal habits that could lead to potential complications has been addressed in previous chapters.

In the set of complex cases (Fig. 5.2) one can encounter patients with severe comorbid conditions

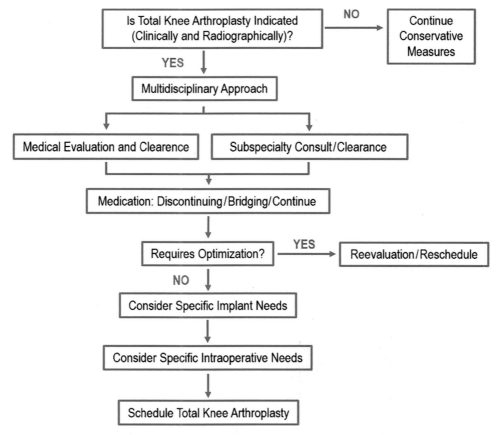

Fig. 5.2 Planning for a medically unstable patients (one or more comorbid conditions).

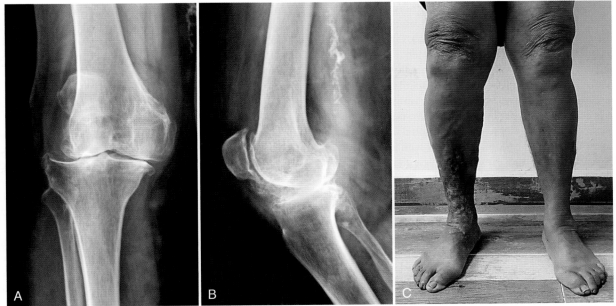

Fig. 5.3 (A) Anteroposterior and (B) lateral radiographic views of a patient's right knee. There is evidence of severe degenerative changes in all three compartments (medial, lateral, and patellofemoral) with marked joint space narrowing and osteophyte formation. Note the tibiofemoral subluxation suggestive of inadequate ligament support (anterior cruciate ligament and posterior cruciate ligament deficiency). There is presence of calcification of the posterior vessels. (C) Clinically, there are prominent varicose veins and important skin changes demonstrating chronic vascular insufficiency. Status of perfusion to the lower extremity is imperative to establish the risk for complications.

that will require evaluation and clearance by a subspecialty physician. These may require specific additional testing such as echocardiogram and stress test for complex cardiac conditions and lower extremity Doppler studies in patients with previous deep vein thrombosis (DVT) or vascular insufficiency (Fig. 5.3). There is an intricate relationship between the patient's medical history and the intraoperative and postoperative planning as certain conditions will demand specific needs. Will this case require the use of specific blood loss prevention tools? Should the anticoagulation therapy be more aggressive due to this condition? Is there a need to prolong antibiotic use for this immunocompromised disorder? Due to the elective nature of TKA, optimization of all possible comorbid conditions will serve the patient better in minimizing the risk for complications during or after the procedure.

PHYSICAL EXAMINATION

The physical examination is the cornerstone of the assessment pyramid. A number of conditions will mimic knee problems and will fool the surgeon into offering surgery to a patient who needs a spine procedure or a hip arthroplasty. Patients should be observed at all times while in the examining room. Careful analysis of the patient getting up from the chair, walking in the room, and getting on the examining table will help the surgeon determine the degree of disability. General appearance and hygiene is to be accounted for; inadequate oral and overall hygiene can lead to potential infection-related complications.[18] The severity of a deformity can be assessed on weight-bearing and during gait. This important part of the assessment can also reveal the overall strength, disability, and discomfort the patient is experiencing as a consequence of the condition.

A detailed examination of the extremity and assessment of the status of the skin (i.e., presence of previous incisions, sites of superficial infection), range of motion, ligament balance, stability, and patellar tracking will relate to the surgeon's ability to estimate technical difficulty, which is essential in the planning process. A large number of prior surgeries or a transverse incision around the knee may be an indication for a plastic surgery consultation. Muscle and rotational flaps need to be considered when encountering this scenario. Peripheral circulation and the presence of vascular insufficiency are important aspects to consider as they can also lead to potential complications. All the examinations need to include a detailed hip examination. The hip should be examined with the patient supine and sitting down. Although spine, hip, and knee disease can coexist, it is important to determine which one to address first. A practical way to determine which joint is responsible for most of the patient's symptomatic presentation is an injection of local anesthetic into the knee or the hip; identifying the location that results in the most positive relief of the patient's symptoms provides a better understanding of the path to take. Although the reports of knee pain can be confirmed, the decision of which condition to be addressed first must be discussed or evaluated in depth to determine what intervention would bring the greatest benefit.

A thorough neurological examination is also needed. It should include the assessment of reflexes, sensation, and presence of clonus or pathological reflexes such as Babinski.

IMAGING

Patient evaluation for TKA requires routine radiographic imaging, which will help assess the severity of the disease and confirm the diagnosis. Weight-bearing anteroposterior (AP), lateral, intercondylar or notch, patellofemoral, and, ideally, long standing weight-bearing views should be performed.

The AP view should be obtained with the patient in a standing position. Assessment of joint space of both the medial and lateral compartments can help determine the amount of cartilage damage. The varus and valgus alignment and degree of the deformity will affect the technical aspects of the procedure. Bone quality, presence of associated osteophytes, and subchondral changes are also to be noted; these can be related to degenerative changes. These findings might not be as evident in patients who present with an inflammatory condition (Fig. 5.4).

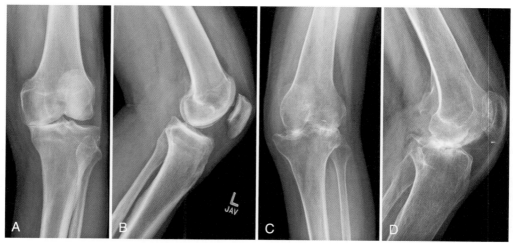

Fig. 5.4 Anteroposterior and lateral short film views that compare radiological changes found due to (A, B) a degenerative condition (osteoarthritis [OA]) and (C, D) an inflammatory process (rheumatoid arthritis [RA]). Predominant differences include asymmetrical (OA) versus symmetrical joint space narrowing (RA). Variable (OA) versus marked (RA) osteoporotic changes. Presence (OA) versus lack (RA) of subchondral sclerosis and osteophyte formation. Variable (OA) versus marked (RA) soft tissue swelling.

Long standing AP weight-bearing views of the lower extremities can help assess the overall mechanical alignment of the lower extremity. The mechanical alignment refers to the angle formed by a line drawn from the center of the femoral head to the medial tibial spine and another line from the tibial spine and the center of the ankle joint.[19] This angle should be approximately 5 to 6 degrees for men and 6 to 7 degrees for women. It is essential to ensure that the patient is in neutral rotation of the legs to obtain the most accurate measurements. This view allows determination of the varus/valgus alignment of the knees, leg length discrepancy, and the presence of extraarticular deformities (i.e., bowing of the femur or tibia). An asymmetrical enlargement of one knee noted on a long standing view suggests the presence of a flexion contracture. This finding must be recorded as it implies the potential for increased difficulty during the procedure and an automatic adjustment in the amount of bone taken from the femur. This hip-to-knee-to-ankle view is key in the complete evaluation of the mechanical axis of the extremity. This view allows the visualization of any coronal curvature in the tibia or femur and any disease in the hip or ankle joints. This curvature on the femur or the tibia will affect the cutting angle on the transverse cuts of both the femur and the tibia when the anatomical axes are used to make the bony resections. At this point, it is important to clarify the difference between the anatomical axis and the mechanical axis of each individual bone as well as the extremity (Fig. 5.5). The mechanical axis is used and represents the static mechanics of the leg. The anatomical axis is used in surgery to make the transverse cuts to both bones, tibia and femur. These cuts are key determinants in the coronal orientation of the extremity. Another important parameter to evaluate in these coronal views is the joint line orientation (Fig. 5.6). Any major deviation of the joint line from the horizontal will result in abnormal kinematics in the gait cycle.

The lateral view (knee with 30 degrees of flexion) also helps in assessing for joint space narrowing, bone quality, presence of associated osteophytes, and subchondral changes of the anterior and posterior aspect of the knee. It aids in determining the extent of disease of the patellofemoral compartment, evaluation of patellar height (Insall-Salvati ratio), tibial inclination, and the presence of loose bodies at the suprapatellar and posterior regions.

The intercondylar view (AP view of the knee flexed at 40 degrees) can aid in assessing for loose body (locked knee) and better delineation of the intercondylar eminence. The change in deformity produced by this view provides the surgeon with a three-dimensional view of the cartilage loss location. The femoral condyles should be free from superimposition with the intercondylar fossa in profile, giving the appearance of a "notch."[20] It will also contribute in determining joint space, bone quality, presence of associated osteophytes, and subchondral changes.

The sunrise view assists in determining the patellofemoral alignment, trochlear grove, and articular surfaces. As on previous images, joint space narrowing, bone quality, presence of associated osteophytes, and subchondral changes can be found. Evidence of inadequate patellar tracking or patellar subluxation should alert the surgeon for lateral release of the patella during the procedure.

The advent of more complex imaging technologies for preoperative planning has failed to provide any major difference in clinical outcomes after TKA when using manual instrumentation.[21] To date, the use of CT, MRI, or bone scanning in the preoperative planning for TKA has been limited and is not advocated by most surgeons. CT and MRI imaging may be necessary in extraordinary conditions such as incidental findings during evaluation that would suggest the presence of a bony lesion (Figs. 5.7 and 5.8), rotational deformities, congenital dislocation of the patella, and posttraumatic severe deformities that require additional technical considerations and preparation.

TEMPLATING

Careful preoperative planning will require an adequate set of radiographic images to ensure appropriate sizing and aligning the cuts. A marker of known dimensions is mandatory if accurate sizing is to be determined. Conventional templating uses printed radiographs to determine the size and position of the implants based on acrylic/acetate sheets with silhouettes of the actual implants with a set magnification.[22] These templates are overlaid on radiographs and are made with a standard 10% to 20% magnification that cannot be adjusted for variations in radiographic technique, potentially increasing the risk for inaccurate measurements.[23] With

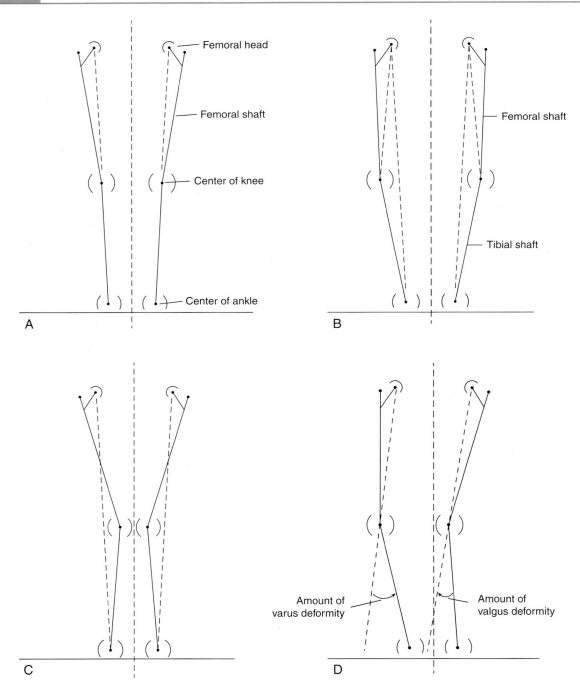

Fig. 5.5 (A) Diagram demonstrating the mechanical axis with interrupted lines and the anatomical axis with complete lines. The deformity is a deviation from a line that goes from the center of the hip to the center of the ankle: (B) varus deformity, (C) valgus deformity, and (D) windswept deformity. From Krackow K. *The Technique of Total Knee Arthroplasty. Mosby. 1990.*

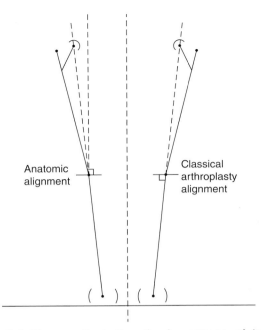

Fig. 5.6 Diagram illustrating the importance of joint line orientation and the two current philosophies used in total knee arthroplasty for cutting both bones. The classical way of making the cuts, which leaves a slightly slanted joint line, and the anatomical way of making the cuts, which yields a horizontal joint line. From Krackow K. *The Technique of Total Knee Arthroplasty.* Mosby; 1990.

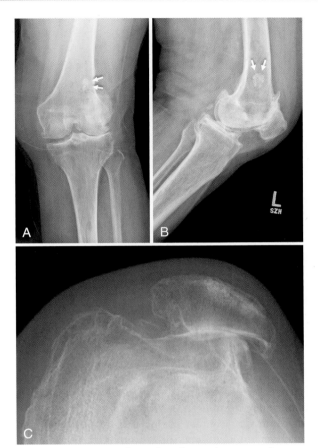

Fig. 5.7 Routine series of radiographs to evaluate a potential knee arthroplasty candidate. Patient demonstrates valgus deformity; medial, posterior, and lateral osteophyte formation; bilateral joint space narrowing predominantly of the lateral compartment; subchondral sclerosis; and patellofemoral subluxation with a hypoplastic lateral femoral condyle. Incidental finding of a bone lesion (*white arrows*) is suggestive of a benign enchondroma. It is appropriate to further evaluate, although there is a low risk of malignant transformation (chondrosarcoma). (A) Short format anteroposterior; (B) lateral view, appropriate for close detail; and (C) sunrise patellar view.

the advent of digital radiography, printing of radiographs in the United States has become a thing of the past. These digital images are obtained using x-rays on receptors that will then create an image of the bony structures. These digital images are viewable on monitors and can be manipulated using a picture archiving and communication system (PACS). These PACS systems allow the surgeon to change resolution, magnification, and picks ablation of every radiograph. Digital templating software packages use accurately digitized images obtained by scanning three-dimensional images of the implants and projecting them into one dimension. The software allows the surgeon to calibrate the images and templates to the correct magnification factor. The appropriate template is selected from a library and digitally overlaid on the image. Several steps are involved in using digital templating. Variable results have been reported with the use of conventional and digital templating for hip and knee arthroplasty. A study by Peek

et al.[24] found that digital templating was a very useful tool and that their experienced resulted within one size (above or below the one measured during preoperative templating) of the implanted prosthesis. Specht et al.[25] showed that digital templating was more accurate in predicting the tibial component size; no differences were

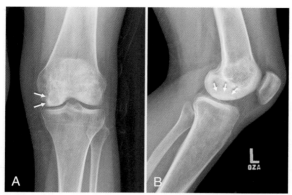

Fig. 5.8 (A) Anteroposterior and (B) lateral radiographic views of the left knee of a patient reporting severe pain. Note the patchy area of radiolucency on the lateral condyle (*white arrows*) and sclerosis surrounding the lesion. There are relatively well-maintained joint spaces. Despite minor surface irregularities, the patient was thought not to have radiographic film consistent with mayor degenerative changes; although the images are suggestive of a bony infarct (osteonecrosis) that requires attention.

found between techniques for the femoral component. In a different publication Hsu et al.[26] highlighted the importance of digital imaging and templating to help reduce errors associated with manipulating radiographs and templates by scaling templates to the actual radiographic magnification.

Initial steps of templating will involve determining the mechanical alignment of the lower extremity by drawing a line on the long standing view from the center of the femoral head to the center of the ankle joint. A neutral mechanical alignment should bisect the center of the knee joint. This will aid in establishing the direction of the deformity (varus or valgus malalignment), and any extraarticular deformities (bowing) should be noted. This is followed by an assessment of the tibiofemoral angle (angle between the anatomical axis of femur with the anatomical axis of tibia). The tibial resection is perpendicular to the mechanical axis of the tibia; whether a gap balancing or a measured resection technique is used for coronal stability, these angle measurements will provide valuable insight to more accurately attain proper femoral component rotation.[27] Posterior slope of the tibia and patellar height are measured on the lateral view. An effort to restore the patient's native posterior tibial slope should be made when using a

cruciate-retaining design. The posterior tibial slope angle influences knee kinematics, knee stability, flexion gap, knee range of motion, and tension of the posterior cruciate ligament (PCL). A study showed that reproduction of the native posterior tibial slope within 3 degrees resulted in better clinical outcomes manifested by gains in range of motion and knee functional outcome scores.[28] In the posterior substituting design the aim is to cut the tibia with minimal posterior slope. The posterior slope increase is directly correlated to flexion gap. In this design, the flexion gap can increase by 2-fold because of (1) PCL removal and (2) excessive slope, leading to posterior flexion instability.[29] Cam-post impingement is a potential problem with this design and can be avoided by keeping a minimal tibial slope inclination.

When the amount of bone resection has been determined, evaluation of how this will affect the ligament balance needs to be done. Restoring the height of the joint line is crucial as it helps optimize knee kinematics. Elevation of the joint line may lead to midflexion instability and patellofemoral problems (equivalent to patella baja). Lowering the joint line can lead to lack of full extension, patellar subluxation, and flexion instability. If any change to the joint line is noted during the planning process, sources of augmentation need to be available (i.e., cement/graft/metal augments).

At the end of the task, femoral and tibial components are sized. Templating is dictated primarily by the coronal dimensions of the femur and tibia. The position of the template on the sagittal plane with the use of a lateral radiograph view is usually a secondary factor. The objective is to avoid complications related to under- and oversizing of the component.

IMPLANTS

Bearing Surface Materials

Currently, knee arthroplasty is being performed in a younger, more active population with an increased functional demand and usually a desire to participate in impact-loading activities.[30] This poses an important challenge for designers. Over the last decade, there have been major improvements in the quality and wear resistance of the materials being used for knee arthroplasty surgery. The accumulation of polyethylene wear debris over time in periprosthetic tissue can lead to particle-induced inflammation and subsequent osteolysis.[31] Free radicals within the plastic used as a bearing material can also lead to oxidative degradation of the polyethylene insert, contributing to abrasive wear. Vitamin E has been introduced as an antioxidant in third-generation highly cross-linked polyethylene to decrease wear rates, but it has not been proven in long-term studies to date.[32]

New bearing materials have also been introduced in the field of arthroplasty. Oxidized zirconium is a relatively new material used for femoral components in knee devices and in femoral heads in hip surgery. This technology involves a process that uses a thermally driven oxygen diffusion and transforms the metallic cobalt-chromium alloy surface into a durable low-friction oxide. It has been suggested that oxidized zirconium provides superior resistance to abrasion without the risk of brittleness or fracture, thereby combining the benefits of metals and ceramics.[33] A study by Ahmed et al.[34] on a series of 303 knee surgeries using oxidized zirconium femoral components found that a survival rate at 10 years postoperatively (assessed using Kaplan-Meier analysis) was 97%. There were no revisions for loosening, osteolysis, or failure of the implant. There was a significant improvement in all patient-reported outcomes and clinical scores. A review by Civinini et al.[35] reported low revision rates at 12.6 years of follow-up, and a survival rate that ranged from 98.7% to 100% at 5 to 7 years to 97.8% at 10 years. They did not find any adverse reactions for this new material.

Knee Implant Designs

Over the years, there have been many implant designs. The modern development of knee arthroplasty implants started in the 19th and early 20th centuries in an effort to overcome the many obstacles encountered with the early materials and techniques. When planning for knee arthroplasty, size and mechanical stability or level of constraint are the two most important parameters. Insert thickness is usually determined in surgery. Mechanical level of constraint needs to be planned and selected before the surgery. Most knee implants can be categorized as (1) nonconstrained, (2) semiconstrained, or (3) constrained.

A nonconstrained TKA design relies primarily on the patient's ligaments and muscles for stability. Under this definition, two designs fulfill the requirements: (1) bicruciate-retaining designs and (2) cruciate-retaining designs. The preservation of all ligament structures can provide a more natural knee movement pattern design (i.e., enhanced kinematics and proprioception) which enhances the shock-absorbing function and reduces transmission of shear forces. Conserving the anterior cruciate ligament (ACL) requires sparing the ACL insertion at the mid aspect of the tibial plateau; this results in a narrowing of the tibial component fixation thus jeopardizing tibial anchoring of the implant. In 2019 Troelsen et al. reported on a radiostereometric analysis of tibial component micromotion and found no differences at 2 years between the bicruciate-retaining and cruciate-retaining implants in terms of fixation, stability, or patient-reported outcomes. They recommended against the routine clinical use of bicruciate-retaining implants as there was an increase in complications when trying to preserve the ACL. In addition, there was no demonstrable benefit to the patient and an increased cost.[36] Additional publications concur with these findings and state that current research has not shown clear indications and guidelines for the value and use of this implant. Although kinematics have been shown to mirror the native knee more closely, the clinical outcomes of bicruciate- versus cruciate-retaining total knee do not differ significantly.[37,38]

The standard treatment of advanced osteoarthritis involves sacrificing the ACL. Cruciate-retaining systems are designed and require a functional PCL to provide stability in flexion, mid flexion, and extension; thus it is not advisable to use this design in patients with preexisting or intraoperatively recognized PCL insufficiency. Advantages of this design include (1) inherent stability, (2) improved proprioception and kinematics, and (3) bone preservation by minimizing distal femoral bone resection.[39] These facts should not obscure the consideration that in certain cases the use of a cruciate-retaining implant may not be feasible. Severe knee deformities will require a more constrained implant. Characteristics that can not be met by a cruciate retaining implant design which requires ligament integrity to provide stability, should guide the surgeon to a more constrained prosthesis.

Semiconstrained or cruciate-substituting prostheses are used when PCL retention is not possible or under circumstances that require a more stable prosthesis. This implant provides a more inherent stability where a transverse metal cam contained in the posterior aspect of the femoral component engages the tibial polyethylene post during flexion. Advantages of this design are that it (1) facilitates soft tissue balancing due to an absent PCL,

(2) reduces axial rotation and condylar translation, and (3) avoids the risk of PCL insufficiency.[39]

Both PCL-retaining and PCL-substituting knee arthroplasties are very successful, with success rates over 95% in 10-year follow-up studies. Multiple metaanalyses have demonstrated satisfactory survivorship and similar outcomes comparing the cruciate-retaining and posterior-stabilized TKA prosthesis designs.

The option of an ultracongruent insert is available in some prosthetic cruciate-retaining implant systems. These inserts are characterized by a higher anterior wall and deeper trough compared with the standard inserts; this compensates for a deficient PCL using increased condylar congruency. In a recent cadaveric study Willing et al.[40] compared the kinematics and laxity limits of cruciate-retaining implants with a PCL to condylar-stabilized implants without a PCL. Overall, there appears to be a reduction in anterior–posterior stability, suggesting that the condylar-stabilized bearing surface design does not adequately compensate for the loss of the PCL. Clinical outcomes have also been measured. Stirling et al. compared early knee function when using cemented TKA with either a cruciate-retaining polyethylene insert or a highly congruent condylar-stabilizing insert. They found that condylar-stabilizing inserts have equivalent patient-reported outcome measures and patient satisfaction at 1 year compared with cruciate-retaining inserts.[41] Similar findings were also reported by Song et al.[42] who stated that the ultracongruent design showed comparable functional outcomes with those of the cruciate-retaining design and provided similar in vivo stability.

Constraint within an implant indicates a limitation in the range of motion in the axial and coronal planes; this can be obtained by using either a linked or a nonlinked design. The constrained nonhinged design continues to be a nonlinked prosthesis. It is derived from the PCL-substituting model and fundamentally uses a larger tibial post and deeper femoral box, yielding more stability and constraint (about 2 to 3 degrees) in both sagittal and rotational planes. Indications include collateral ligament attenuation or deficiency, flexion gap laxity, and moderate bone loss. Weaknesses of this design include a greater risk for early aseptic loosening, as there are higher transmission forces to the fixation interfaces, and the requirement of extensive femoral bone resection to accommodate the components.

The constrained hinged design is composed of linked femoral and tibial components. Rotating hinge options allow the tibial bearing to rotate around a yoke that theoretically mitigates the risk of aseptic loosening at the expense of increasing levels of prosthetic constraint. They are used when the knee is highly unstable and the ligaments will be unable to support other types of prostheses. Constrained prostheses are reserved for severely damaged knees. Typically they are used in the revision setting after a failed primary procedure or complication. Because of the higher amount of mechanical stress put on hinged prostheses, they are not expected to last as long as other less-constrained designs. Fixed hinged designs implanted in the middle of last century led to a high failure rate, and new modular designs with rotational systems were developed to address this issue. Important improvements in these designs, such as the ability of the implant to rotate and the introduction of metal wedge augmentation and modular fluted stems with variable offset to improve the alignment and allow cementless fixation, have yielded positive results.

REFERENCES

1. Newton-John T, McDonald A, Pain management in the context of workers compensation: A case study. *Transl Behav Med.* 2020;2(1):38–46. doi:10.1007/s13142-012-0112-0.
2. Desmeules F, Dionne CE, Belzile E, Bourbonnais R, Fremont P. The burden of wait for knee replacement surgery: Effects on pain, function and health-related quality of life at the time of surgery. *Rheumatol (Oxf).* 2010;49(5):945–954.
3. Desmeules F, Dionne CE, Belzile EL, Bourbonnais R, Fremont P. The impacts of pre-surgery wait for total knee replacement on pain, function and health-related quality of life six months after surgery. *J Eval Clin Pract.* 2012;18(1):111–120.
4. Lizaur-Utrilla A, Martinez-Mendez D, Miralles-Munoz FA, Marco-Gomez L, Lopez-Prats FA. Negative impact of waiting time for primary total knee arthroplasty on satisfaction and patient-reported outcome. *Int Orthop.* 2016;40(11):2303–2307.
5. Bourne RB, Chesworth BM, Davis AM, Mahomed NN, Charron KD. Patient satisfaction after total knee arthroplasty: Who is satisfied and who is not? *Clin Orthop Relat Res.* 2010;468(1):57–63.
6. Noble PC, Conditt MA, Cook KF, Mathis KB. The John Insall Award: Patient expectations affect satisfaction with total knee arthroplasty. *Clin Orthop Relat Res.* 2006;452:35–43.

7. Bedard NA, Pugely AJ, Elkins JM, Duchman KR, Westermann RW, Liu SS, et al. The John N. Insall Award: Do intraarticular injections increase the risk of infection after TKA? *Clin Orthop Relat Res.* 2017;475(1):45–52.

8. Alcerro JC, Lavernia CJ. Stem cells and platelet-rich plasma for knee osteoarthritis: Prevalence and cost in south Florida. *J Am Acad Orthop Surg.* 2019;27(20):779–783.

9. Duivenvoorden T, Brouwer RW, van Raaij TM, Verhagen AP, Verhaar JA, Bierma-Zeinstra SM. Braces and orthoses for treating osteoarthritis of the knee. *Cochrane Database Syst Rev.* 2015;(3):CD004020.

10. Van Ginckel A, Hall M, Dobson F, Calders P. Effects of long-term exercise therapy on knee joint structure in people with knee osteoarthritis: A systematic review and meta-analysis. *Semin Arthritis Rheum.* 2019;48(6): 941–949.

11. Bedard NA, Pugely AJ, Westermann RW, Duchman KR, Glass NA, Callaghan JJ. Opioid use after total knee arthroplasty: Trends and risk factors for prolonged use. *J Arthroplasty.* 2017;32(8):2390–2394.

12. Manalo JPM, Castillo T, Hennessy D, Peng Y, Schurko B, Kwon YM. Preoperative opioid medication use negatively affect health related quality of life after total knee arthroplasty. *Knee.* 2018;25(5):946–951.

13. Demiralp B, Koenig L, Nguyen JT, Soltoff SA. Determinants of hip and knee replacement: The role of social support and family dynamics. *Inquiry.* 2019;56 46958019837438.

14. Keswani A, Tasi MC, Fields A, Lovy AJ, Moucha CS, Bozic KJ. Discharge destination after total joint arthroplasty: An analysis of postdischarge outcomes, placement risk factors, and recent trends. *J Arthroplasty.* 2016;31(6):1155–1162.

15. Fang M, Noiseux N, Linson E, Cram P. The effect of advancing age on total joint replacement outcomes. *Geriatr Orthop Surg Rehabil.* 2015;6(3):173–179.

16. Lavernia CJ, Sierra RJ, Baerga L. Nutritional parameters and short term outcome in arthroplasty. *J Am Coll Nutr.* 1999;18(3):274–278. https://doi.org/10.1080/07315724.19 99.10718863.

17. Lavernia CJ, Villa JM, Iacobelli DA, Rossi MD. Vitamin D insufficiency in patients with THA: Prevalence and effects on outcome. *Clin Orthop Relat Res.* 2014;472(2): 681–686.

18. Howard JL, Morcos MW, Lanting BA, Somerville LE, McAuley JP. Reproducing the native posterior tibial slope in cruciate-retaining total knee arthroplasty: Technique and clinical implications. *Orthopedics.* 2020;43(1): e21–e26.

19. Abdel MP, Ollivier M, Parratte S, Trousdale RT, Berry DJ, Pagnano MW. Effect of postoperative mechanical axis alignment on survival and functional outcomes of modern total knee arthroplasties with cement:

A concise follow-up at 20 years. *J Bone Jt Surg Am.* 2018;100(6):472–478.

20. Lampignano J, Kendrick LE, Bontrager's. *Textbook of Radiographic Positioning and Related Anatomy.* 9th ed. Elsevier; 2017. ISBN: 9780323399661.

21. Karas V, Calkins TE, Bryan AJ, Culvern C, Nam D, Berger RA, et al. Total knee arthroplasty in patients less than 50 years of age: Results at a mean of 13 years. *J Arthroplasty.* 2019;34(10):2392–2397.

22. Lavernia CJ, Alcerro JC, Contreras JS. Knee arthroplasty: Growing trends and future problems. *Int J Clin Rheumatol.* 2010;5:565–579. https://doi.org/10.221/ ijr.10.49.

23. Heal J, Blewitt N. Kinemax total knee arthroplasty: Trial by template. *J Arthroplasty.* 2002;17(1):90–94.

24. Peek AC, Bloch B, Auld J. How useful is templating for total knee replacement component sizing? *Knee.* 2012;19(4):266–269.

25. Specht LM, Levitz S, Iorio R, Healy WL, Tilzey JF. A comparison of acetate and digital templating for total knee arthroplasty. *Clin Orthop Relat Res.* 2007;464:179–183.

26. Hsu AR, Kim JD, Bhatia S, Levine BR. Effect of training level on accuracy of digital templating in primary total hip and knee arthroplasty. *Orthopedics.* 2012;35(2): e179–183.

27. Dennis DA, Komistek RD, Kim RH, Sharma A. Gap balancing versus measured resection technique for total knee arthroplasty. *Clin Orthop Relat Res.* 2010;468(1):102–107.

28. Kucukdurmaz F, Parvizi J. The prevention of periprosthetic joint infections. *Open Orthop J.* 2016;10:589–599.

29. Sierra RJ, Berry DJ. Surgical technique differences between posterior-substituting and cruciate-retaining total knee arthroplasty. *J Arthroplasty.* 2008;23(7 Suppl): 20–23.

30. Huijbregts HJ, Khan RJ, Sorensen E, Fick DP, Haebich S. Patient-specific instrumentation does not improve radiographic alignment or clinical outcomes after total knee arthroplasty. *Acta Orthop.* 2016;87(4):386–394.

31. Gallo J, Goodman SB, Konttinen YT, Wimmer MA, Holinka M. Osteolysis around total knee arthroplasty: A review of pathogenetic mechanisms. *Acta Biomater.* 2013;9(9):8046–8058.

32. Wilhelm SK, Henrichsen JL, Siljander M, Moore D, Karadsheh M. Polyethylene in total knee arthroplasty: Where are we now? *J Orthop Surg (Hong Kong).* 2018;26(3). 2309499018808356.

33. Good V, Ries M, Barrack RL, Widding K, Hunter G, Heuer D. Reduced wear with oxidized zirconium femoral heads. *J bone Jt Surg Am volume.* 2003;85-A(Suppl 4): 105–110. https://doi.org/10.2106/00004623-200300004- 00013.

34. Ahmed I, Salmon LJ, Waller A, Watanabe H, Roe JP, Pinczewski LA. Total knee arthroplasty with an oxidised zirconium femoral component: ten-year survivorship analysis. *Bone Joint J*. 2016;98-B(1):58–64. https://doi.org/10.1302/0301-620X.98B1.36314.

35. Civinini R, Matassi F, Carulli C, Sirleo L, Lepri AC, Innocenti M. Clinical results of oxidized zirconium femoral component in TKA. A review of long-term survival: Review article. *HSS J*. 2017;13(1):32–34.

36. Troelsen A, Ingelsrud LH, Thomsen MG, Muharemovic O, Otte KS, Husted H. Are there differences in micromotion on radiostereometric analysis between bicruciate and cruciate-retaining designs in TKA? A randomized controlled trial. *Clin Orthop Relat Res*. 2019;2020(478):2045–2053.

37. Baumann F. Bicruciate-retaining total knee arthroplasty compared to cruciate-sacrificing TKA: What are the advantages and disadvantages? *Expert Rev Med Devices*. 2018;15(9):615–617.

38. Osmani FA, Thakkar SC, Collins K, Schwarzkopf R. The utility of bicruciate-retaining total knee arthroplasty. *Arthroplasty Today*. 2016;3(1):61–66.

39. Song SJ, Park CH, Bae DK. What to know for selecting cruciate-retaining or posterior-stabilized total knee arthroplasty. *Clin Orthop Surg*. 2019;11(2):142–150.

40. Willing R, Moslemian A, Yamomo G, Wood T, Howard J, Lanting B. Condylar-stabilized TKR may not fully compensate for PCL-deficiency: An in vitro cadaver study. *J Orthop Res*. 2019;37(10):2172–2181.

41. Stirling P, Clement ND, MacDonald D, Patton JT, Burnett R, Macpherson GJ. Early functional outcomes after condylar-stabilizing (deep-dish) versus standard bearing surface for cruciate-retaining total knee arthroplasty. *Knee Surg & Relat Res*. 2019;31:3. https://doi.org/10.1186/s43019-019-0001-7.

42. Song EK, Lim HA, Joo SD, Kim SK, Lee KB, Seon JK. Total knee arthroplasty using ultra-congruent inserts can provide similar stability and function compared with cruciate-retaining total knee arthroplasty. *Knee Surg Sports Traumatol Arthrosc*. 2017;25(11):3530–3535.

Issues and Considerations on the Day of Surgery

6

Setting Up an Outpatient or Same-Day Discharge Total Knee Arthroplasty (TKA) Program

Travis Eason, MD, Patrick Toy, MD, and William M. Mihalko, MD, PhD

INTRODUCTION

When the first edition of this book was released, primary total knee arthroplasty (TKA) was a procedure that had a mean length of stay of around 7 days. Dr. Krackow was a pioneer and advanced the issues pertaining to length of stay throughout his career. Advances in operative techniques, anesthesia, and perioperative analgesia have allowed same-day TKA to become a reality. Outpatient total joint arthroplasty has become more popular, with goals to decrease costs while still providing high-value care. To ensure an efficient, effective, and safe outpatient TKA program, it is imperative to establish appropriate protocols. A multidisciplinary team, including the surgeon, anesthesiologist, nurses, operating room (OR) staff, and therapists, is required to set up a successful and safe outpatient total joint program.

Historically, TKA has been performed in the inpatient setting with a 5- to 10-day hospital stay. Patients remained in the hospital to be monitored for postoperative acute blood loss anemia, pain control, and mobilization with physical therapy. Improvements in pharmacological and surgical techniques have markedly reduced the operative blood loss, and fewer patients are requiring postoperative transfusions for anemia. Multimodal pain control has minimized postoperative pain, allowing earlier mobilization and early discharge. The many innovations in total joint arthroplasty and perioperative care have contributed to the successful transition of TKA to the ambulatory setting.

An estimated 680,000 TKAs were performed in the United States in 2014 and this number is expected to increase to 1.26 million by 2030 according to 2000 to 2014 trends.[1] Policies have been instituted that have incentivized patients and physicians to reduce the cost of TKA. The most effective ways to reduce costs are by reducing the lengths of stay, complications, and readmissions. Outpatient total joint arthroplasty procedures, as a whole, have the potential to save up to $7000 per procedure compared with the inpatient setting.[2] Medicare pays for approximately 55% of TKAs in the United States.[3] In 2018 TKA was removed from the Medicare inpatient-only list. Since that time, there has been a marked increase in the number of TKAs done on an outpatient basis. According to Medicare Fee-for-Service Part A claims data, TKA claims went from 0.2% outpatient coding in 2017 to 36.4% in 2019.[4]

It should be noted that there are major differences between performing a TKA in the hospital setting with the intent to discharge the patient on the same day and performing one at a stand-alone ambulatory surgery center (ASC). Even though TKA in a stand-alone ASC may be considered safe for most patients, this type of program requires a team approach from anesthesia, OR support staff, physical therapists, and nurses, with appropriate measures to account for the possible need for a 23-hour overnight stay, which may not be possible at all centers.

Multiple studies have concluded that there are no increased risks of adverse events or complications with a shorter length of stay with outpatient TKA. In a metaanalysis comparing complication rates between inpatient and outpatient total joint arthroplasties there was no increased risk of major complications, readmissions, deep venous thromboses (DVTs), urinary tract infections, pneumoniae, or wound complications with outpatient TKA.[5] These studies suggest that arthroplasty surgeries can be performed safely in an ASC in appropriately selected patients without increased risks of complications.[6-8] Kelly et al.[9] found that patients who had surgery performed in the ASC had higher patient satisfaction scores in pain management, staff interaction, and preparedness for discharge. Thus reducing discharge delays and improving patient satisfaction scores are paramount considering the financial incentives provided by the Centers for Medicare and Medicaid Services.[2,9]

PATIENT SELECTION

Outpatient TKA may not be feasible or safe for all patients. In the same manner as for traditional TKA patients should be evaluated by their primary care physician preoperatively to note any ongoing medical problems. The first three chapters in this book focus on understanding the comorbidities of patients and how to optimize them. This is important when deciding whether a patient is a good candidate for a same-day discharge or a procedure to be done in an ASC. Patients should be medically optimized for a total joint arthroplasty by correcting modifiable risk factors. An evaluation should be performed by both the surgeon and the anesthesiologist before surgery to determine whether the patient would be a good candidate for TKA at an ASC.

Patients who have specific comorbidities, such as coronary artery disease, diabetes, body mass index (BMI) >40, peripheral vascular disease, chronic obstructive pulmonary disease (COPD), congestive heart failure, cirrhosis, chronic kidney disease, preoperative opioid use, advanced age, higher American Society of Anesthesiologists (ASA) score, and higher Charlson Comorbidity Index, have a higher risk of failure to be discharged or a higher risk of readmission.[3,10-17] Patients with these comorbidities may not be good candidates for TKA in an ASC.

Some common criteria used for determining eligibility of patients for outpatient total joint replacement are age <70 years, ASA score I or II, primary total joint arthroplasty, hemoglobin >10 preoperatively, assistance at home, preoperative independent ambulation, and BMI <40. Some exclusion criteria commonly used are coronary artery disease, COPD, congestive heart failure, cirrhosis, chronic kidney disease, HIV positive, preoperative opioid consumption, and chronic pain syndromes (fibromyalgia). These criteria can be used as a guide, but ultimately it should be a joint decision by the patient, surgeon, and anesthesiologist.

Chart	
Inclusion Criteria	**Exclusion Criteria**
Age <70 years	Chronic obstructive pulmonary disease
Primary total knee arthroplasty	Coronary artery disease
Body mass index <40	Preoperative hemoglobin <10 g/dL
Independent ambulation preoperatively	Preoperative pain syndrome or opioid dependence
ASA score I or II	Congestive heart failure
Appropriate assistance at home	Chronic renal disease

ASA, American Society of Anesthesiologists.

When it is determined that TKA in the ASC is appropriate for a patient, it is important to adequately prepare the patient for what will be involved in the preoperative, perioperative, and postoperative settings. It is imperative that appropriate patient education be relayed not just to the patient but also to family members. A video or class that educates the patient on the importance of the preoperative steps and the postoperative risks and physical therapy guidelines can be productive. The literature presents conflicting data on preoperative education with regard to patient satisfaction,[18-20] but the potential benefits and minimal harm of patient education will likely improve patient expectations.[21] DeCook[22] suggested multiple elements to consider with regard to patient preparation (Table 6.1).

ANESTHESIA AND PREOPERATIVE BLOCKS

Advances in anesthetic techniques and postoperative pain control have allowed earlier mobilization and reduced opioid consumption. Controlling pain in the early postoperative period has a profound effect on postoperative recovery in patients with TKA. Reduced pain allows more aggressive therapy and range of motion exercises in the early postoperative period, which can improve recovery and facilitate an early discharge home. Combining a neuraxial anesthetic approach, an adductor canal block, and periarticular

TABLE 6.1 Patient Considerations for Outpatient TKA
1. Medical optimization
a. Medical and cardiac clearances (include anesthesia input and review)
b. Review of home medications
c. Establishment of a deep venous thrombosis (DVT) prophylaxis regimen
d. Screening for methicillin-resistant *Staphylococcus aureus* (MRSA)
2. Setting patient expectations and education
a. Location of recovery and postoperative therapy
b. Pain expectations, including discussion of multimodal pain management
c. Ambulation and driving expectations
d. Return-to-work expectations
3. Caregiver expectations
a. Identifying and educating the designated caregiver
4. Pathway for patient communication postoperatively during business hours and after hours (establishing a total joint hotline)

injection can be an effective approach to minimize postoperative pain.

Multimodal Pain Control

Postoperative pain control in patients with TKA has traditionally been a challenge. Advances in techniques and implementation of a multimodal approach to pain control have been used to maximize postoperative pain control while minimizing the side effects, particularly of opioid medications. Multimodal pain control is a comprehensive strategy for postoperative pain control that has been shown to reduce opioid consumption, adverse drug events, and lengths of stay and improve patient outcomes.[23]

A typical multimodal pain control regimen consists of acetaminophen, a COX-2 inhibitor (celecoxib), and gabapentin to help reduce overall opioid consumption. An effective multimodal protocol begins in the preoperative period. It has been shown that preemptive administration of medications in conjunction with peripheral nerve blocks and moderate opioid doses will offer greater anesthesia than the administration of these medications postoperatively. A reasonable preoperative oral regimen on the morning of surgery may consist of 1000 mg of acetaminophen, 400 mg of celecoxib, and 300 to 600 mg of gabapentin. These medications, in addition to regional blocks, can greatly reduce pain and total opioid consumption.[24]

In the postoperative period scheduled acetaminophen, celecoxib, and gabapentin are continued and supplemented with oral opioid analgesia. The use of tramadol for postoperative analgesia is popular, and it can be given as a scheduled dose. This is a centrally acting analgesic that acts on the opioid receptors and blocks reuptake of both norepinephrine and serotonin. Tramadol has been shown to have a lower potential for abuse, less constipation, and less respiratory depression than traditional opioids,[25] but it comes with an increased risk of serotonin syndrome and seizures.[26]

Oral opioids are used for ongoing pain control and breakthrough pain. Some have advocated scheduled opioid administration, with an additional dose available for breakthrough pain during the first 48 to 72 hours after surgery. Most immediate-release opioids need regular dosing every 4 to 6 hours to be most effective. When these medications are prescribed as needed, a delay in dosing such as skipping a dose overnight can cause a subsequent increase in pain. Common side effects of opioids are constipation, nausea/vomiting, and sedation. To help with these side effects, patients are also given a bowel regimen and antiemetic medications in the postoperative period.[27]

Neuraxial Versus General Anesthesia

TKA can be performed with neuraxial techniques, such as spinal or epidural anesthesia, or general anesthesia. The reported advantages of neuraxial anesthesia for TKA generally outweigh those of general anesthesia. A metaanalysis of 29 studies showed a significantly shorter length of stay with neuraxial anesthesia compared with general anesthesia, and neuraxial anesthesia is the preferred method if not contraindicated.[28] This was further supported by Pu et al.,[29] who showed similar results of shortened length of stay and decreased nausea with spinal anesthesia compared with general anesthesia. Neuraxial anesthesia also has been associated with reduced 30-day morbidity and mortality, lower frequency of transfusions, lower risk of pneumonia, less acute renal failure, and fewer superficial wound infections.[30] General anesthesia carries risks of respiratory and hemodynamic complications that spinal anesthesia avoids. In comparison to neuraxial anesthesia, general anesthesia was found to have increased risks of postoperative ventilator usage, unplanned reintubation, stroke, and cardiac events.[31] General anesthesia can affect postoperative cognitive function and increase delirium in elderly patients. Neuraxial anesthesia has risks of its own, including epidural hematoma, epidural abscess, hypotension, and urinary retention. In 2019 the International Consensus on Anesthesia-Related Outcomes After Surgery (ICAROS) recommended neuraxial over general anesthesia for hip and knee arthroplasty. They found an increased risk of urinary retention but a decreased risk of mortality, pulmonary complications, acute renal failure, DVT, infections, and blood transfusions with use of neuraxial anesthesia compared with general anesthesia.[32] Memtsoudis et al.[33] looked at 191,570 inpatient TKAs and compared rates of inpatient falls: 10.9% received neuraxial anesthesia, 12.9% received combined general/neuraxial anesthesia, and 76.2% received general anesthesia. In conclusion, both general and neuraxial anesthetic techniques can be implemented in same-day TKA, with a preference for neuraxial anesthesia.

Regional Anesthesia: Adductor Canal Versus Femoral Block

Advances in peripheral nerve block techniques have led to significant improvement in postoperative analgesia, and nerve blocks are a vital portion of multimodal pain control. Regional blocks have traditionally been underused, but they are an important aspect of pain control in successful outpatient total joint arthroplasty. Initially, lower extremity regional blocks (femoral and sciatic nerve blocks) were used for pain control. These blocks provide marked pain control but result in loss of motor function in the operative extremity.

Newer techniques provide isolated sensory blocks, sparing motor function to the operative extremity. The motor-sparing properties of these blocks are essential for early postoperative mobilization and reduction of fall risk.[33] The adductor canal block provides similar pain relief as a femoral nerve block without sacrificing quadriceps muscle function. Many rapid recovery pathways have phased out femoral blocks in favor of the adductor canal block.[34,35] The adductor canal is located where the medial border of the sartorius muscle meets the medial border of the adductor longus and extends to the adductor hiatus where the saphenous nerve exits. The adductor block is performed using sonography to inject local anesthetic into the adductor canal, deep to the vastoadductor membrane adjacent to the superficial femoral artery. Similarly, further analgesia

for TKA can be provided by ultrasound-guided lateral femoral cutaneous nerve block.[36]

Another regional block technique that is fairly new is block of the Interspace between the Popliteal Artery and Capsule of the posterior Knee (IPACK).[37] This is performed by injecting local anesthetic under ultrasound guidance in the area between the popliteal artery and the posterior femoral condyles. This blocks the nerves to the posterior capsule of the knee and can offer additional analgesia compared with an adductor canal block alone. The IPACK block is typically combined with an adductor canal block and periarticular injection for complete analgesic coverage of the knee joint.

Local Infiltration

Periarticular injection is a popular analgesic modality administered by the surgeon into the operative site. Typical injections have included bupivacaine or ropivacaine, morphine, ketorolac, and epinephrine.[38] This solution is typically injected into the posterior capsule, collateral ligaments, capsular incision, quadriceps, and subcutaneous tissues. Some studies have advocated liposomal bupivacaine for a longer-lasting local analgesic effect and early discharge readiness.[39] A recent prospective, randomized, controlled trial demonstrated no significant differences between liposomal bupivacaine and standard periarticular injections for regional anesthesia,[40] but other reports have shown it to be more beneficial than a femoral nerve block.[41]

AMBULATORY SURGERY CENTER VERSUS HOSPITAL SETTING

From a facility standpoint, there are numerous differences in performing outpatient TKA in the ASC versus the hospital setting. The most obvious difference is the overall limitation in space. DeCook et al.[22] noted that the physical space of the ASC must be assessed from an instrumentation and implant standpoint. Whereas hospitals have ample space for various trays, revision instrumentation, and various sizes of implants, the ASC in general may not have the same capabilities to house the same amount of equipment found in the hospital setting. Therefore it is imperative during the surgical planning for outpatient TKA to have proper communication among the surgeon, vendors, and OR personnel to ensure that the proper instruments and implants are available on the day of surgery.

OPERATING ROOM STAFF AND THE TEAM APPROACH

A successful TKA requires a team approach whether it is conducted in an inpatient or an outpatient setting. The surgeons, primary care physicians, anesthesiologists, nurses, OR staff, and therapists are all vital in a successful total joint arthroplasty program. For a same-day TKA program to be successful, the multidisciplinary team approach is imperative.

Surgical scrub technicians play a vital role in the efficient flow of the operation during TKA. Surgical technicians who are experienced in ASC procedures may not be well acquainted with the instruments or the typical flow of total joint arthroplasty surgery. Before starting an outpatient arthroplasty program, it is advisable to educate any surgical staff on protocol and specialized equipment in the hospital setting or conduct a walkthrough with a mock ASC setup. An experienced, well-trained surgical technician is an important factor in creating an efficient operation and should not be overlooked.

The anesthesia team, composed of an anesthesiologist and often a certified registered nurse anesthetist (CRNA), plays an important role in the success of outpatient TKA. The team has an integral effect on controlling the patient's pain and nausea, which can be a limiting factor for discharge. The anesthesia team should be well versed in general anesthesia, spinal anesthesia, and regional blocks. Optimally, anesthesia allows quicker recovery on the day of surgery, allowing the patient to mobilize and be safely discharged home while minimizing pain, nausea, and other undesired side effects of anesthesia. Good communication between the surgeon and the anesthesia team allows adequate planning and optimal outcomes.

Physical therapy in the immediate postoperative period is a cornerstone for safe discharge in same-day surgery. Therapists should be trained for total joint arthroplasty therapy and should understand the goal of patients meeting their therapy milestones and safely being discharged home the same day. The implementation of motor-sparing regional blocks, periarticular injections, and improved surgical techniques have allowed early mobilization. Physical therapy protocols for outpatient total joint arthroplasty focus on safe transfers into and out of bed, ambulation for a specified distance, and sometimes stair walking. Inquiries should be made into the conditions present at the patient's site of convalescence so that appropriate patient education can be provided on navigating special circumstances.

DEVELOPING STANDARDS AND CARE PATHS

Development of accelerated care pathways and standardized protocols has been shown to expedite discharge across many procedures, including TKA. Care pathways facilitate coordination among the patient, surgeon, anesthesiologist, nursing staff, and physical therapist. A successful care pathway for TKA is an essential tool for accelerated recovery and same-day discharge. Protocols are developed with the goals of accelerated recovery for the patient through surgical techniques and optimal control of nausea, hypotension, pain, and anxiety.

Enhanced Recovery After Surgery (ERAS) protocols have been implemented for numerous surgeries across many specialties, with pathways developed specifically for TKA. These protocols encourage patients to drink clear fluids up to 2 hours before surgery. Several studies have shown decreased lengths of stay, lower complication rates, and lower total costs but no changes in 30-day readmission rates with the implementation of accelerated recovery pathways.[42–45]

The ERAS Society released consensus recommendations for total joint arthroplasty protocols.[46] They gave these "strong" recommendations:

1. Patients should routinely receive preoperative education and counseling.
2. Controllable risk factors (e.g., smoking cessation, alcohol abuse cessation, correction of anemia) should be optimized before surgery.
3. Clear fluids should be allowed up to 2 hours before surgery and solids up to 6 hours before surgery.
4. Both general anesthesia and neuraxial techniques can be used.
5. Local infiltration is recommended for TKA as part of multimodal pain management.
6. Patients are given multimodal nausea and vomiting prophylaxis postoperatively.
7. Tranexamic acid is recommended to reduce perioperative blood loss.

8. Multimodal regimens should include acetaminophen and nonsteroidal antiinflammatory drugs for patients without contraindications.
9. Body temperature should be maintained both preoperatively and postoperatively.
10. Patients should receive systemic antimicrobial prophylaxis intraoperatively.
11. Patients should receive venous thromboembolism prophylaxis in line with local policy.
12. No recommendations for surgical approach.
13. Fluid balance should be maintained to avoid both overhydration or underhydration.
14. Patients should have an early return to normal diet postoperatively.
15. Patients should undergo mobilization as early as they are able.
16. Objective discharge criteria should be used.
17. There should be routine review and improvement of care pathways.

Standardized accelerated recovery protocols should be implemented at all institutions to give clear guidance to the perioperative care of TKA patients in the outpatient setting. Care pathways advise all parties to aid in the rapid recovery of patients and allow safe discharge home the same day of surgery. Implemented protocols should be routinely examined and improved.

PERIOPERATIVE CARE

Intravenous (IV) antibiotic prophylaxis of cefazolin should be administered within 1 hour of incision for TKA. Two grams of cefazolin should be given for patients who weigh 80 to 120 kg and 3 g should be administered for patients over 120 kg. For patients who are allergic to penicillin, 900 mg of clindamycin IV or 15 mg/kg of vancomycin IV antibiotics can be given. Modest decreases in surgical site infections have been shown with a combination of cefazolin and vancomycin in patients at high risk of methicillin-resistant *Staphylococcus aureus* (MRSA) infection or with a positive MRSA nasal swab.[47] In the inpatient setting patients may receive 24 hours of antibiotic prophylaxis after TKA. Tan et al.[48] evaluated 20,682 total joint arthroplasties and found a periprosthetic joint infection rate of 0.6% (27 of 4523) in patients receiving a single dose of prophylactic antibiotics compared with 0.88% (142 of 16,159) in patients who received the complete 24-hour regimen. This study suggests that

additional antibiotics after skin closure may not be needed in primary total joint arthroplasty.

Tranexamic acid (TXA) has been shown to decrease postoperative blood loss and transfusions in TKA. The American Academy of Orthopaedic Surgeons recommends administration of TXA for all patients undergoing TKA who do not have contraindications, such as history of thromboembolic or ischemic events. TXA has been administered orally, topically, and intravenously, all showing effective decreases in blood loss compared with placebo. Fillingham et al.,[49] in a network metaanalysis on TXA use in TKA, reported a mean difference in blood loss between 225 and 331 mL with the use of TXA compared with placebo. No differences in blood loss were found between the various administration routes or the number of doses given. They found a statistically significant decrease in blood loss and postoperative transfusions when a single IV dose was administered before incision compared with a single IV dose given after incision. In the ASC TXA should be used in all TKA patients who do not have contraindications.

Skin Preparation and Tourniquet Pros and Cons
Skin Preparation

Surgical skin preparation is essential in reducing the risk of early postoperative infection. Skin can be sterilized with an aqueous-based scrub (i.e., povidone-iodine, alcohol, hexachlorophene, or chlorhexidine) and/or an alcohol-based solution. Most surgeons scrub with an aqueous-based skin preparation (i.e., povidone-iodine or chlorhexidine), followed by an alcohol or combination type skin preparation (i.e., chlorhexidine-alcohol).[50] Shaving the surgical site should be delayed until immediately before surgery.[51] There is some conflicting evidence about the use of various skin preparations, with some studies showing superiority of chlorhexidine gluconate to povidone-iodine[52] and others reporting a slightly decreased risk of deep infection with iodine-alcohol skin preparation (0.5%) compared with chlorhexidine-alcohol (1.8%).[53]

Preadmission skin preparation has been shown to decrease infection rates. Kapadia et al.[54] conducted a randomized controlled trial testing the use of preadmission chlorhexidine skin preparation in total joint arthroplasty. In 539 patients prosthetic infection rate decreased from 2.9% in the standard-of-care cohort to

0.4% in patients who had a chlorhexidine skin cleansing the night before their operation. Preadmission chlorhexidine cleansing should be strongly considered in all total joint programs.

Tourniquet Use

A thigh tourniquet has traditionally been used in TKA to improve visibility and reduce intraoperative blood loss; however, recent studies show that there may be some negative consequences of thigh tourniquet use. Dennis et al.,[55] in a randomized trial involving patients who had bilateral TKA, compared one knee in which a tourniquet was used to the contralateral limb with no tourniquet or limited tourniquet use for cementation. They found diminished quadriceps muscle strength in the tourniquet group up to 3 months after surgery. A randomized controlled trial of tourniquet use in TKA for full surgery compared with use in the second half of surgery showed a decrease in multiple inflammatory factors, decreased limb swelling, less pain, and faster recovery with shorter duration tourniquet use.[56] The benefits of tourniquet use are improved visualization, shorter operative times, and decreased blood loss, but it is not known whether these benefits outweigh the negative effects on quadriceps muscle strength, pain, risk of thrombosis, and potential wound complications. The literature is not clear on whether or not a tourniquet should be used.[57]

DISCHARGE CRITERIA

Standardized discharge criteria should be established when transitioning to TKA in the ASC setting. These criteria may differ between institutions, but the same principles apply. Patients should be able to tolerate oral intake without significant nausea. Pain should be well controlled on oral pain medications. Patients should work with physical therapy for gait training, transfers, and stairs if these are present in the patient's home. Physical therapy specific mobilization goals may include ambulating 100 feet, transferring with minimal assistance in and out of bed, and using the restroom. Some patients may be required to stair-walk the equivalent number of stairs that are required to enter the patient's home. A single episode of controlled voiding should be demonstrated before the patient leaves the facility. A list of common discharge criteria are outlined in Table 6.2.[6,58]

TABLE 6.2   Common Discharge Criteria for Outpatient/ASC TKA Patients

1. Ambulate 100 feet with minimal assistance
2. Transfer from bed to standing and to the restroom with minimal assistance
3. Climb equal number of stairs as are required to enter the patient's home
4. Able to tolerate oral intake of fluids and solids with minimal nausea
5. Hemodynamic stability
6. Voiding without assistance
7. Discharge to a safe environment with appropriate support

The American Academy of Hip and Knee surgeons listed predictable delays to discharge: blood pressure abnormalities (i.e., hypotension and hypertension), pain, oversedation, postoperative urinary retention, postoperative nausea and/or vomiting, and social support issues.[59]

CONCLUSION

Same-day discharge TKA can be safely performed in properly selected patients with major cost savings to the healthcare system. Specific considerations discussed in this chapter should be taken into account when starting an outpatient TKA program. Standardized accelerated care pathways should be implemented to expedite safe discharge and decrease complications. A team-based approach allows surgeons, anesthesiologists, nurses, OR staff, physical therapists, and vendors to work together to facilitate a successful surgery, recovery, and discharge of patients in the outpatient setting.

REFERENCES

1. Sloan M, Premkumar A, Sheth NP. Projected volume of primary total joint arthroplasty in the U.S., 2014 to 2030. *J Bone Joint Surg Am.* 2018;100(17):1455–1460.
2. Aynardi M, et al. Outpatient surgery as a means of cost reduction in total hip arthroplasty: a case-control study. *HSS J.* 2014;10(3):252–255.
3. Lovald S, et al. Patient selection in outpatient and short-stay total knee arthroplasty. *J Surg Orthop Adv.* 2014;23(1):2–8.
4. Barnes CL, et al. An Examination of the adoption of outpatient total knee arthroplasty since 2018. *J Arthroplasty.* 2020;35:S24–S27.

5. Xu J, et al. Comparison of outpatient versus inpatient total hip and knee arthroplasty: a systematic review and meta-analysis of complications. *J Orthop.* 2020;17:38–43.

6. Toy PC, et al. Low rates of adverse events following ambulatory outpatient total hip arthroplasty at a free-standing surgery center. *J Arthroplasty.* 2018;33(1): 46–50.

7. Goyal N, et al. Otto Aufranc Award: a multicenter, randomized study of outpatient versus inpatient total hip arthroplasty. *Clin Orthop Relat Res.* 2017;475(2): 364–372.

8. Darrith B, et al. Inpatient versus outpatient arthroplasty: a single-surgeon, matched cohort analysis of 90-day complications. *J Arthroplasty.* 2019;34(2):221–227.

9. Kelly MP, et al. Inpatient versus outpatient hip and knee arthroplasty: which has higher patient satisfaction? *J Arthroplasty.* 2018;33(11):3402–3406.

10. Hoffmann JD, et al. The shift to same-day outpatient joint arthroplasty: a systematic review. *J Arthroplasty.* 2018;33(4):1265–1274.

11. Courtney PM, Boniello AJ, Berger RA. Complications following outpatient total joint arthroplasty: an analysis of a national database. *J Arthroplasty.* 2017;32(5): 1426–1430.

12. Sher A, et al. Predictors of same-day discharge in primary total joint arthroplasty patients and risk factors for post-discharge complications. *J Arthroplasty.* 2017;32(9, Supplement):S150–S156.e1.

13. Fleisher LA, Pasternak LR, Lyles A. A novel index of elevated risk of inpatient hospital admission immediately following outpatient surgery. *Arch Surg.* 2007;142(3): 263–268.

14. Warth LC, et al. Total Joint arthroplasty in patients with chronic renal disease: is it worth the risk? *J Arthroplasty.* 2015;30(9, Supplement):51–54.

15. SooHoo NF, et al. Factors that predict short-term complication rates after total hip arthroplasty. *Clin Orthop Relat Res.* 2010;468(9):2363–2371.

16. Johnson DJ, et al. Risk factors for greater than 24-hour length of stay after primary total knee arthroplasty. *J Arthroplasty.* 2020;35(3):633–637.

17. Keulen MHF, et al. Predictors of (un)successful same-day discharge in selected patients following outpatient hip and knee arthroplasty. *J Arthroplasty.* 2020;35:1986–1992.

18. Noble PC, et al. The John Insall Award: patient expectations affect satisfaction with total knee arthroplasty. *Clin Orthop Relat Res.* 2006;452:35–43.

19. Culliton SE, et al. The relationship between expectations and satisfaction in patients undergoing primary total knee arthroplasty. *J Arthroplasty.* 2012;27(3):490–492.

20. McDonald S, et al. Preoperative education for hip or knee replacement. *Cochrane Database Syst Rev.* 2014(5):CD003526.

21. Rutherford RW, Jennings JM, Dennis DA. Enhancing recovery after total knee arthroplasty. *Orthop Clin North Am.* 2017;48(4):391–400.

22. DeCook CA. Outpatient joint arthroplasty: transitioning to the ambulatory surgery center. *J Arthroplasty.* 2019;34:S48–S50.

23. Hebl JR, et al. A Pre-emptive multimodal pathway featuring peripheral nerve block improves perioperative outcomes after major orthopedic surgery. *Reg Anesth Pain Med.* 2008;33(6):510–517.

24. Cullom C, Weed JT. Anesthetic and analgesic management for outpatient knee arthroplasty. *Curr Pain Headache Rep.* 2017;21(5):23.

25. Beakley BD, Kaye AM, Kaye AD. Tramadol, pharmacology, side effects, and serotonin syndrome: a review. *Pain Physician.* 2015;18(4):395–400.

26. Hassamal S, et al. Tramadol: understanding the risk of serotonin syndrome and seizures. *Am J Med.* 2018;131(11):1382.e1–1382.e6.

27. Amundson AW, Panchamia JK, Jacob AK. Anesthesia for same-day total joint replacement. *Anesthesiol Clin.* 2019;37(2):251–264.

28. Johnson RL, et al. Neuraxial vs general anaesthesia for total hip and total knee arthroplasty: a systematic review of comparative-effectiveness research. *Br J Anaesth.* 2016;116(2):163–176.

29. Pu X, Sun JM. General anesthesia vs spinal anesthesia for patients undergoing total-hip arthroplasty: A meta-analysis. *Medicine (Baltimore).* 2019;98(16):e14925.

30. Memtsoudis SG, et al. Perioperative comparative effectiveness of anesthetic technique in orthopedic patients. *Anesthesiology.* 2013;118(5):1046–1058.

31. Basques BA, et al. General compared with spinal anesthesia for total hip arthroplasty. *J Bone Joint Surg Am.* 2015;97(6):455–461.

32. Memtsoudis SG, et al. Anaesthetic care of patients undergoing primary hip and knee arthroplasty: consensus recommendations from the International Consensus on Anaesthesia-Related Outcomes After Surgery group (ICAROS) based on a systematic review and meta-analysis. *Br J Anaesth.* 2019;123(3):269–287.

33. Memtsoudis SG, et al. Inpatient falls after total knee arthroplasty: the role of anesthesia type and peripheral nerve blocks. *Anesthesiology.* 2014;120(3):551–563.

34. Hanson NA, et al. Continuous ambulatory adductor canal catheters for patients undergoing knee arthroplasty surgery. *J Clin Anesth.* 2016;35:190–194.

35. Jæger P, et al. Adductor canal block versus femoral nerve block for analgesia after total knee arthroplasty: a

randomized, double-blind study. *Reg Anesth Pain Med.* 2013;38(6):526–532.

36. Sogbein OA, et al. Ultrasound-guided motor-sparing knee blocks for postoperative analgesia following total knee arthroplasty: a randomized blinded study. *J Bone Joint Surg Am.* 2017;99(15):1274–1281.

37. Niesen AD, et al. Interspace between Popliteal Artery and posterior Capsule of the Knee (IPACK) Injectate Spread: A cadaver study. *J Ultrasound Med.* 2019;38(3):741–745.

38. Kerr DR, Kohan L. Local infiltration analgesia: a technique for the control of acute postoperative pain following knee and hip surgery: a case study of 325 patients. *Acta Orthop.* 2008;79(2):174–183.

39. Dysart SH, et al. Local infiltration analgesia with liposomal bupivacaine improves early outcomes after total knee arthroplasty: 24-hour data from the pillar study. *J Arthroplasty.* 2019;34(5):882–886.e1.

40. Hyland SJ, et al. Liposomal bupivacaine versus standard periarticular injection in total knee arthroplasty with regional anesthesia: a prospective randomized controlled trial. *J Arthroplasty.* 2019;34(3):488–494.

41. Surdam JW, Licini DJ, Baynes NT, Arce BR. The use of exparel (liposomal bupivacaine) to manage postoperative pain in unilateral total knee arthroplasty patients. *J Arthroplasty.* 2015 Feb;30(2):325–329.

42. Zhu S, et al. Enhanced recovery after surgery for hip and knee arthroplasty: a systematic review and meta-analysis. *Postgrad Med J.* 2017;93(1106):736–742.

43. Vendittoli PA, et al. Enhanced recovery short-stay hip and knee joint replacement program improves patients outcomes while reducing hospital costs. *Orthop Traumatol Surg Res.* 2019;105(7):1237–1243.

44. Deng QF, et al. Impact of enhanced recovery after surgery on postoperative recovery after joint arthroplasty: results from a systematic review and meta-analysis. *Postgrad Med J.* 2018;94(1118):678–693.

45. Auyong DB, et al. Reduced length of hospitalization in primary total knee arthroplasty patients using an updated enhanced recovery after orthopedic surgery (ERAS) pathway. *J Arthroplasty.* 2015;30(10):1705–1709.

46. Wainwright TW, et al. Consensus statement for perioperative care in total hip replacement and total knee replacement surgery: Enhanced Recovery After Surgery (ERAS®) Society recommendations. *Acta Orthop.* 2020;91(1):3–19.

47. Schweizer ML, et al. Association of a bundled intervention with surgical site infections among patients undergoing cardiac, hip, or knee surgery. *JAMA.* 2015;313(21):2162–2171.

48. Tan TL, et al. Perioperative antibiotic prophylaxis in total joint arthroplasty: a single dose is as effective as multiple doses. *J Bone Joint Surg Am.* 2019;101(5):429–437.

49. Fillingham YA, et al. The efficacy of tranexamic acid in total knee arthroplasty: a network meta-analysis. *J Arthroplasty.* 2018;33(10):3090–3098.e1.

50. Illingworth KD, et al. How to minimize infection and thereby maximize patient outcomes in total joint arthroplasty. *J Bone Joint Surg Am.* 2013;95(8):e50.

51. Mishriki SF, Law DJ, Jeffery PJ. Factors affecting the incidence of postoperative wound infection. *J Hosp Infect.* 1990;16(3):223–230.

52. Noorani A, et al. Systematic review and meta-analysis of preoperative antisepsis with chlorhexidine versus povidone-iodine in clean-contaminated surgery. *Br J Surg.* 2010;97(11):1614–1620.

53. Peel TN, et al. Chlorhexidine-alcohol versus iodine-alcohol for surgical site skin preparation in an elective arthroplasty (ACAISA) study: a cluster randomized controlled trial. *Clin Microbiol Infect.* 2019;25(10):1239–1245.

54. Kapadia BH, Elmallah RK, Mont MA. A randomized, clinical trial of preadmission chlorhexidine skin preparation for lower extremity total joint arthroplasty. *J Arthroplasty.* 2016;31(12):2856–2861.

55. Dennis DA, et al. Does tourniquet use in tka affect recovery of lower extremity strength and function? A randomized trial. *Clin Orthop Relat Res.* 2016;474(1):69–77.

56. Cao Q, et al. Effects of tourniquet application on Enhanced Recovery After Surgery (ERAS) and ischemia-reperfusion post-total knee arthroplasty: full- versus second half-course application. *J Orthop Surg (Hong Kong).* 2020;28(1):2309499019896026.

57. Arthur JR, Spangehl MJ. Tourniquet use in total knee arthroplasty. *J Knee Surg.* 2019;32(8):719–729.

58. Berger RA, Cross MB, Sanders S. Outpatient hip and knee replacement: the experience from the first 15 years. *Instr Course Lect.* 2016;65:547–551.

59. The American Association of Hip and Knee Surgeons Hip Society, Knee Society, American Academy of Orthopaedic Surgeons Position Statement on outpatient joint replacement. *J Arthroplasty.* 2018;33(12):3599–3601.

7

Surgical Procedure

Audrey M. Tsao, MD

Primary total knee arthroplasty (TKA) starts with the surgical approach and then moves to a step-wise approach, which includes bony preparation, osteophyte removal, soft tissue balancing, and implant placement. This chapter details an in-depth discussion of soft tissue balancing, and techniques related to the proper exposure of the knee. A generic discussion of different prostheses and instrumentation systems is also included. This material supplements the step-by-step instructions of the typical manufacturers' surgical techniques. It is anticipated that the final decision of the implant choice and related specific techniques will remain with the surgeon. There is also a wide variability in the sequence of the surgical procedure that is dependent on the use of a cruciate-retaining or -sacrificing implant systems, so each anatomical area of bone resection will be handled individually. Although this discussion is appropriate for the resident or other novice in the area of TKA, the more experienced surgeon may find the discussion of the various surgical approaches, the management of the extensor mechanism, and some of the general discussion of the drawbacks and pitfalls of the instrumentation informative. Any discussion in the first person reflects a combination of the opinion of the original author (Dr. Krackow) and the current author's experiences.

One common safety protocol that has been established is the surgical marking of the operative extremity, and it is advocated by the American Association of Orthopaedic Surgeons. Many hospital systems require a preprocedure safety discussion with the surgeon, anesthesiologist, any operative personnel, and all active participants to confirm patient identity, operative site, and procedure. This safety standard before the initiation of any surgical procedure, especially to confirm laterality and the description of the procedure, has become

common practice. In the early 1990s Dr. Krackow initiated many of the standard surgical markings and timeout procedures that are used today, as any fellow or resident who rotated with him are well aware.

SURGICAL EXPOSURE

The initial aspects of surgical exposure with respect to placement of the skin incision and deeper capsular incision offer several alternatives (Fig. 7.1). They may be narrowed somewhat according to the specifics of the case at hand. Of special importance is the presence of prior skin incisions, which may influence the particular incision line to be chosen. A previous medial parapatellar incision will likely dictate that the same line be used for the upcoming TKA (Fig. 7.2). It is usually safe to cross prior transverse incisions that were placed for patellar fracture fixation or high tibial osteotomy. If a perpendicular angle is not possible, at least a 60-degree angle when crossing a prior skin incision will often allow appropriate healing. The greatest danger arises with placement of essentially parallel incisions and the creation of areas of "isolated" skin bridges. This kind of occurrence is potentiated by previous relatively long incisions.

The surgeon can usually incorporate a prior incision even if it is not in the favored location. Relatively short, 1½-inch to 3- or 4-inch previous incisions, which are among the common ones, are not especially troublesome. A prior incision on the opposite aspect of the knee can usually be avoided by moving in a more medial and occasionally lateral direction to avoid a narrow skin bridge. Where possible, 8 cm of distance from an old incision using the most usable lateral old incision is generally recommended because of the medial circulation of the soft tissue flap in the knee. In a situation where

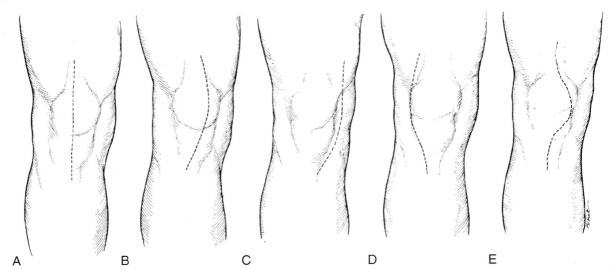

Fig. 7.1 Alternative elective total knee arthroplasty incisions. (A) Longitudinal midline. (B) Median parapatellar with gentle curve close to midline. (C) Medially positioned, median parapatellar incision. (D) Lateral parapatellar incision. (E) Sharply curving median parapatellar incision, generally not preferred.

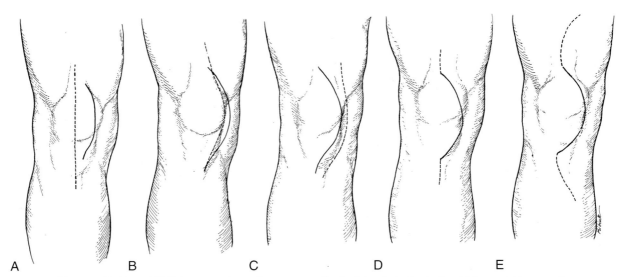

Fig. 7.2 (A, B, and C) Prior curved median parapatellar incision is indicated, which would be unsafe to combine with total knee incision. Relatively thin or small areas of potentially poorly vascularized skin shown in cross-hatching. (D and E) More permissible proximal and distal extensions that, while representing larger incisions, should permit adequate exposure without as much concern for skin flap viability.

multiple prior incisions exist and a concern is raised for soft tissue viability consultation with a plastic surgeon to consider potential tissue necrosis and local flaps can occur before the actual surgical procedure.

Beyond the regard for prior skin incisions, surgeons have several different capsular exposure options. Features of each will be described, but the most common capsular incisions are variations of median parapatellar and medial capsular exposures.

Lateral Exposure

TKA can be performed through a lateral skin incision in at least two ways. One is simply a modification of the more standard median parapatellar approach; namely, a lateral incision is made. However, the capsular incision is made after medial undermining and is made in a manner identical to those described in discussions that follow.[1] This lateral skin and medial capsular exposure may have some theoretical advantages with regard to skin healing, sensation, and potential neuromata formation. It is also used to better protect the main capsular closure because this is not directly under the skin incision. The surgeon may feel that the advantages are purely conjecture and are outweighed by the potential disadvantages of a more difficult exposure. Even if the surgeon prefers this approach, its use in patients with obesity would definitely be more difficult. Here the presence of a medial or even a lateral skin flap involves a much more troublesome exposure (Fig. 7.3).

A lateral skin incision paired with a lateral parapatellar arthrotomy may be considered, especially in the presence of severe valgus deformity. This may have some advantages for skin healing and skin innervation. It may also maintain both superior medial and inferior medial

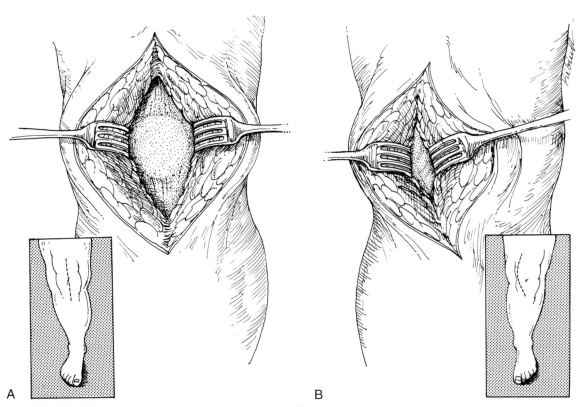

Fig. 7.3 (A) In a patient with obesity straight midline incision can be retracted without obligate eversion of medial or lateral edges. (B) Medially or laterally based flap requires eversion for adequate exposure. In the patient with obesity this eversion can be nearly impossible.

blood supplies to the patella and the general integrity of the medial tissues to obviate certain problems of lateral patellar subluxation.

In this approach special attention to the patellar tendon and more difficult access to the distal end of the femur can be anticipated because of the relative lateral position of the tibial tubercle. This point appropriately introduces an exposure wherein a lateral parapatellar incision is combined with a small tibial tubercle osteotomy.[2] The approach was described for facilitating lateral collateral and other lateral soft tissue release in patients with severe valgus deformity. True lateral parapatellar approaches have a presumed advantage of effecting good lateral retinacular release and providing direct exposure for a lateral collateral release or pie-crusting technique.

Medial Exposure

Medial exposure of the knee joint for TKA may be done through a variety of skin incisions ranging from centrally oriented, straight longitudinal ones to curved incisions directed as far medially as the medial femoral condyle and/or epicondyle. Almost anything in between, straight or curved, may be used as well (see Fig. 7.1A–C. If the very unusual expectation of needing some type of auxiliary lateral incision were to be considered, then a more medially positioned skin exposure may be appropriate to allow an adequate 8-cm skin bridge. The alternative option is to plan a full thickness skin and subcutaneous tissue flap to allow access to the lateral retinaculum and capsule.

In the case of morbid or super obesity a strong argument can be made for a straight midline incision, because it can be very difficult to evert the subcutaneous and skin tissue flap in these patients. An asymmetrical collection of the subcutaneous mass in anything other than a midline incision in the patient with obesity presents a major obstacle, first to exposure and second to approaching the knee with the prosthetic instruments (see Fig. 7.3). Often in those patients where the subcutaneous tissue is actually a barrier to the procedure, this layer can be mobilized from the fascia on the lateral side of the knee to allow this layer and the patella to actually "tuck" under the more superficial layer and remove the soft tissue block.

Medial exposures involve midline or slightly medial incisions in both the quadriceps and patellar tendons and are typically considered the "standard" median parapatellar incision. Another approach is the subvastus or "southern" form of incision that avoids any cut in the quadriceps mechanism directly (Fig. 7.4A–C). This medial approach proceeds along the inferomedial border of the vastus medialis muscle. Its obvious advantage would be the avoidance of direct surgical trauma to the extensor mechanism. Its disadvantages include some tendency to less extensive exposure and the fact that at the time of closure the capsular layer just anterior and proximal to the medial collateral ligament is quite thin and closure can be incomplete. This drawback would have to be considered in terms of adequate exposure in the especially difficult cases or in those with obesity and/or proximal tibial deformity such as what occurs after proximal tibial osteotomy. A variation of this approach is the midvastus split that follows this approach and extends about 1 to 2 cm proximally. It does involve a slight split of the vastus muscles in line with the muscle fibers (Fig. 7.4D and E).

The medial parapatellar approach, for most orthopedic surgeons in the United States, is a very familiar one that gives relatively good and easy exposure for a given length of incision even in the more difficult cases. This is because of the relatively lateral position of the tibial tubercle and the longitudinal incision in the quadriceps mechanism. This latter point allows the respective medial and lateral aspects of the quadriceps musculature to fall to each side, thus facilitating overall exposure. Its possible disadvantage includes considerations of patellar circulation, especially if extensive lateral release is to be performed; possible failure of the superior medial capsular repair; and development of lateral patellar subluxation. Compromise of the patellar circulation with the possibility of inducing avascular necrosis of the patella is an infrequent complication but is a valid concern in the event of patellar fracture. It is possible to dissect the lateral superior geniculate vessels to the patella if an extensive lateral release is required to preserve the blood supply. Preservation of the fat pad is also a consideration to preserve patellar circulation if an extensive lateral release is anticipated.

Full discussion of the approaches and the pertinent anatomy can be found in most orthopedic surgical approach textbooks. The following discussion is in the context of a medial arthrotomy and difficult cases where the greater level of exposure involves techniques for handling the quadriceps mechanism.

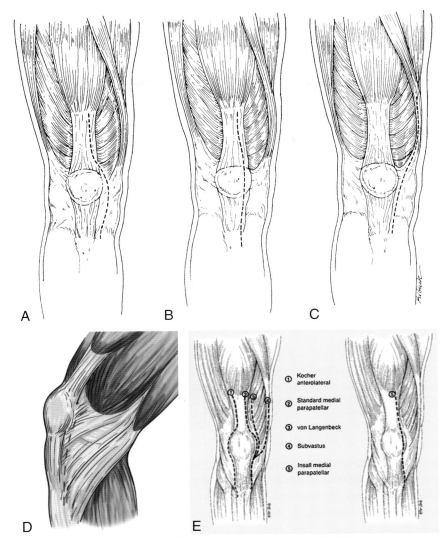

Fig. 7.4 Three different forms of medial capsulotomy/arthrotomy. (A) Standard approach involving longitudinal incision and quadriceps tendon at the junction of central and medial one-third, swinging medial to patella and staying medial to patellar tendon. (B) Midline incision splitting both quadriceps and patellar tendons and elevating tissue from patella. (C) "Southern" exposure elevating vastus medialis and entering capsule adjacent to midmedial patella and femur under the surface of vastus medialis. Before entering the joint per se, vastus medialis muscle is retracted well laterally so that deep capsule and synovial incision is made more centrally than the margin of vastus medialis originally presents. (D & E) Surgical approaches in total knee arthroplasty: standard and minimally invasive surgery techniques.

Tibial Tubercle Osteotomy and Quadriceps Turn Down

In patients who have a stiff preoperative knee with limited flexion, or those with patella baja, mobilization of a contracted anterior extensor mechanism may need to be incorporated into the exposure to allow adequate flexion of the knee and mobilization of the patella. This can be more important in the patient who is morbidly obese.

Insall Quadriceps Snip

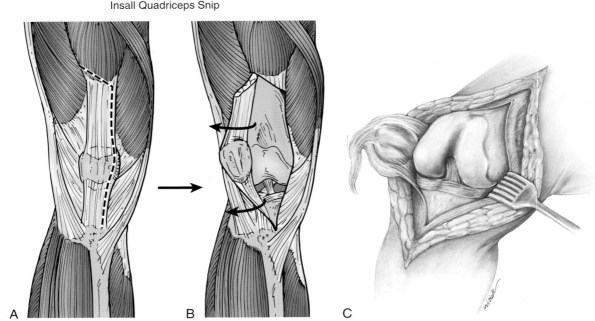

A   B   C

Fig. 7.5 (A) Coonse-Adams lateral quadriceps turndown technique. Diagrammatic relationship between main medial capsulotomy and proximal lateral oblique incision (Springer in Surgical Techniques in Total Knee Arthroplasty pp. 149–154). (B) Anteromedial capsulotomy is shown with minimal dissection necessary to achieve proximal lateral incision. (C) Exposure present after performing proximal lateral turndown. (A) (From Garvin, KL, Aberle, NS. Quadriceps Snip Techniques in Revision Hip and Knee Arthroplasty. 2015; 40–44.)

Occasionally, despite excellent attempts to achieve adequate surgical exposure, the surgeon is unable to do so or they find themselves relatively more compromised than desired. The situation is usually simplified by "disconnecting" the quadriceps mechanism. This disconnection may be accomplished either proximally or distally and may be viewed as analogous to trochanteric osteotomy during exposure of the hip.

Proximal Quadriceps Tendon[3,4]

The quadriceps snip, which extends a standard median parapatellar approach across the proximal quadriceps tendon, can be done easily and often does not require a more extensive dissection. A 45-degree angle cut in line with the vastus lateralis muscle is performed (Fig. 7.5A).[5]

A more extensile exposure is the Coonse-Adams turn down, which facilitates exposure in some especially difficult cases (Fig. 7.5B–C). Performance of this technique requires subcutaneous dissection along the proximal

lateral aspect at the capsular plane or, more accurately, the plane of the quadriceps tendon and the vastus lateralis. An oblique incision is then made across the lateral portion of the quadriceps muscle and is directed in a distal lateral direction. This incision will generally allow sufficient mobilization of the lateral extensor tissues. One may question the adequacy of circulation remaining to the patella and the basic requirements for protection of the repair of this incision postoperatively. It can be noted immediately that the tissue involved in the repair is strong and that it should provide a scaffold for strong suturing techniques. In consideration of this approach one is directed to the report concerning the use of this auxiliary incision as part of a V-Y quadricepsplasty.[6]

In comparison to a tibial tubercle osteotomy, which is described in the next section, the Coonse-Adams turn down does not provide as great a degree of extensor mechanism mobilization. However, it may be easier to perform and to repair.

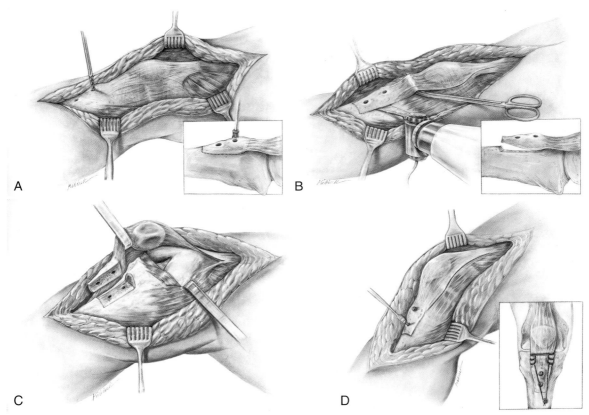

Fig. 7.6 Technique of tibial tubercle osteotomy. (A) Fixation holes are predrilled and prepared with countersink instrument. (B) Osteotomy is performed with saw and includes, if possible, proximal contouring so that proximal migration could only be achieved with anterior displacement. (C) Tibial tubercle has been removed, and general exposure is evident. (D) Tubercle has been replaced and fixed with screws. *Inset,* After screw fixation, the reinforcing ligament suture has been placed in the edges of the patellar tendon. It can be tied to screw, staple, or any other distally secure structure.

Tibial Tubercle Osteotomy

Osteotomy of the tibial tubercle offers wide exposure, but it has potential drawbacks. The surgeon has to be primarily concerned about the possibility of postoperative avulsion, that is, failure of fixation. This fact is of special concern in knee arthroplasty surgery because immobilization in extension by bracing postoperative protection will affect the knee motion and outcome. Avulsion is a realistic concern, as the patient setting is typically one in which flexion is limited from the beginning. If poor bone quality compromises fixation, then the surgeon may prefer a proximally extended exposure option.

A specific technique of tibial tubercle osteotomy is shown in Fig. 7.6. Efforts are made to achieve a suitably thick piece of bone without undermining the residual strength of the proximal tibial area. The bone fragment is made long enough to provide room for two or three fixation screws, and provision is attempted for contouring the bone proximally so that there is a step cut that will prevent proximal migration as long as the fragment remains opposed to the tibial base. The osteotomy can also be contoured to anteriorize the extensor mechanism and realign the patellar tendon for lateral subluxation of the mechanism if needed. The fragment is elevated using a bone saw with a thin blade. Fascia and muscle that attach to the fragment laterally are maintained in continuity as well as possible.

If fixation is to be achieved by screws, then predrilling these holes along with tapping and countersinking before osteotomizing the tubercle fragment can be done as long as the surgeon plans to avoid the baseplate keel. However, if there is a planned change for antero-medialization of this fragment, this should not be done. These maneuvers protect the resulting fragment, ensuring that it is large enough to receive the screws and that no damage will occur during drilling or tapping of the screws. The fragment is reapplied with AO malleolar screws (4.5-mm lag screws). These automatically provide a lag effect without proximal over-drilling. Furthermore, location of the distal cortex is relatively easier owing to the pointed shape of the screw tips and the self-tapping nature of the screw threads. Alternatively, or in combination, fixation may be achieved by wiring as shown in Fig. 7.7.

Fixation can be augmented by placing a screw and washer proximal to the tibial tubercle fragment. This practice provides a post that is an obstacle to proximal migration failure. Additionally, fixation can be further enhanced by the use of at least one heavy ligament suture, which is restrained by a screw head or staple distally, or the use of a bone anchor. As with trochanteric fixation at the hip, the best opportunity for this approach is at the time of original surgery and not as a revision procedure. Therefore the tubercle is securely reattached by whatever number of screws, wires, sutures, or staples

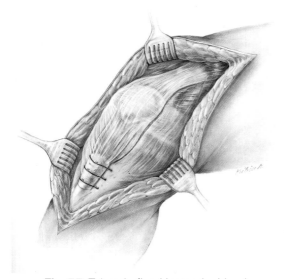

Fig. 7.7 Tubercle fixed instead with wires.

are required. Any bulky, prominent hardware can be removed after the tubercle is healed.

Postoperative management of both the tibial tubercle osteotomy and the Coonse-Adams turn down is described in the postoperative rehabilitation section. Briefly, patients protect such repairs with removable knee immobilizer splints. They are permitted active flexion to tolerance out of the splint and very gentle passive flexion that is commonly done with gravity-assisted knee bending. Also, they can dangle the extremity with instruction to the therapist to perform no forced flexion or extension against resistance. For patients who have had a V-Y type of turn down, there is initial permission to do straight leg raising exercises with the knee immobilizer in place, but they are not permitted to perform active knee extension out of the splint for the first 6 weeks after surgery.

Exposure Details

The details of exposure discussed in this section are particular to the general anteriomedial exposure. This section reflects the personal opinions and experience of the original and current authors so that the true novice should have a minimal number of questions remaining about a technique that works. The technique has evolved from a large operative experience, where a great emphasis has been placed on technical facility, a proper combination of speed, efficiency, gentleness of tissue handling, accuracy of hemostasis, and care in the accuracy of ligament balance and bone cutting. Efficiency in the operative procedure to decrease time of open exposure of the knee has also been shown to decrease complications and infection. The development of the smooth performance of an operation, without wasted time and with good facility, becomes worthwhile when the technically difficult cases are approached.

Capsular Exposure

Fig. 7.8A illustrates a relatively straight, very slightly medially positioned incision; a longitudinal midline approach is used in patients with obesity (see Fig. 7.1A). A slightly curved, relatively more medially positioned incision is used when tightening of the medial collateral ligament is planned (see Fig. 7.1C).

Incision length should avoid the traumatic stretching incisional margins, especially at the inferior apex, to avoid any wound healing issues. Relatively larger incisions are particularly indicated in patients with obesity.

Except when large, subcutaneous venous varicosities are encountered, no major bleeding points are present

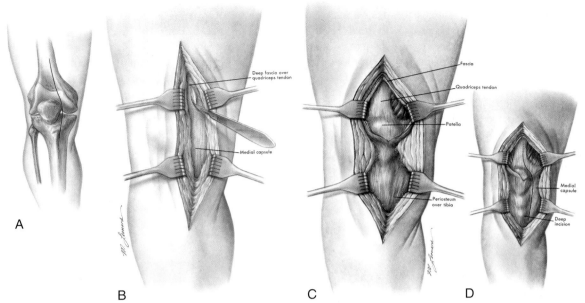

Fig. 7.8 Anteromedial exposure. (A) Incision. (B) Incision made to level of deep fascia over quadriceps tendon and to capsule medially. (C) Incision made through fascia proximally and then through fat overlying quadriceps tendon. It has been carried to level of periosteum of tibia distally. (D) Exposure completed along surface of medial capsule working from tibial area proximally. Deep incision is marked. (E) Relationship of deep fascia and capsule of knee joint. It should be appreciated that one is crossing from more superficial plane distally to deeper aspect proximally. Fascia overlies fat of quadriceps tendon and actually blends to become most superficial layer of capsule more distally. Incision through fascia proximally puts the surgeon at a deeper level than the typical level of dissection about capsule distally. As distal dissection is brought proximally or as proximal dissection extends distally, these different planes must merge. Fascia is typically crossed at the mid or slightly proximal aspect of joint capsule. Again, "crossing" is such that fascia is divided. It remains with subcutaneous fat and is retracted in upper half of wound, and it remains on capsule in the lower half of the wound.

down to the level of the capsule. Once the capsular area is well defined, the two- or three-member team may focus its attention on hemostasis in the subcutaneous region.

On incising the subcutaneous fat in the suprapatellar region, one is directed to identify the deep fascia that overlies the fat investing the quadriceps tendon (Fig. 7.8B). The purpose of making this identification relates principally to wound closure, because specific repair of this deep fascia can be accomplished and provides strength and good approximation while avoiding strangulation of large amounts of subcutaneous fat with sutures. The fat underlying this fascia leads directly to the quadriceps tendon. Also, the identification of this deep fascia improves understanding of the tissue planes as they relate to the exposure of the medial aspect of the joint capsule.

Exposure is carried deeper to the level of the quadriceps tendon in the proximal one-third of the wound, to the capsular tissue over or adjacent to the patella in the middle one-third, and distally to the periosteum over the anteromedial flare of the tibia (Fig. 7.8C). Specifically, incision into the prepatellar bursa at the anterior aspect of the knee or into the paratenon overlying the patellar tendon itself is avoided.

Definition of the capsular plane is performed next from distal to proximal (Fig. 7.8D). As dissection proceeds from the area of the distal, medial aspect of the capsule and the medial tibial flare, it comes to a soft tissue plane, which is superficial to the level of the quadriceps tendon. This is because the fascia overlying the quadriceps tendon, which was mentioned earlier and which has been incised, is in the proximal aspect of the wound, superficial to the level of dissection. In the distal aspect it is the layer contiguous with the distal capsule and actual periosteum. Incising this fascia proximally puts the surgeon at a deeper level in the proximal aspect of the wound than in the distal aspect. As the distal plane of dissection is taken proximally, it is necessary to incise this fascia to connect the two levels of dissection (Fig. 7.8D, inset).

Sufficient medial capsular space is uncovered to allow the medial capsular incision adjacent to the patella and enough edge to effect good repair at the time of closure. Enough exposure of the anterior extracapsular surface of the patella to allow the use of any patellar fixation clamps or cutting jigs needed in the procedure can be done at this stage. In the patient with obesity this layer can be mobilized in a full thickness layer of skin and subcutaneous tissue to allow the fascial layer to sublux below without tethering to allow exposure.

Arthrotomy

The incision is begun in the quadriceps tendon approximately at the junction of the central and medial one-third. It proceeds distally close to the patella but allowing enough retinacular/capsular attachment for closure, and it sweeps around the proximal medial margin of the patella, staying close enough to the patella so that tendinous tissue is present on the medial side. The capsular incision then proceeds distally and medially at first, so that there is enough capsule to suture on each side. This incision ends 1½ to 2 inches below the joint line, adjacent or distal to the tibial tubercle (Fig. 7.9).

Joint Exposure

After completion of the arthrotomy, care is directed to uncovering the proximal tibial margins (Fig. 7.9B). Capsule and periosteal tissue are elevated medially.

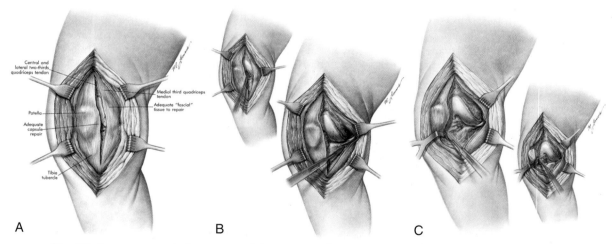

Fig. 7.9 Deeper aspect of anteromedial exposure. (In this series distinction of deep fascia and superficial capsular layers of Fig. 7.8 is not emphasized.) (A) Arthrotomy is being completed. Incision is made at junction of central and medial one-third of quadriceps tendon and has progressed close to vastus medialis at patella, but an attempt is made to save suitable tissue on muscle (medial) side for later closure. Dissection then moves medially from patella to allow even more adequate soft tissue on each side of incision for later closure. Dissection continues down across joint line medial to patellar tendon and ends either at level of tibial tubercle or slightly distal and typically about a centimeter medial. (B) Exposure of medial tibial epiphyseal and metaphyseal area. Medial edge of capsulotomized tissue is retracted further medially. Ligament securing remaining medial meniscus is divided sharply with a knife and facilitates better retraction of medial or capsular margin. Careful dissection along medial tibial bone just below the joint line allows better retraction and exposure of area. (C) Lateral tibial exposure retraction of fat pad and careful dissection of the anterior and anterolateral tibia is undertaken. It is not typically necessary to excise much fat pad. Care is taken to free tissue attached to the periphery of the tibia in this area and to the intercondylar notch and not to the joint surface aspect of tibia.

Careful attention should be paid to freeing the attachments of the coronary ligaments at the inferior margin of the medial meniscus. This maneuver allows free retraction and separation of the remaining medial meniscal remnant and/or capsular margin at the joint line. It is relatively easy to perform a sharp subperiosteal elevation just below the joint line in keeping the medial soft tissue sleeve intact. A Hohmann or Z-type retractor or a periosteal elevator can be used and turned perpendicular to the surface to create a gap to clear soft tissue attachments right at the joint line itself and at the inferior margin of the medial osteophytes. An assistant can also externally rotate the tibia to allow greater exposure of the proximal posteromedial tibia for further exposure and release if needed at this stage.

Detachment of the anterior horn of the lateral meniscus with an intraarticular radial cut to detach it and then placement of a Hohmann or similar retractor allows further lateral joint line exposure as needed. This exposure becomes more critical in the valgus knee. The major challenge is retracting the fat pad and reaching far enough laterally. A partial fat pad resection can be done at this stage for exposure and for better visualization of the patellar tendon to better protect it during the case (Fig. 7.9C). To retract the fat pad anteriorly, laterally, and inferiorly, any synovial strands, such as the ligamentum patellae, going to the intercondylar notch are released. To preserve blood supply to the patella and also because fat is a better periarticular tissue than fibrous tissue, it is recommended to leave as much of the fat pad as possible and to only occasionally remove the deepest synovial layer when performing a synovectomy. A worthwhile point to keep in mind while exposing the margins of the proximal tibia release any soft tissue attachments at the margins. Therefore the soft tissue clearing at the margin of the tibia just below the joint line should be as complete as possible. All of these exposures can be performed with the knee in about 20 to 40 degrees of flexion. This is generally easier than working in either full extension or at 90 degrees of flexion.

As the proximal tibial exposure is first undertaken, the surgeon can pause and pull the tibia distally, distracting the tibia away from the femur. This maneuver gives an intraoperative preliminary assessment of the degree of fixed deformity. If it is clear that the varus is markedly fixed, then the surgeon can proceed along the anteromedial and medial aspects of the proximal tibia to perform a more generous medial capsular ligamentous release. Also, medial marginal osteophytes can be removed at this stage. When the lateral tightening characteristic of fixed valgus is seen, the anterolateral dissection is undertaken more vigorously along the crest of the tibia. After the knee is flexed and the patella is retracted laterally, blunt spreading scissors dissection is carried out in the direction of the posterolateral corner to achieve exposure of the lateral collateral ligament and the posterolateral capsular complex. Developing this degree of lateral exposure at this early stage is not absolutely essential. However, it is another example of exposure that will need to be achieved later and exposure that, when achieved early, makes visualization of this important aspect of the joint much easier. This is especially true because visibility in valgus cases tends to be suboptimal, and surgeons find themselves struggling with the TKA instruments in the early parts of the case.

The patella can be retracted anterolaterally (Fig. 7.10) into the lateral "gutter," which is palpated for synovial plica and to examine the general freedom of the patella, that is, the tightness of the lateral patellar retinaculum. One usually encounters a lateral patellar plica, which can be divided longitudinally; this area is best exposed with the knee in full extension. The surgeon can perform the necessary patellar retraction using their nondominant hand. Note that the patella is pulled or retracted in the peripheral anterolateral direction and not everted at this point. Also, particular attention to the lateral femur and lateral patellar osteophytes is necessary. Occasionally these may be a source of difficulty in achieving free patellar eversion. If they are, they should be removed early, because they will need to be removed later anyway. Once the knee is initially flexed, retraction with or without everion of patella is facilitated by dividing the lateral synovium and deep capsular tissue as shown in Fig. 7.11.

If a synovectomy is indicated, one should beware of progression of the synovectomy beyond the lateral and medial recesses to avoid injury to the origins of the medial and lateral collateral ligaments. Their first protection is derived simply from careful thought about just how they are coursing deep to the visible synovial surface, almost within the synovial layer itself. Note that each originates approximately two-thirds of the way toward the posterior margin of the femoral condyle and that each actually originates from its respective femoral epicondyle, which is almost visible and just barely palpable. In cases with densely contracted synovial spaces and near or true obliteration of the suprapatellar pouch sharp dissection directed between the femur and overlying quadriceps will be necessary. Additionally, the surgeon inspects to

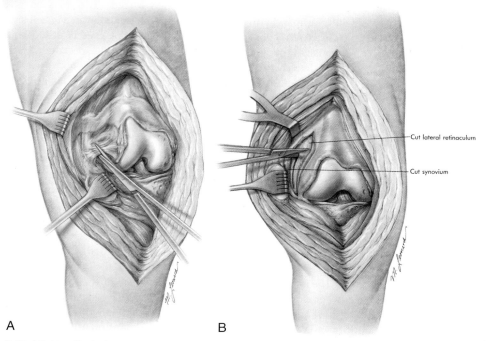

A   B

Fig. 7.10 (A) Patella is being retracted manually in the anterior lateral and peripheral directions. Knee is in full extension. Inspection is made for lateral patellar plicae that are typically present, and these are cut as necessary to facilitate patellar mobilization. (B) Technique of lateral release. Patella is retracted anteriorly, laterally, and peripherally. Synovium is incised longitudinally. Denser capsular and even iliotibial band fibers are divided in longitudinal direction. Care is taken to avoid, where possible, inferior lateral and superior lateral circulation to patella. In some cases adequate lateral release will require interruption of this blood supply.

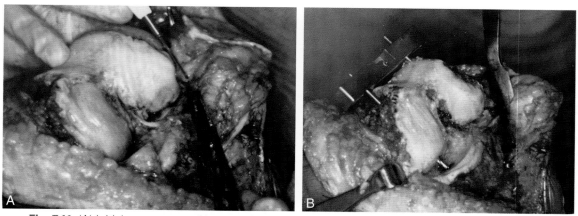

Fig. 7.11 (A) Initial appearance of knee on flexing. Next the capsular tissue from the lateral border of the patella running to the anterolateral tibial margin is divided. This maneuver facilitates further lateral retraction of the patella without representing much lateral release or interruption of blood supply. (B) Better access to distal femur. Patella is retracted laterally, and the anterior cruciate ligament is being removed from femur.

see that the proximal lateral and medial undersurfaces of the quadriceps mechanism are free to retract away from their respective sides (Fig. 7.12).

Further flexion of the knee and general mobilization anteriorly of the tibia are facilitated by resecting the anterior cruciate ligament. If the planned procedure is for a posterior cruciate substituting knee, division of the posterior cruciate ligament can also be done at this time. Removal of the meniscal fragments can be done after the distal femoral and proximal tibial resections have been performed to allow adequate exposure in either flexion

or extension with the joint placed in tension, which can be facilitated by a laminar spreader.

In TKA, as in most other orthopedic operations, exposure is key. Furthermore, the benefits of adequate exposure should not be underestimated. It is advised that attention be paid early to the soft tissue aspects and the exposure of the knee is because this will affect the ease of the remainder of the entire case. Excellent exposure allows one to see important aspects of the joint and to check instrument position; it also allows easier seating of implants and fixation of cutting blocks and facilitates the later step of clearing extruded cement at relatively posterior bone prosthesis margins.

USE OF KNEE SYSTEM INSTRUMENTS

The surgeon is now ready to begin using their chosen system instruments. Effective application of these instruments will require careful retraction of ligaments and other periarticular soft tissues. Two points of caution deserving emphasis are in order. First, potentially osteopenic bone should be considered; this is particularly likely on the least affected nondeformity side of a varus or valgus deformity (e.g., the lateral side in the case of varus). In such patients it is quite easy to lever retractors right through soft cortical bone. The second point especially if the assistant is unable to fully view the surgical field. One must take good care, during ligament retraction, to place the retractor so that it protects at the necessary level. That is, a medial retractor generally will not protect the medial collateral ligament along its entire length. It is necessary for the retractor to be continually repositioned opposite the femur or tibia as the focus of dissection and, particularly, saw position change.

It is appropriate to make a final check of anatomical landmarks before any bone is removed. In extension the surgeon notes the position of the tibial tubercle, which is normally slightly lateral; the position of the intermalleolar axis; and the foot progression angle when the knee is held in a neutral or stimulated weight-bearing fashion. Also, the appearance of the distal femoral trochlear groove is noted in extension. In flexion with the soft tissues retracted, the outline of the femur, the presence of osteophytes, the position of trochlear groove, and other items are all quickly noted. It is recommend that the surgeon assess in flexion the patient's deformity to better understand that effect on the remainder of the procedure and to make note of any rotational deformity and its potential accommodation.

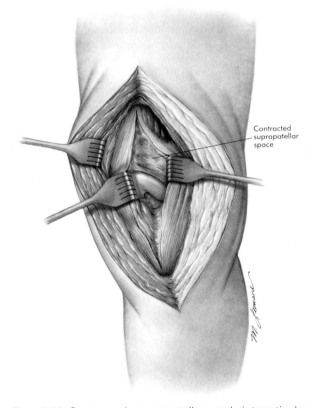

Contracted suprapatellar space

Fig. 7.12 Contracted suprapatellar and intraarticular space. This situation prevents anterolateral and anteromedial retraction and displacement of quadriceps mechanism. It is necessary to divide along this area at the undersurface of the quadriceps mechanism. Basically, this is division through fibrotic joint lining tissue to a region typically of fat overlying femur and separating bone from the undersurface of quadriceps muscle. After this division has been performed, the quadriceps mechanism can be better retracted to each side.

The next sections discuss the bone resections involved in knee arthroplasty. The order of these cuts does not affect the ultimate goal of the resection, but the order of resection can be quite variable. Patellar resection can be done first to avoid eversion and give greater exposure for the remainder of the surgical procedure, but the remnant needs to be protected if this is the preferred sequence. For posterior cruciate–sparing knee arthroplasties, distal femoral resection followed by proximal tibial resection is often preferred for exposure. In a posterior cruciate–sacrificing system, the tibia can often be subluxated anteriorly to allow adequate resection without doing the distal femoral resection.

Tibial Resection

The tibial resection will affect varus-valgus alignment and the flexion-extension gaps. Tibial cuts made perpendicular to the overall tibial shaft axis are common in the classical planned posterior cruciate–sacrificing knee system. When a cut is perpendicular to the longitudinal axis of the bone, there is no need to worry about the rotational position of the bone at the time the cut is made. In addition, proper varus-valgus and flexion-extension attitudes are automatically achieved if indeed, the cut is accurately perpendicular to the long axis of the tibia.

Today, an increasing number of instrument systems direct the surgeon to make a tibial cut that is not perpendicular to the long axis. The goal may be a posteriorly sloped cut to facilitate the flexion and extension balance of the knee. When a nonperpendicular cut is to be made, it is necessary to establish a reference of neutral rotation before the jigs are set to make this cut. Also, sufficiently good exposure is necessary for the varus-valgus and flexion-extension attitudes of the cut to be set properly.

In all TKA systems there exists some freedom to perform the tibial resection at different levels. This happens, first, because all manufacturers supply tibial components of different thicknesses and, second, because wear patterns in the proximal tibia and deformity situations will affect the level of tibial resection.

Several considerations need to be made regarding the thickness of the tibial resection (i.e., the depth of the tibial cut). In the case of a symmetrical tibial joint surface (i.e., one that parallels the expected cut line in the medial and lateral compartments) a minimum thickness tibial cut is the most appropriate. In a flexion-extension gap, using a classical technique would result in the absolute thinnest proximal tibial resection.

In the presence of fixed varus or valgus deformity there are several possibilities that may tend to confuse the selection of the thickness of the tibial cut (Fig. 7.13). One aspect is the relative distance from the end of the femur to the proximal tibial cut level in

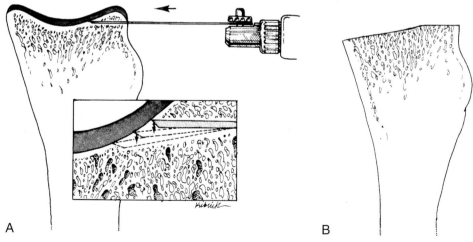

A   B

Fig. 7.13 Cut-away of the phenomenon described as "deep skiving." Although properly positioned at the cutting block or cutting slot, the saw blade entrapped under dense subchondral bone may be seen to "deep deflect" rather than cut its way into harder bone. This is analogous to skiving, which is visible quite frequently at total knee arthroplasty. However, it is occurring within bone and is not visible until resection is completed.

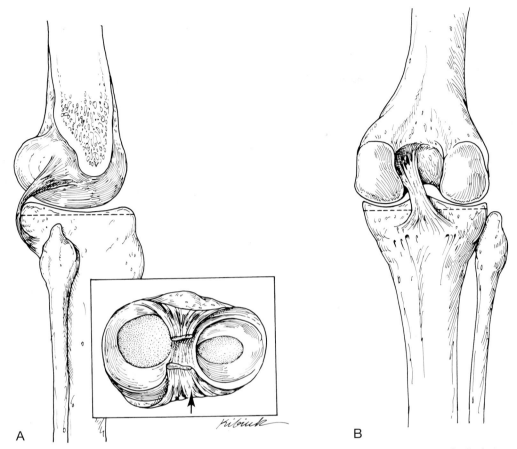

Fig. 7.14 Posterior cruciate relationships at tibia. (A) Posterior cruciate ligament typically inserts distal to joint line posteriorly at tibia. (B) It is frequently possible to perform minimum thickness tibial resection and not disturb posterior cruciate ligament attachment in any significant way. It is not then necessary to mark off "bone island" to preserve posterior cruciate insertion. (***Continued***)

both flexion and extension, as the distance relates to the release of deformity. As medial or lateral soft tissue releases are performed, the tibia will be at a greater distraction point from the end of the femur in extension and flexion. In a matched resection technique the tibia is cut at a 2- to 3-mm resection depth from the worn articular side (medial in varus and lateral in valgus deformity), and the gaps can be equalized after soft tissue balancing.

Another feature of the depth of tibial resection relates to the attachment of the posterior cruciate ligament. It can be seen in Fig. 7.14AB that the majority of insertion of the normal posterior cruciate ligament is located just below the joint line. Because of this, it is typically safe to perform a minimum thickness cut across the top of the tibia without great concern about disconnecting the posterior cruciate ligament attachment (Fig. 7.14CD). However, with posterior sloping of the cut, and especially if this cut is made any deeper than minimum thickness, the necessity of protecting a bony attachment point with a osteotome or retractor is recommended for the posterior cruciate–retaining systems (Fig. 7.14EF). However, the primary protection is the avoidance of the posterior cruciate ligament by the surgeon during the tibial resection saw-cut.

If the posterior cruciate ligament has become detached, conversion to a posterior sacrificing implant or a deep dished tibial insert with a high-wall anterior

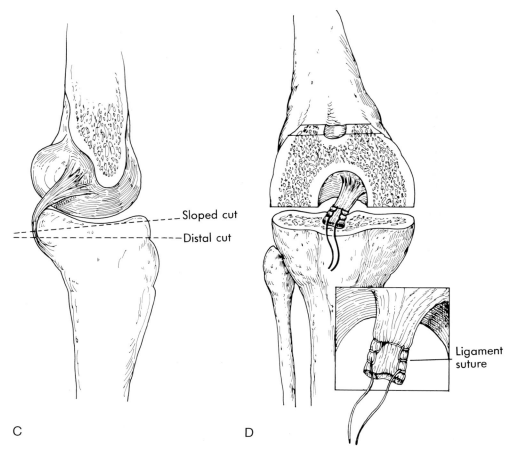

C   D

Fig. 7.14 (**Continued**) (C) However, with deeper cuts and/or posteriorly sloped cuts likelihood of detaching posterior cruciate insertion on tibia will increase. (D) Reinforcement/reattachment.

lipped liner can usually be done within the same system. For a posterior cruciate–sacrificing implant system, additional femoral cuts and use of a tibial post insert and femoral box with a cam may be used. Rarely will an adjustment of the anterior tibial resection to decrease the posterior slope need to be done. In a planned posterior cruciate–sacrificing implant system an increased flexion gap may be noted, and the surgeon should anticipate ways to stabilize the flexion gap if this occurs.

Fixation of many tibial cutting blocks and instruments requires placing drills or pins into the proximal tibial bone. This may be difficult when the lateral tibial bone is worn or otherwise close to the tibial tubercle level, as is the case after proximal tibial osteotomy. If the jig is placed too far anteriorly, a longer lever arm for the tibial resection can result in inaccuracy of the tibial resection because the cutting jig is further away from the proximal

tibia. Placement of pins thru, rather than under, the patellar tendon is preferable to avulsing the tendon in an attempt to retract it sufficiently. The cutting assembly can also be pushed into an abnormal varus position by underlying soft tissue if too much interference is seen with the patellar tendon being overly retracted.

Careful checking of jig orientation is particularly important with respect to the tibial cutting block. The decision about the use of intramedullary versus extramedullary alignment instruments on the tibia has become a matter of preference of the surgeon. Use of computer-assisted surgery has been shown to potentially decrease the variability of the proximal tibial jig placement. However, all current systems require good visibility of the proximal tibia, accurate knowledge of the position of the ankle, and an accurate appreciation of the overall axis of the tibial shaft, along with any tibial

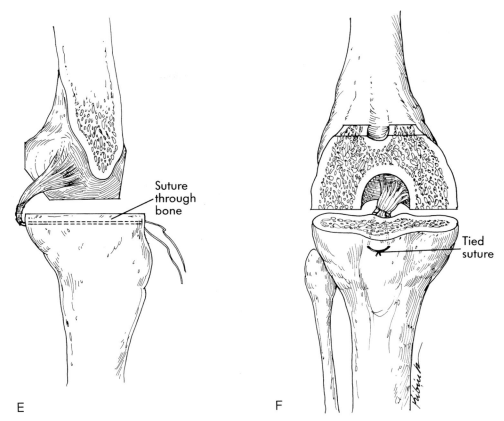

E

F

Fig. 7.14 (***Continued***) (E and F) Heavy ligament suture is placed in stump of posterior cruciate ligament and "tails" of this suture are easily brought through drill holes placed across top of tibia before placement of final components.

deformity of the shaft or proximal joint line. The goal of the jig placement is to allow the planned tibial resection in both the varus-valgus and anteroposterior planes to center the weight-bearing line through the center of the ankle joint. The typical landmarks used to check jig placement are the medial third of the tibial tubercle and the second metatarsal space if there is no anatomical patient variation of the tibia, ankle, or foot. This means that padding or leg positioner that obscures landmarks of the distal tibia, ankle, and foot should be avoided. The entire calf, ankle, and foot areas are routinely prepared and are covered by a plastic stockinette with a light overwrap of aseptic padding before being placed into a leg holder and secured by an ACE wrap or similar dressing, which allows good outline and palpation of the anatomy.

One must avoid erring on the side of abnormal varus tilt and also extension of the tibial component (i.e., an anterior slope). Excessive varus and abnormal slope are associated with premature prosthetic failure. If the surgeon is giving consideration to an anatomical varus position, then that technique is generally paired with a correspondingly more valgus distal femoral cut; the overall resulting tibiofemoral angle should be proper if both proximal tibia and distal femoral cuts are made at the stated orientation for the given system. Anterior slope of the tibial resection can also lead to potential difficulty with flexion and extension balancing. The previous author and Dr. Krackow does cite cases in special consultation, all of which looked perfect in every technical sense, except for just such a cutting error. Each progressed to component fixation failure within 12 months by exactly the same mode, which was excessive anterior force with component subsidence and obvious early loosening.

The actual performance of the tibial cut is relatively straightforward. There are several tips worth mentioning. There is the judicious use of peripheral ligament soft tissue retractors, which must be held properly at the cutting level. Also, there should be the realization of the important aspect of feeling the bone as the saw blade is being used. This point is especially pertinent at the tibial cut because the proximal tibia is typically attached to soft tissue throughout its entire anterolateral, posterolateral, posterior, and even some posteromedial aspects. The surgeon has to be more careful not to direct the saw recklessly deep into this soft tissue, especially as the width of the blade and the mechanical excursion of the saw will increase the effective mechanical cutting width that is hidden during a portion of the actual resection. In addition, the surgeon should protect the bone island of the posterior cruciate ligament if that is intended. There is another relatively uncommon cutting error that can be seen when addressing hard subchondral bone. This phenomenon is a reverse skiving or an inverted deepening of the cut as the saw blade, trapped under a dense subchondral bone, is deflected deeper while the cut is being made. This is not an insurmountable problem; it is just mentioned to foster understanding of its possible occurrence. Listening to the vibrational sound can also assist the surgeon in understanding when this occurs and supplements the tactile feedback through the saw. It is best heard and felt when the saw is operated at consistent full power; this assists in the efficacy of all aspects of the sawing technique.

Access to the anterolateral tibial margin and the posterior margin will usually require removal of the tibial cutting jig and possibly even drill bits or pins, especially those protruding anteromedially because they block access to the anterolateral edge of the tibia. It is almost always possible to cut across the proximal tibia so that the resulting cut bone is free. The exception is when the tibia is so large that the saw blade will not reach across it or in cases where peripheral or posterior osteophytes block free movement of the tibial bone fragment. In performing this cut the surgeon can create a slotted tibial cut jig with the patient's native bone based on the initial accuracy of the tibial cut. The achievement of a complete cut can usually be judged if the surgeon has developed the ability to feel the bone with the saw.

The loose tibial bone is further mobilized by prying it upward with a broad osteotome. It is then gripped with two towel or Lahey clamps and removed in a rotational fashion. Facile removal of the cut tibial surface can be an elusive basic maneuver of TKA. It requires attention to the points just stated.

The flatness of the tibial cut is checked, and specific instrumentation or improvised techniques should be used to recheck that the angular orientation of the cut is proper. Most implant systems have an alignment rod that can be attached to the spacer block and/or tibial trial baseplate to check the alignment of the tibial cut to the ankle distally. As the surgeon seeks access to the proximal tibial surface for trial baseplate positioning, it is easier to present this surface by hyperflexion of the knee and drawing the proximal tibia forward.

Femoral Resection

The exact sequence of cuts for femoral preparation is variable according to the system instruments in use. Only basic technical points will be emphasized here. Further discussion, especially relevant to this aspect of the procedure, may be found in sections dealing with intraoperative assessment of alignment and with specific instrumentation systems. The use of intramedullary guided femoral jigs is the most common method of instrumentation. Computer-assisted guides using the rotational hip center and standard femoral anatomical landmarks are an alternative. The choice of guide is left to the surgeon's preference.

Regardless of whether an "anatomical" or "classical" resection is to be performed at the distal femur, rotational orientation is important as discussed previously on the chapter for instrumentation. When using anatomical or mechanical axis alignment and an intramedullary alignment rod to perform the distal femoral cut, the surgeon should decide on the distal valgus cut angle from a long-standing radiograph. When using the mechanical axis of the femur, the angle between the anatomical and mechanical axes of the femur will be used during the procedure. The distal jig is then pinned at this angle, and the distal resection is made.

The major conceptual variation with respect to femoral preparation depends on whether the surgeon is dealing with a flexion-extension gap technique or a measured resection technique. Because the distal femoral cut in either case is not perpendicular to the femoral shaft axis, some attention needs to be paid to the rotational orientation of this cut. Identification of the epicondylar axis and Whitesides line are commonly used surgical landmarks. A neutral anteroposterior or mediolateral axis needs to be established. It is suggested that, as a rule, the surgeon may also reference the posterior femoral condyles for this

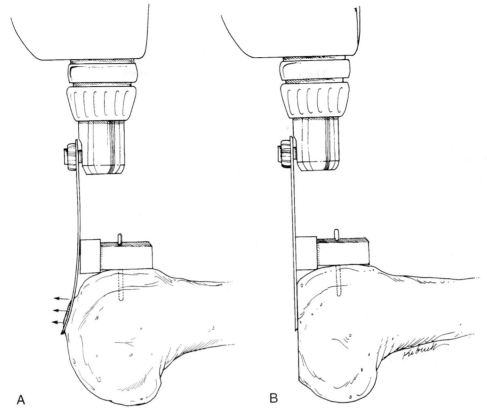

Fig. 7.15 There is almost always increased potential for skiving with one or more femoral cuts. Saw blade is approaching a sometimes relatively dense bone at an angle. (A) Skiving at distal femur. (B) Proper, flat cut.

purpose, planning either to parallel them or, in the case of classical alignment, to make a specific 2- to 3-degree alteration based on posterior condylar deformity.

Once the external rotation is determined, it is possible to use the sizing jig of the implant system to properly size and place femoral cutting jigs to remove the appropriate predetermined amount of bone from any of the surfaces. In performing the posterior femoral cut for an anatomical system neutral anatomical rotation indicates that an essentially equal amount of bone needs to be resected. In a classical system rotating the femoral cutting jig 2 to 3 degrees externally will often lead to a planned resection of 1 to 3 mm more from a normal medial femoral condyle to balance the tibial resection. The distal femoral cut can be made as one of the first bone cuts and before the proximal tibial cut to allow the surgeon additional exposure of the tibia. Adjustment of the order of resection is left up to the surgeon.

The first cut made on the femur will, without question, present a curved, angled bone surface to the saw blade and will carry with it a relatively increased chance of skiving (Fig. 7.15). The same concept applies throughout the remaining femoral cuts. If a measured resection was initially performed, than the spacer block can be used at this time to check correction of deformity and overall alignment in both flexion and extension. In a gap-balancing technique the cutting jigs are typically set so that the femoral cuts are performed to ensure limb alignment.

Other technical points to consider at the time of femoral preparation relate to careful checking of the cut accuracy if press-fit components are to be used. If the instrumentation allows, this is done well by checking with a flat surface to see that the resulting cut surface is properly positioned (Fig. 7.16). Emphasis on this point is important because of the complexity of fit at the femur. On the tibial and patellar surfaces, the surgeon needs to

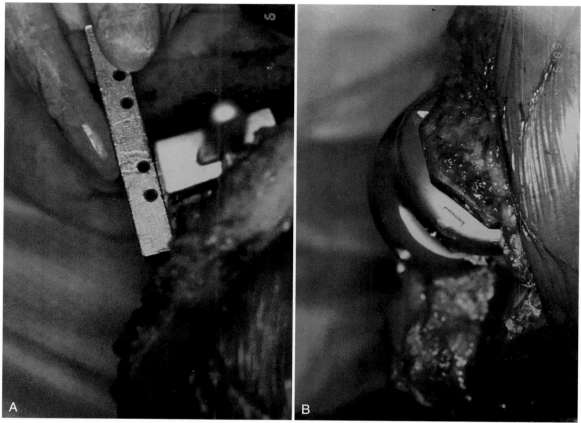

Fig. 7.16 (A) Surgeon may check accuracy of cut by applying a flat-surfaced implement to the surface of the cutting jig. (B) Appearances of essentially imperfect femoral component fit as result of inaccurate bone preparation.

achieve only a flat cut to get perfect approximation. On the femur, the surgeon seeks perfect approximation to at least three, typically five, surfaces (Fig. 7.17). demonstrates typical appearances of a femoral component that is not seating properly because of failure to remove adequate bone. Excessive bone removal leads to space that is visible under the component.

Perhaps the most curious appearance of poor fit is seen with apparent space under the medial and/or lateral aspect of the femoral component at the distal cut. This situation is caused by centrally prominent bone. It is relatively common, and its definitive detection involves checking the flatness of the distal cut.

The importance of accurate cutting at the femoral chamfer areas and any patella-femoral notch resections should be appreciated as this will affect the ultimate fit and seating of the femoral component. Deep cuts will not interfere with seating of the major anterior, posterior, and distal cuts. However, "proud" cuts, or inadequate bone resection, will lead to poor fit, and the cause may not be so obvious. To modify cuts, the cutting jigs in the previously established pin sites can be replaced. Examination of the security of pin sites should be examined as well so as not to alter the needed accuracy of the cutting jig and to avoid a suboptimal position; free hand cuts may occasionally be required.

An additional concern with the femoral preparation is the area of the posterior femoral condyles. Removal of loose bodies and osteophytes is important for allowing full extension and eliminating potential problems of a mechanical nature from overlooked fragments. Additionally, it is wise to remove bone extending at the

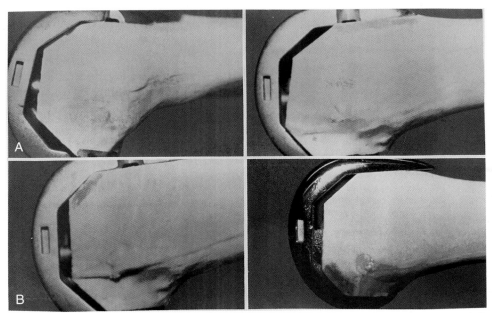

Fig. 7.17 Appearance of femoral component being impacted on after improperly prepared distal femoral surfaces. (A) Excess bone remaining posteriorly. Component tilts toward hyperextension. (B) Extra bone remaining anteriorly. Femoral component tilts into flexion. (C) Extra bone remaining at anterior chamber area. Component fails to impact full distance. Contact is evident at anterior chamber, not at posterior chamber. (D) Bone remaining at posterior chamber area. Component fails to impact fully. Gap is present distally and at anterior chamber. (Reprinted with permission Lenox DW, Cohn BT, Eschenroeder HC Jr. The Effects of Inaccurate Bone Cuts on Femoral Component Position in Total Knee Arthroplasty. *Orthopedics*. 1988;11(2):257.)

posterior cut surface proximal to the margin of the posterior femoral condyles of the prosthesis (Fig. 7.18A, B). Bone remaining at this location can be expected to block flexion as the tibial component glides posteriorly on the condyles. It can be difficult to feel such bone with the trials in place. An alternative can be to measure on the trial component with a ruler and then measure the corresponding distance back from the distal margin of the posterior cut. A mark can then be made, and the overlapping bone can be removed with a curved osteotome or saw. Caution is in order because the superior lateral or medial geniculate vessels could possibly be disrupted with an overexuberant technique. Such injury would be relatively close to the vessels' origins and could be expected to bleed vigorously. Owing to the poor exposure of this area, the bleeding is difficult to control. With reasonable care, however, the chance of this problem occurring should be minimal. Use of a pituitary rongeur to remove loose posterior osteophytes and loose bodies can be effective.

Patellar Resection

Proper patellar resection may be much more difficult to perform than one would expect. The bone is relatively small; it may be hard to hold securely. Reliable jigs are not often available in many implant instrument sets, and the bone is quite firm and frequently hard to cut. Different from the other femoral and tibial cuts that require careful varus or valgus flexion extension, or even rotational orientation, certain aspects of the patellar cut may seem to be more straightforward.

Surgical exposure is usually not a problem. The surgeon has the choice of working with the patella when the knee is extended or flexed. When working with the knee flexed and the patella everted, the bone is naturally secured and does not have to be held so firmly during the cutting process. In either position it is helpful to clear the surrounding synovial tissue by sharp dissection and removal of any remaining osteophytes that potentially interfere with the implant itself.

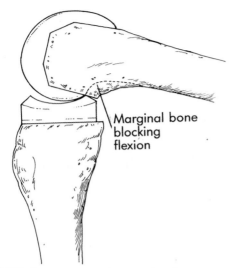

Fig. 7.18A Importance of posterior femoral marginal debridement. Residual posterior osteophytes can tent posterior capsule and contribute to creation or persistence of a flexion contracture.

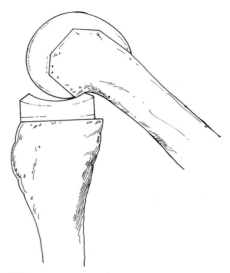

Fig. 7.18B Importance of posterior femoral marginal debridement. Residual bone at posterior femoral cut. Bone extends farther cephalad than margin of condyle at prosthesis and can abut the margin of the tibial component as the knee is being brought into flexion.

When planning a patellar cut, several choices are possible. There is freedom regarding the depth of the cut and the flexion-extension and mediolateral tilt to the cut. This discussion is concerned mainly with the technical challenge of performing the cut. From a practical standpoint, the goal is to resect the minimal amount of bone that will serve to excise the facets sufficiently and create a flat surface for the seating of the component without overstuffing the anterior compartment and leaving 12 mm of bone to protect it from possible periprosthetic fracture. The technique that has been found to be extremely useful is to define the mediolateral tilting orientation of the cut by starting just below the level of the medial patellar facet and aiming for just below the articular surface along the lateral facet. The flexion-extension tilt can be adjusted with another skim cut if needed. In this way the two cut lines form a plane of resection that is consistent with the desired mediolateral and flexion-extension orientation. A caliper can be used to measure the overall thickness of the native patella before any bone resection and again after resection. To prevent patellar fracture and leave adequate bone stock for fixation, excessive resection of patellar bone over and above what is necessary to achieve a flat surface for component seating is not recommended.

The overall consideration is the relative position of the quadriceps mechanism after prosthetic arthroplasty compared with its position before surgery. If the patellar button surface and the femoral implant trochlear groove are not placed back into their original positions, then this tethering can be expected for the patellar component, especially if the femoral implant and resurfaced patellar button exceed the amount of bone removed from these respective areas.

It is difficult to appreciate the position of the superficial surface of the patella while the cut is being made. Thus it is important that the patella be palpated and inspected carefully before and after the cut is made. In this manner the surgeon can determine the orientation of the cut surface relative to the superficial surface, feeling for areas of unusual thinness or thickness.

Patellar preparation can be made difficult by the presence of very hard bone. This is fairly common. The section on saw technique provides recommendations for handling this problem. An additional challenge is present when excessive wear occurs such that one facet, usually the lateral one, is seen to be nearly or actually too thin to work with.

If the patella is very thin and there is a concern for a fixation peg perforating the superficial cortical surface, several possibilities exist for handling this matter. The plastic pegs can simply be trimmed shorter with a knife or saw, or a smaller resection depth can be used as long as less than 4 mm is added to the thickness of the resurfaced patella.

The previous discussion clearly relates to patellar components that are placed onto a flat, saw-cut surface. Some systems guide preparation of an inset patellar fixation surface by way of a holding clamp and reamer and drill instrument. Although such an approach avoids the choices of directing specific saw cuts, one should still think of the orientation of the prepared surface and the ultimate thickness of both the prepared bone and the combined bone and prosthetic patella.

In all systems the challenge is to provide a solid and congruent good bony interface, proper alignment, and adequate bony support that avoids excessive iatrogenic thickening of the patellar construct.

Trial Reduction

During the process of preparing a femur, tibia, or patella, it may be helpful to perform trial component placement to assess fit, seating, and accuracy of cuts. What is being addressed in this section is the final trial reduction step or the combined trial reduction when all components are examined together. The purpose of such a step is to assess individual component fit and seating. However, the surgeon is principally addressing the issue of tibial component thickness, varus or valgus and anteroposterior stability, patellar tracking, range of motion, and, possibly, rotational orientation of the tibial and femoral components. In the case of press-fit uncemented applications and in the presence of profound osteopenia the surgeon must be careful to avoid damage to bone during the trial process especially if the press-fit trials are difficult to remove. Recognition of the problem and development of efficient means for manipulating the trial components without damaging bone are important steps.

In cemented arthroplasties bone surfaces should be prepared so that trial components go over and onto bony surfaces easily. Fixation holes should be widened and anteroposterior femoral cuts adjusted so that all the components slip on easily. If this condition is not met, then it is potentially impossible to know when components are seated to their desired level against the respective bone surfaces. This is particularly true with the patella and tibia and may also be true at the femur. A femoral component that sits "proud" by 2 mm distally

introduces as much difference in extension tightness as is seen when an 11-mm tibial component is selected instead of a 9-mm one. In addition, an asymmetrical error where the component sits proud on one condyle only introduces an alignment error at least equal in degree to the number of millimeters of displacement. One millimeter of asymmetrical displacement of a femoral or tibial component at the medial or lateral margin introduces approximately a 1-degree varus or valgus error. This is relatively easy to remember if one thinks of it as an application of the dictum familiar in proximal tibial osteotomy surgery: "1 mm per degree."

In performing a trial reduction to assess ligament stability several suggestions are offered. Regardless of how happy the surgeon may be with the original choice of tibial component thickness, trying one size larger and, if possible, one size smaller (thinner) can ensure an optimal fit. The surgeon should also be mindful of the tendency to introduce a flexion contracture. A thicker tibia may seem to provide better collateral stability, but it is important to make certain that this does not occur at the expense of creating a flexion contracture. If the stability in flexion is really needed and if a flexion contracture of importance is being introduced, then a more posterior soft tissue release may be necessary or movement of the distal femoral cut more proximally needs to be considered.

Of concern during the trial step in some systems is the estimation of tibial rotation. Care needs to be directed toward the relative position of the trial tibia and the orientation of the tibial tubercle, the intramalleolar axis, and the foot. In such systems a mark or alignment indicator needs to be established after determining proper tibial component rotational position. The surgeon can allow the tibial component to float and can allow the natural motion of flexion and extension to help address the rotational alignment and assess the implant position. The surgeon can generally check the medial tibial implant position to ensure it is appropriately placed on the bony tibia based on the previous assessment of tibial implant sizing.

During the trial step and before the hemostasis step described later, patellar tracking needs to be checked and patellar realignment undertaken as appropriate.

Patellar Stability and Tracking

The highly disabling nature of patellar maltracking requires strict attention to any propensity for lateral subluxation during the trialing stage. The conditions routinely associated with patellar instability include marked

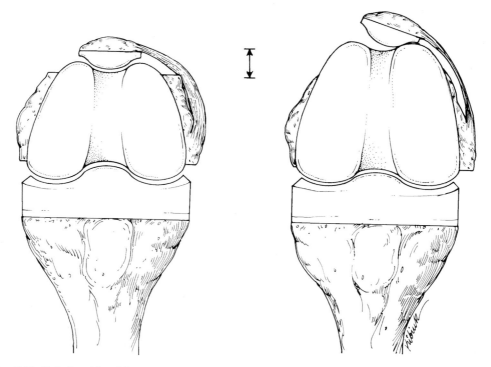

Fig. 7.19 Relationship of femoral component size and patellar tracking. **(A)** Smaller femoral component with centrally tracking patella. **(B)** Larger femoral component leading to lateral soft tissue tethering and lateral displacement of the patellar component.

valgus deformity or relative external tibial torsion, with lateral positioning of the tibial tubercle. It is sometimes possible early in the case to detect the presence of a relatively tight lateral retinaculum. This possibility was discussed in the section Surgical Exposure. Additionally, the influence of femoral component size and rotational position on patellar tracking should be considered. Any situation where there is excessive replacement of anterior femoral bone (i.e., replacement by more prosthesis than there was bone removed) and where the patellar component replaced exceeds the amount of bone resected introduces the possibility of creation of a lateral tether (Fig. 7.19).

During the trial step, with regard to patellar tracking, the patellar component is simply relocated with the trial femur and tibia in place, and the tracking of the patella is observed throughout the entire range of motion. Ideally, the component stays well located within the trochlear groove without any lateral finger pressure ("no thumbs"). The mildest amount of medially directed pressure may be consistent with satisfactory long-term function and stability. However, moderate pressure and the requirement for closing the capsule temporarily to achieve tracking stability are conditions that are highly suspect. The tourniquet can tether the proximal mechanism and should be deflated before any releases are performed if there is evidence of patellar maltracking.

When frank instability or relative tightness is noted, the lateral retinacular capsular area is examined by palpation, and release is performed first in the area that feels tightest. A common practice is to perform such release from inside the joint, first dividing synovium to get to the retinacular structures. Other surgeons routinely use an extraarticular approach. Ideally, a sufficient lateral release is performed until the patella tracks without any requirement for moderately directed force or certainly without excessive force. The extent of release required is variable, depending on causative factors for the case at hand. In the extreme one can imagine release from the region of Gerdy tubercle to and including the tendon of the vastus lateralis. When patellar maltracking is present during trialing, the surgeon should reassess the external rotation of both the femoral and tibial components to make certain these are in proper position.

In terms of the potential problems to be expected from excessive lateral release, probably the greatest concern centers around preservation of adequate circulation to the patella. It is certain, however, that most surgeons interrupt two avenues of circulation at the proximal medial and distal medial quadrants. With extensive proximal lateral and distal lateral release, two additional sources of circulation can be interrupted. It is open to argument whether sufficient circulation exists by the proximal and distal attachments through the quadriceps and patellar tendons and associated synovium, as is the consideration of revascularization (i.e., the possibility that an initially devascularized patella could go through a postoperative revascularization process).

An attempt to preserve the superior lateral circulation to the patella when possible is certainly warranted, but it is not always possible to preserve such vessels and provide sufficient release. My practice and that of many others on this point is to sacrifice such circulation, when necessary, in favor of recreating proper patellar tracking. The incidence of patellar complications that are most likely associated with avascularity is reported, but the incidence is small enough to assume that devascularization is not a major problem in many of these cases. The performance of a lateral patellar release is shown in more detail in Fig. 7.20. Once this

has been accomplished, checking the tracking using the "no thumbs" technique should be done. In rare situations the possible need for medial plication during closure can be assessed here. The section concerning tibial tubercle osteotomy may be consulted in the rare case where medialization is necessary to achieve stability. A lateral release can injure blood vessels, which would cause a major postoperative hemorrhage if left unnoticed. For this reason, patellar tracking ought to be handled before the final check of hemostasis.

The Hemostasis Step

The increasing use of tranexamic acid in joint arthroplasty has been a recent change copied from the experience of our cardiac and obstetrical gynecological surgeon colleagues. The recommended pharmaceutical dose is off-label, but it is typically 10 mg/kg intravenous (IV) over 30 minutes before inflation of a tourniquet with a second dose to be administered 3 hours after the first dose and the maximal dosage not to exceed 3900 mg per day orally (PO) or 40 mg/kg per day IV.[7] The orthopedic literature has not set a standard for the need for a second dose and has not determined whether the efficacy of IV, oral, or topical applications is similar as of this writing. We can state that its use in any form has dramatically decreased intraoperative and postoperative blood loss in the knee arthroplasty patient. This medication along with the change in hemoglobin levels that would trigger the accepted need for a blood transfusion has led to a marked change in modern day transfusions for this patient group. However, no one can argue

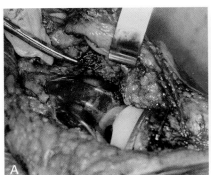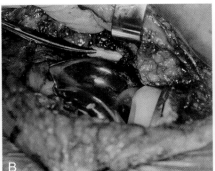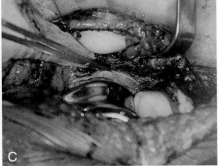

Fig. 7.20 Lateral patellar release. **(A)** Patella is retracted anteriorly, laterally, and peripherally. Synovium is incised longitudinally. **(B)** Denser capsular and iliotibial band fibers are divided in longitudinal direction. Care is taken to avoid, where possible, inferior lateral and superior lateral circulation to patella. In some cases, adequate lateral release will require interruption of this blood supply. **(C)** More complete lateral release.

the merits of hemostasis as a general principle. The following discussion is warranted for those surgeons who advocate a tourniquet-less knee arthroplasty or do not deflate the tourniquet before closure of the wound.

The average reader is urged to establish a specific hemostasis protocol and use it as needed. It has become a matter of debate whether the tourniquet is deflated to check the knee for major bleeding points before complete closure. However, the following are areas for the surgeon to focus on hemostasis. The incisional area, the suprapatellar region, and other relatively superficial surfaces are inspected for bleeding points, and hemostasis is achieved with electrocautery. Attention is directed only to the more major bleeders and not to every small pinpoint vessel. Bleeding is generally more profuse if an anterior synovectomy has been performed. Probably the most consistent superficial, relatively accessible bleeding can be seen in the region of the inferior medial geniculate vessels at the lower margin of the cut medial meniscus and slightly distal. Another major point to inspect in the posterolateral corner is the region of the inferior lateral geniculate artery. This vessel, which is frequently divided, courses between the popliteus tendon and the lateral collateral ligament at the approximate level of the meniscus. It is probably the single most frequently present major bleeding point in TKA. Specific attention should be paid after meniscal resection. Electrocautery can be used to achieve hemostasis immediately after resection. In both the posteromedial and posterolateral regions there may be smaller bleeding points to cauterize. Especially with prostheses that required sacrifice of the posterior cruciate ligament, attention must be directed toward controlling the intermediate geniculate at the midline. In the case of the lateral gutter these locations are the paths of the superior lateral and inferior lateral circulation to the patella. When an extensive lateral release has been performed, it may be necessary for one surgical member to clamp a synovial edge to provide accurate retraction, which will allow exposure of the bleeding point. If lateral patellar release has not been performed, relevant bleeding from the lateral gutter is almost never encountered.

In the event that there is concern for excessive bleeding, the knee can be systematically packed and examined in the following manner. The knee is brought to full extension to check carefully for bleeding points. Tension is placed across the joint by pulling on the tibia. A gentle valgus force is created along with the tension, and a regular 4 × 4 inch sponge is placed in the posteromedial corner of the knee. The tibia is then held with a varus attitude, and a second sponge is placed posterolaterally. A third sponge is placed in the lateral gutter (i.e., lateral to the patella in the area of the lateral patellar release). Care is taken to make certain that these sponges are positioned well posteriorly so that they place pressure in the respective areas where they have been inserted. In the case of knee systems that use intramedullary alignment rods or otherwise have created large intramedullary holes separate packing or plugging of these areas is appropriate. This maneuver will keep intramedullary bleeding from interfering with the hemostasis steps in the packed areas. Each area, the lateral gutter and the posterolateral and the posteromedial corners, should be inspected. Detailed examination can also occur in the setting of the difficult primary knee or the revision knee where a second tourniquet inflation is needed for cemented arthroplasty.

The hemostasis step just described in detail may be the only time or the most likely period when the extremity is manipulated extensively in a highly unstable state. In other words, the femoral condyles and proximal tibia have been excised, and no trial implants are in place between the bone ends to provide stability. The knee is completely lax and, as such, the bony ends and the surrounding soft tissues deserve additional attention and protection. This is a time when one could easily stretch a peroneal nerve, damage a calcific popliteal artery, or damage an osteopenic bone surface. Such an extremity must not be lifted solely by upward force at the ankle or even moved into a varus or valgus attitude by force at the ankle alone. It should be moved only while support is being provided under the knee and, generally, with some degree of tension being applied across the joint (Fig. 7.21).

Intraoperative Cautions Concerning Instrumentation

Although this chapter deals with the broad and detailed subject of surgical procedure, it is appropriate to point out proper surgical handling of knee system instruments. In particular, those features of instrumentation that require special attention and those areas where errors frequently occur are emphasized.

Both intramedullary and extramedullary alignment guides need to be monitored for wear. Anteroposterior

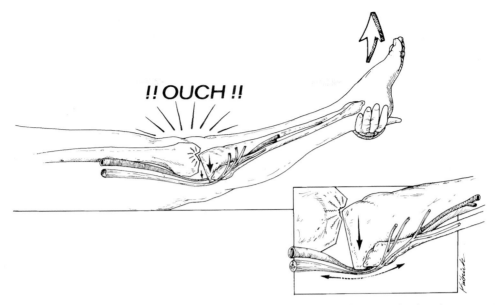

!! OUCH !!

Fig. 7.21 Inadvertent flexion and varus-valgus stress with joint surfaces excised and no components in place is to be avoided. Such movements may not only damage cut bone surfaces but also would appear possibly to stretch and damage important neurovascular structures.

and mediolateral differences in entry point for the intramedullary rods affect flexion-extension and varus or valgus positions, respectively. Parallax error and other general aiming errors with extramedullary systems also cause trouble. Pins, drill bits, or other pegs used to stabilize cutting jigs can wander off target as they are being placed in bone and cause marked alignment and component position errors. All of the problems being considered really relate to the existence of play in any instrumentation system. One should inspect the instruments, have some idea about the interlock stability of various pieces of the instrumentation, and generally look for obvious sources of such error.

It is appropriate to develop ways of checking the orientation of cuts before they are made, whether or not checking steps are a part of the given instrumentation. Especially in uncemented arthroplasty, checking the accuracy and flatness of cuts against the intended standard from the jig is necessary. It is much easier to check the cut with the jig in place and adjust it right then. Two or three steps later, when the femoral trial does not fit properly, is not the best time to be reexamining the accuracy of the femoral cuts. No cutting guides or techniques, surfaces, slots, rotary planers, are error free.

Also, one is cautioned to check component (especially tibial) rotation with the knee in extension and flexion. Abnormal internal or external rotation may occur during flexion. It is wise to reassess the position of the tibial tubercle, foot, and ankle with the knee extended and the foot held in a neutral, plantigrade attitude.

Final Trial Component Reduction

Before final bone surface preparation and component implantation, the surgeon will usually perform a trial reduction to confirm final component position, knee balancing, and patellar tracking.

If the surgeon is not using a modular tibial implant, the final decision for this implant will be determined by the trial reduction. Any uncertainties regarding size and fit must be resolved. Confirmation of the final selected implants is usually confirmed by surgeon, operating personnel, and an implant company representative by careful reading of labels.

PROSTHETIC COMPONENT PLACEMENT

Placement of Cemented Components

Between the time that each component is impacted in final position and the time at which the cement is

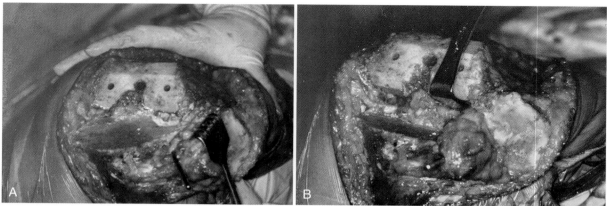

Fig. 7.22 (A) View of proximal tibia with knee hyperflexed and anterior drawer motion. (B) View of image A with femur lifted upwards. Hyperflexion anterior drawer maneuver in most cases will present the proximal aspect of the tibia for inspection, débridement, and placement of tibial instruments. Lifting femur creates better flexion space, but it also pulls the tibia posteriorly and can make access actually more difficult than one would expect.

satisfactorily cured, the components must be held steady in relation to the bone. Even though cement clearing does not begin until the marginal cement is nearly hard and even if it is cleared quickly and efficiently, one is still faced with additional "holding time" to allow hardening of the cement. Furthermore, in the latest stages of curing, one may be tempted to try to stretch or position the knee in various ways to expose recesses where cement is hidden.

The surgeon should be aware of two potential problems during this phase of the procedure. First, hyperflexion of the knee to access the posterior recesses may lead to anterior or distal displacement of the femoral component (Fig. 7.22 and 7.23). This would be occurring at the stage where it would probably not be safe simply to push the component back against the femur. To do so might create a relatively poor cement interface because of micromotion and disturbance of an adequate cure of the cement; this can lead to early loosening.

The second caution is in regard to taking the knee out to full extension. This maneuver is rather attractive, as it provides substantial compressive force between the tibial and femoral components and across the respective femoral and tibial interfaces. It is even used by some surgeons to enhance trabecular cement intrusion. The concern is that in some knees there is a tendency for eccentrically directed force to cause the tibial and/or femoral components to "lift off" the bone posteriorly

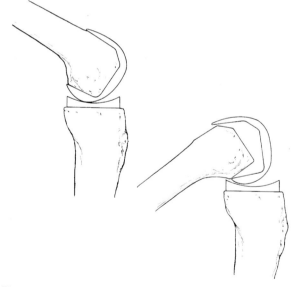

Fig. 7.23 With hyperflexion, the surgeon may dislodge the femoral component during cementing stage. This phenomenon is seen as result of wedging or squeezing that can occur in a tight posterior compartment. This tendency may be demonstrated during trial reduction. Special care must be taken in cementing during the final component placement so as not to provoke displacement. Thought may be given, if such displacement is seen at time of trial reduction, to increasing the posterior slope of the tibial cut.

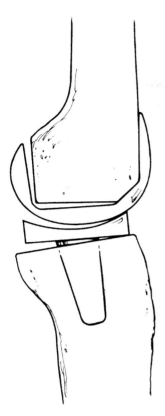

Fig. 7.24 When less than rigid fixation exists at the femoral and/or tibial component, occasionally eccentric anterior loading at the time of cementing in extension can lead to component "lift off." The phenomenon may not be apparent from the anterior aspect of a fully extended knee. This liftoff may lead to inappropriate tightness during flexion and relatively inadequate cement-bone prosthesis interface.

(Fig. 7.24). This may go unnoticed without specific attention to its possibility. The liftoff is not readily apparent from the anterior aspect when the knee is at the level of the table. This situation can compromise the bone-cement prosthesis interface and can lead to varus or valgus alignment error if there is asymmetrical mediolateral liftoff. It can also lead to excessive ligamentous tightness in flexion, because the liftoff tends to occur posteriorly. It is not, strictly speaking, wrong to take the knee out into extension during the final cementing step. However, this maneuver must be done carefully, with attention directed toward the possibilities mentioned. One can occasionally extend the knee for the principal

purpose of exerting some additional compression and also to assess that the joint, indeed, comes to full extension. When there is a question of liftoff, cementation in 20 degrees of flexion can be used instead.

Placement of Uncemented Components

Techniques of final implantation of uncemented components vary according to individual systems and individual methods of fixation. Furthermore, some considerations may not be applicable to certain systems.

The principal message is to provide special care during final component implantation so that fixation stability is maintained. I think that surgeons should handle uncemented tibial components just as if they were cemented. That is, after careful impaction and final fixation, great care is taken, while addressing the femur, not to bump or otherwise stress the tibial component in a way that might loosen it.

The surgeon needs to be certain at this stage, based on provisional or trial reductions, that the femoral component is going to fit properly. There is risk of dislodging the tibial component and/or damaging femoral bone if it is necessary to remove the final femoral component once it has been impacted into place.

A patella secured by multiple studs may be the component most susceptible to the problem of fixation instability by preliminary removal of the true component.

Local Injection

Local injection has been popularized in combination with regional anesthetic techniques as a part of multimodal pain control regimen. The choice of a local nerve block with possible neuraxial or general anesthesia has become more predominant. The localized intraarticular injection given by the surgeon can be a powerful adjunct to the postoperative multimodal pain control for the patient, especially as the move toward outpatient joint arthroplasty becomes more prevalent. There are many combinations of compounded injectables, but the primary goal is to assist locally with multiple different pain receptors. A general recommendation is to use a short and longer acting local anesthetic, epinephrine or clonidine, to locally prolong the effect and to use a nonsteroidal antiinflammatory drug or, when not possible, substitute a corticosteroid to enhance the antiinflammatory effect of the injection. These injections are also technique dependent, and injection along the posterior aspect of the femur and tibia along the joint line after the initial bone cuts have been made can be done with a long spinal needle. Injections are also recommended along the capsular area where the meniscal resection has occurred while avoiding the peroneal nerve and in the apexes of the incision at the fascia and skin. The surgeon can also apply medication medially along the incision and across the anterior aspect of the knee to assist with a block.[8]

Wound Closure

Orthopedic literature has advocated for the discontinuation of the use of closed suction drainage systems to control and decrease postoperative blood loss. When a closed wound suction drainage is used, the tubes are placed in the suprapatellar intraarticular space and along the gutters, and they are checked to ensure they can be extracted freely at a later date. It is also recommended to cut the drains between the holes with the theory that if a portion of drain were to remain lodged within the knee, it would like break through the holes at the weakest link of the drain.

It is sufficient to close the capsule and the tendinous layer without a separate deeper synovial closure. Personal preference dictates suture type and exact stitching technique in terms of interrupted versus running sutures and other factors.

In patients with moderate and gross obesity attention should be given to the deep fascia that overlies the quadriceps tendon and that can be readily identified during initial exposure. Specific suturing of this fascial layer provides excellent wound approximation. Additional aspects of subcutaneous tissue to minimize the dead space and potential seroma or hematoma collection postoperatively is also recommended. Skin closure is also a matter of personal preference. One is, however, cautioned to understand the importance of careful and accurate skin approximation in this type of wound. The surgeon

is dealing with a large collection of foreign material that, in some examples, can be on the order of only 1 cm deep to the superficial surface of the skin. Furthermore, the joint itself produces synovial fluid, and the wound must withstand the stresses inherent in range-of-motion exercises. Provision of the most optimum situation for early healing is critical because benign drainage can definitely lead to late, deep infection.

REFERENCES

1. Muller W. *The knee: form, function, and ligament reconstruction*. New York: Springer-Verlag; 1983.
2. Keblish PA. Valgus deformity in total knee replacement—the lateral approach. Scientific exhibit 3322, at the fifty-fourth annual meeting of the American Academy of Orthopaedic Surgeons, San Francisco, 1987.
3. Coonse K, Adams JD. A new operative approach to the knee joint. *Surg Gynecol Obstet*. 1943;77:344.
4. Insall JN. Surgical approach to the knee. In: Insall JN, ed. *The knee*. New York: Churchill Livingstone; 1984.
5. Garvin KL, Scuderi G, Insall JN Evolution of the quadriceps. *Clinical Orthopaedics and Related Research*. 1995;321:131–137
6. Scott RD, Siliski JM. The use of a model V-Y quadricepsplasty during total knee replacement to gain exposure and improve flexion in the ankylosed knee. *Orthopedics*. 1985;8:45.
7. Fillingham YA, Ramkumar DB, Jevsevar DS, et al. Tranexamic Acid in Total Joint Arthroplasty: The Endorsed Clinical Practice Guides of the American Association of Hip and Knee Surgeons, American Society of Regional Anesthesia and Pain Medicine, American Academy of Orthopaedic Surgeons, The Hip Society and The Knee Society. https://www.aaos.org, Guidelines and Reviews.
8. Busch CA, Shore BJ, Rakesh G, et al. Efficacy of periarticular multimodal drug injection in total knee arthroplasty. *JBJS Amer*. 2006;88:959–963.

8

Bone-Cutting Technique

Audrey M. Tsao, MD

Dr. Krackow was a stickler for precision, and he was relentlessly thinking about how to make his bone-cutting techniques more reproducible and precise. This chapter on bone-cutting technique and accuracy is inspired from much of the teaching and direction he provided to countless residents and fellows over the years.

SAW TECHNIQUE

Accurate, safe, and efficient use of a power bone saw has become a basic task in modern orthopedic surgery. This section discusses those aspects of equipment and technique that relate to the development of an ability to make accurate and efficient bone cuts. The use of slotted cutting jigs will assist in limiting the error margin for saw cuts and can dictate the thickness of the saw blade. It is useful for the surgeon to understand the basic principles of cutting on an open block versus a slotted jig and the technical considerations for selecting this power tool, which is intimately involved throughout the procedure and has a direct effect on the achievement of the success of the case. For the novice, placing the saw at full power to observe the excursion distance of the tip of the saw is worthwhile to understand the width of the effective cutting arc compared with the physical saw blade. For similar reasons, observation of the distance between the saw's cutting edge and the handpiece to understand changes in the angle along the length of the sawblade due to lifting off the cutting jig that would affect over- or underresection is a worthwhile exercise.

SAW BLADES

At least five characteristics of saw blade design and manufacture relate to cutting properties at total knee arthroplasty: metal quality, tooth arrangement, blade length, blade width, and blade thickness. Although intuitively obvious, it is worth pointing out that the oscillating saw cuts at the end not at the sides of the blade, and a reciprocating blade cuts along the edge of the blade and can cut at the tip depending on the configuration of the saw blade. Selection of the saw blade will have a direct effect on the technique used to complete the surgical procedure.

Metal hardness, the metal's ability to take and hold a good edge with respect to maintaining sharp saw teeth, is a characteristic that is difficult to assess, especially as it is not routinely supplied by manufacturers. Certain saw tooth configurations provide relatively sharp cutting action but introduce interesting control problems, see Fig. 8.1. If one approaches the bone eccentrically or asymmetrically using principally one side of the saw blade, then this blade strongly tends to kick toward the opposite direction because of the angular orientation of the saw teeth. The saw tooth arrangement creates a form of ratchet or barb effect. Avoidance of this blade behavior is achieved by approaching with the saw so that the blade is centered within the arc of travel over the bone encountered by the blade.

The next point concerning saw tooth design relates to a superior/inferior splaying of saw teeth and the significance of this for some press-fit applications. Fig. 8.2 shows how this aspect of tooth arrangement causes the cut surface to be produced some distance "deep" to the surface of a cutting guide. This is not a realistic problem in the vast majority of cases. It is, however, a detail that should be recognized, especially if one is shown new saw blades with greater variation in the angulation and/or greater length to the angled teeth, a condition that also would accentuate this deep cutting effect.

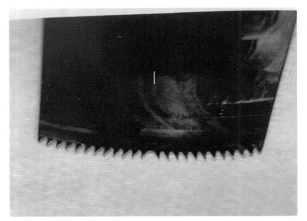

Fig. 8.1 Asymmetrical arrangement of teeth in this saw blade causes the blade to kick to the right or left, if the left or right aspect of blade encounters bone alone. If the blade approaches bone at the center of its arc, the tendency is minimized.

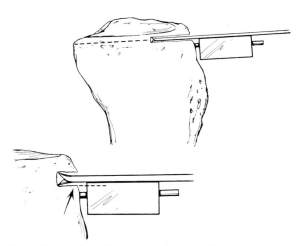

Fig. 8.2 Splaying of the sawblade teeth can produce a cut that is deeper than the surface of the cutting jig.

For the same tooth design and sharpness, functionally the thinner and narrower blade will appear to be sharper and will cut more easily. Note that at this point no consideration has been given to the control of the direction of the cut, hence the blade's accuracy or its tendency for any skiving is due to the blade's potential for increased flexibility. However, the blade may seem to be more difficult to control when trying to achieve a flat cut and the saw blade flexibility has caused a nonuniform flat cut due to the arching of the blade. Consideration of completing the saw cut and then returning to the cut

with a heavier less flexible blade as described below and creating a new edge for the bone cut under direct visualization can solve this problem.

The last size characteristic to analyze is blade length. One can regard either the size of the bone front or the issue of moment arm to see that although a long blade may reach farther, it is less powerful in its cutting role and has a wider excursion at the cutting end. Because of the fixed arc of oscillation, the longer blade traverses a greater linear distance of arc and therefore can encounter a proportionately larger area of bone front. The resistance to oscillation applied at the saw blade edge has a proportionately greater moment because of the longer moment arm of the longer blade itself. Thus sclerotic bone, due to its increased hardness, can at times be more effectively cut using a thinner, shorter blade.

One can expect the sharpest, most effective cutting of hard bone while using short, thin, and narrow blades. However a shorter and narrow blade does not create the smoothest and most accurate cut and can affect the accuracy of the bone cut.

CUTTING EFFICIENCY

Several variables regarding bone density, direction of cut, and pressure of cut may be altered to improve the efficiency of cutting.

An overall factor to be regarded is cutting pressure, that is, how hard one leans on or pushes the saw into the bone. Developing the sensitivity to manual feedback with the saw will allow the surgeon to continually adjust both pressure and direction. Tactile sensitivity is necessary when one is making blind cuts, such as when cutting the lateral condylar surface of the tibia or the posterior condyles of the femur. The most obvious sense of ineffective bone cutting is imparted as greater saw pressure leads to a greater sense of vibration in the handpiece with a decreased advancement forward of the saw; this can bind the blade against the bone. Excessive vibration in the handpiece means that the saw blade is not moving fully at the cutting, bone front, and the oscillation of the motor is then being transferred to the handpiece rather than to the saw tip. This is generally accompanied by a change in the sound of the saw similar to when a reamer is in contact with cortical bone when placed in a tight intramedullary shaft. The opposite extreme occurs when the saw is working at full oscillatory rate and inadequate vibration is felt in the handpiece as minimal; this may indicate the presence of the saw tip within soft tissue. The sense of pushing the blade forward and "feeling" the bone is also important from the standpoint of protecting surrounding soft tissues and producing complete cuts. Feeling the bone refers to the practice of using the end of the moving saw blade as a gauge to determine that it is still against bone, as opposed to being outside the bony margin or having cut through the bone so that the blade is working against soft tissue with the potential for soft tissue damage. The sense is analogous to feeling the distal cortex of diaphyseal bone when drilling holes for fixation screws. One drills through the near cortex and then carefully advances the drill deeper, varying the forward pressure until the far cortex is palpated. Then one responds quickly to the giving-way sensation, anticipating it and guarding against it as the drill goes through the distal cortex.

This sense with a bone saw is similar to what one encounters in removing a plaster cast. An oscillating saw is used to cut completely through the cast. With experience, care is taken to "feel" when the cut is through the cast to avoid plunging the saw blade unnecessarily deep and, at the same time, to be certain that the cast is cut entirely.

The last aspect of bone-sawing efficiency to be considered is what can be thought of as the "whittle" principle. In wood carving as a wider, relatively flat surface develops, the carver finds themselves trying to cut a lot larger front of wood, and it becomes difficult, perhaps impossible, to make headway. Cutting becomes more effective when the board is approached at an angle approximating 45 degrees; this allows the entire energy of the sawing effort to be directed toward a relatively smaller dimension of wood. Even as the cut is deepened, a much smaller surface is attacked than would be encountered if the saw blade was laid flat against the longer side of the board. In surgery entrapping the sawblade will decrease the oscillating movement of the saw and will not allow movement of bone debris away from the cutting teeth. This can be avoided with the whittling technique. This front becomes more formidable as it gets wider and/or the bone is harder. One can use an awareness of these factors as a more effective means to facilitate the task of cutting hard bone. Fig. 8.3 indicates how one can use this change in direction to diminish the size of the bone front and increase the effectiveness of the cutting. The directional change should not be made in a haphazard way but with a specific eye toward achieving the whittle effect.

Most commonly, really hard, dense bone is encountered in patients with compartmental overload caused by varus or valgus deformity. Whereas such patients have hard bone at the concave, overloaded side of the knee, the bone at the convex aspect is relatively soft, possibly even absolutely osteoporotic. The trick here is not to expend the entire saw blade effort against hard bone only. The cut should be started in the soft area and should venture into the hard area a little at a time. In some cases it feels almost as if one is sequentially shaving or chipping away at the more sclerotic side to use the energy of the saw against the smaller, less resistant front of bone.

The effective sharpness and cutting efficiency is also directly affected by the speed of the oscillation of the bone saw. The cutting power of the saw is affected by the size and strength of the motor but also affected by the extend of the blade oscillation excursion and how rapid the oscillation of the blade is further modified by the angular extent of the blade oscillation and the frequency of that oscillation. In general, use of the saw at full power to ensure that it is working at peak performance is advocated. The friction in hard dense bone can cause heat generation and binding of the blade by not allowing the saw to work at its full oscillation excursion; this will decrease the efficiency of the blade. Because the actual work performed is directly proportional to the amount of bone that is contacted and cut by the business end of the saw blade, it may be necessary to allow the bone debris to clear from the cutting end of the saw. A technique that allows the surgeon to release the pressure against the edge of the bone in short bursts instead of a using constant direct forward pressure with the saw can improve the efficiency of the cutting action.

ACCURACY

It is necessary, first, to select a method of ensuring cut accuracy. The choices available are (1) careful visual attention to the position of the saw blade against the cutting block, or one side of a cutting slot, with adjustments in the pressure, direction, and bend of the saw blade as necessary; (2) reliance on the confining boundaries of a cutting slot; (3) application of a tool to hold the saw blade in position against a cutting guide; and (4) use of a modified cutting slot.

As the cut is started, the saw should be activated with the blade in position on the cutting guide; the

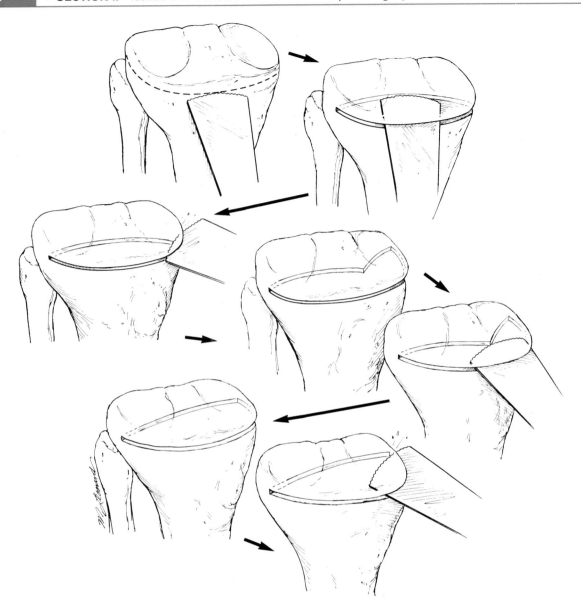

Fig. 8.3 As the saw is approaching the bone a cutting front is created along the entire extent of the bone. As the progress slows, the blade can be withdrawn and angled 10-45 degrees to allow a different smaller bone front against the sawblade to allow greater power directed against a smaller cutting surface. This can be done as needed and also allow the saw blade to be angled away from vital soft tissue structures. Care should be taken to make sure the throw of the blade is not outside the edge of the bone.

saw blade is held flush against the instrument but 1 or 2 mm away from the bone. Generally, the saw should be activated to full power. The surgeon can try to use local pressure to control any up-down whip that is present in the saw blade and then advance the blade to cut the periphery of the bone. A surgical assistant can help visualize this and give feedback as necessary.

If the saw is activated with the blade contacting the bone, then the blade is usually thrown out of position abruptly, and it is necessary to reposition and start over. As the bone is approached, the surgeon watches for resistance caused by hardness and tries to alter direction or location to provide a smaller or softer bone front, as described previously. As the cut is being initiated, the surgeon should try to complete the close, near aspect of the cut all the way across the bone surface before going into the depth of the bone in any one area, in essence creating their own bony slotted jig initially. The surgeon can retreat to the more superficial area within this slot when cutting into a new section of bone before going deeper to progress the cut. For example, in cutting the tibia the procedure works better if the cortical cut is completed across most of the anterior cortex before going deeper into a single compartment. Going all the way into the cut on one side alone tends to create two different cut levels in the medial versus lateral compartment, which need to be adjusted. This principle may need to be varied if the surgeon is taking advantage of differential bone density. In this case the cutting proceeds deeper into the soft bone; then the hard bone is approached gradually from its "softer" direction (Fig. 8.4).

The initiation of certain cuts is particularly difficult with regard to skiving, which causes a raised cut on harder bone. Once the bulk of the bone has been removed, the surgeon can return to the cutting jig and, using a gentle hand, create a front from the softer bone surface and push across the edge of the front to make flat and nonraised cut. A relatively thick, wider saw blade usually works well as it has less tendency to bend. There are typically limited areas of bone that need adjustment, and the bone front is often not the entire length of the cut surface and often limited to one area at a small change in depth.

The next point of technique is the most obvious but is possibly the most frequently ignored. The surgeon ought to use the jig for the full length of the saw blade or up to the point at which the cut is completed. Many times, cutting guides prevent the completion of a cut, because the saw blade does not seem to be long enough. The instruction here is for the surgeon to make sure that all the bone possible has been cut and full use has been made of the jig before removing it.

Special care in completing cuts is needed when the cutting guides have been removed. The surgeon should try to use the previously cut surface as a cutting guide to direct the completion of the deeper aspect of the cut. When working freehand, it is safer to approach from the far side of the proud aspect and create an edge to work against, as shown in Fig. 8.5. Starting with the blade at the

Blade entrapment

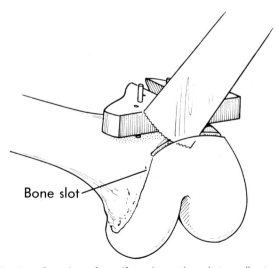

Fig. 8.4 Creation of a self made cutting slot can "entrap" the saw blade while maximizing the contact of the saw blade against the cutting jig. The direction of the saw-blade can be modified as needed to achieve the cut.

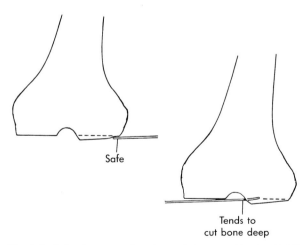

Fig. 8.5 Adjusting a previously made bone cut by approaching from the higher side can assist in modifying the cut. If using the previously cut deeper side, care should be taken to avoid blade lift off or arcing the sawblade to avoid over or under resection of the previous cut surface.

deep side of the offset invites the possibility of removing excess bone as the surgeon follows the direction indicated by what is at first the deeper, less proud surface. The most difficult, hence most hazardous, maneuver is to approach the margin of any relatively high bone freehand without the aid of any cutting block.

My approach is to start with the most accurate blade (i.e., the thicker, wider, and longer one) and then to adjust the size variables as necessary according to the variable quality of bone being cut. Bone may not be hard, and thickness may not be necessary to prevent skiving. A surgeon may be dealing with excision of posterior condylar bone or trying to preserve a posterior cruciate tibial bone island. In these cases a narrower saw blade may be necessary, not just preferable. Also, it is only in really large knees that the longest saw blades available make a real difference.

The last points to be covered in this section on accuracy involve final checking of the cuts. The surgeon can frequently use a flat instrument or even a saw blade through a slot to check the accuracy of a cut. This surface can be laid against the cutting guide and advanced toward the cut surface of bone, rather than spanning the cut surface and the guide to begin with. Movement of the flat surface being used to check accuracy as it advances away from the cutting jig across the length of the bone surface will allow the surgeon to feel high and low spots.

This chapter details a basic aspect of total knee arthroplasty and describes the difference between finesse and struggle in bone-cutting techniques. Excellent component fit and accurate limb alignment are facilitated by the combination of surgeon awareness, attention to detail and technique, and use of an efficient workflow. These basic principles will aid the novice and may also give some insight for the more experienced surgeon.

TKA Balancing

Arun Mullaji (Bipin), MChOrth, FRCSEd, MS Orth, DNB Orth, MB, D Orth

INTRODUCTION

Knee arthroplasty was in its infancy in India in the 90s, when I returned from overseas having done hundreds of fairly straightforward cases, to start practice in India. I was accosted with patients with profound knee deformities, and I was desperately in need of guidance! That's when a colleague suggested I read Ken's book. However, in the early "90s," in the sprawling metropolis of Mumbai, there was just one copy of The Technique of Knee Arthroplasty by Ken Krakow. It took a month of searching to track down this elusive copy, in the library of one of the medical colleges, but that book transformed my entire concepts about knee arthroplasty and Ken immediately became a superstar in my eyes. I met my idol Ken at the Current Concepts in Joint Replacement meeting in Orlando in December 1995 and since then, first as a participant and then as a faculty for 15 years, I would quiz him at every opportunity about the problems I faced. That's when I realized what a perfectionist he was, how meticulous and precise was his thinking. I also saw another side, an ardent photographer, he was the only one permitted to amble around in the aisles and during the faculty dinner to take hundreds of photos (only a few lucky ones got to see them!). He was also the most prepared for any eventuality wherever he went—he always carried spare batteries, a laser pointer, a torch, a whistle, and some tools with him! A model of sartorial elegance, he would inspect carefully my watch and attire and share his views on how to match shoes and accessories. About 5 years ago, I tried convincing him that he needed to publish an updated version of his book which was sold out and nearly impossible to get. He said he had made several notings on pieces of paper so I suggested to him that we could capture these on camera and organize them, and that I would be only too happy to

help in this endeavor. Annually, I would beseech him to update his book. Finally, a few years ago, he relented and said that Bill Mihalko would spearhead the project. It is such a delight that I have been able to contribute to this book as my tribute to one of the finest thinking surgeons that it has been my privilege to meet!

Both alignment and balancing are critical for the optimal functioning of a total knee arthroplasty (TKA) and are rendered more challenging in the face of deformity. In the first edition this chapter[1] was prefaced by the statement that deformity correction involved "a combination of philosophy and hypothesis" (p. 249). Since its publication, many of these concepts have been substantiated by cadaveric, computational, finite element analyses, and clinical studies, whereas others have been supplemented and a few have been replaced by newer developments. It is pertinent to allude to these advances at the outset while reaffirming certain established tenets; both are equally and extremely germane to and set the stage for the vital aspect of soft tissue balancing.

FUNDAMENTAL CONCEPTS

Kinematics of the knee refers to the relative motion between the femur and the tibia. The knee can move in different directions, and these are known as degrees of freedom. There are three translations and three rotations that are possible. The three translations are in the anterior-posterior, medial-lateral, and proximal-distal directions. The three rotations are flexion-extension, varus-valgus, and internal rotation-external rotation. Kinematics of the prosthetic knee are governed by the implant factors (principally the design), patient factors (such as knee extensor-flexor muscle strength), and surgical factors (such as soft tissue balancing).[2]

Unlike the intrinsically more stable ball-and-socket configuration of the hip joint, stability is conferred upon the knee by static stabilizers, such as ligaments, menisci, and capsule, and less by shape of the articulating surfaces. In addition, there are dynamic stabilizers that are the muscles and tendons around the knee such as the quadriceps, gastrocnemius, hamstrings, and the iliotibial tract (IT).

Soft tissues have an initial tension and stiffness. *Tension* refers to two forces pulling in directly opposite directions. Tension in a ligament controls the boundaries of laxity. *Laxity* refers to translation or rotation occurring in a particular direction when a force or torque is applied. *Stiffness* is the ability of soft tissues to resist elongation when a load is applied and shows a typical curve with an initial toe-in region, linear region, and the failure region. *Ligament stiffness* is defined as the force (in newtons, Nm) needed to stretch the ligament by 1 mm and is the slope of the linear region.[3] *Strain* refers to the resulting deformation that occurs.

The superficial medial collateral ligament (MCL) complex has been reported to have a stiffness value of 80 N/mm, 42 N/mm for the deep MCL complex in cadaveric knees,[4] and 58 N/mm for the lateral collateral ligament (LCL).[5] In osteoarthritic (OA) knees undergoing TKA stiffness of the soft tissue envelope was greater in cruciate-retaining (CR) knees (80.9 and 80.8 N/mm, in flexion and extension respectively) than posterior-stabilized (PS) knees (64.3 and 68.5 N/mm, respectively), with no differences because of age or sex and no differences between extension and flexion within CR and PS groups.[6] Stiffness in full extension was 28 N/mm for the medial compartment (not just the MCL) and 20 N/mm for the lateral compartment.[7]

The stabilizing structures around the knee are not symmetrical in terms of anatomy and function medially and laterally nor anteriorly and posteriorly. The MCL is isometric, whereas the LCL is anisometric. Also, the articulating surfaces of the medial side of the knee differ from the lateral side in terms of shape and hence congruity and stability. The medial side of the knee is more stable, and the lateral side is more mobile; the lateral femoral condyle translates further posteriorly with flexion.[8]

The key restraints in different directions are as follows. Valgus rotation is principally resisted by the superficial medial collateral ligament (sMCL) and varus rotation by the LCL. One-fifth of medial and lateral restraint at 5 degrees of knee flexion is conferred upon by the cruciates.[9] Anterior translation is resisted by the anterior cruciate ligament (ACL) and MCL; posterior translation is resisted by the posterior cruciate ligament (PCL), posterior oblique ligament (POL), and posterior lateral structures (popliteus and popliteofibular ligament [PFL]). External rotation is resisted by the MCL and posterior lateral structures; internal rotation is resisted by the LCL, POL, and posteromedial capsule. Hyperextension is prevented by the oblique popliteal ligament (OPL), which is the largest ligament in the posterior capsule. The IT controls varus and internal rotation of the knee. The anterolateral ligament has been added as an additional and distinct ligament. It originates from near the popliteal tendon attachment on the lateral femoral epicondyle and courses to its tibial attachment midway between Gerdy tubercle and the fibular head.[10,11] It resists anterior tibial translation but possesses much weaker tensile properties.[12]

Flexion and extension also bring into action different restraints. For example, in flexion the posterior structures are relaxed, and therefore the main stabilizers are the medial and lateral structures. In extension the posterior structures and the medial and lateral structures provide restraint. The anterior fibers of the MCL confer more stability in flexion because of their anatomy.

Normal and osteoarthritic (OA) knee kinematics show continuous and smooth femoral external rotation with knee flexion. Maximum femoral external rotation and condylar posterior translation occur in normal knees, followed by OA knees, and the least in knees with an arthroplasty. Posterior-stabilized TKA (PS-TKA) consistently display an abnormal anterior femoral translation during the first 60 degrees of flexion; screw-home motion has not been observed in OA knees or in knees after TKA during passive motion.[13]

INSTABILITY AND BALANCE

Alterations or damage, due to congenital, developmental, traumatic, pathological, or surgical reasons, to the bony articulating surfaces, soft tissues, and muscles can result in changes in stability of the knee. These must be carefully assessed preoperatively as they have a direct bearing on the restoration of stability when a TKA is performed. The vastus muscles and gastrocnemius are the primary contributors to the knee joint forces during gait, followed by the rectus femoris, gluteus maximus, soleus, and hamstrings.[14]

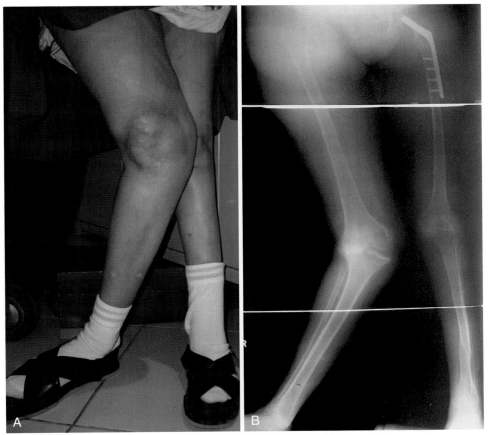

Fig. 9.1 Severe instability but no pain in a (A) patient with poliomyelitis and (B) the corresponding radiograph.

Instability is a symptom experienced by the patient. It can be simply described as a feeling of abnormal knee movement during normal activities. Instability may or may not be accompanied by pain. For example, a patient who has poliomyelitis (Fig. 9.1) may experience instability but no pain; a patient who has OA may have both instability and pain.

Balancing refers to the art and science of restoring stability to and improving kinematics of the patient's arthritic knee during TKA so that there is ligament stability throughout the functional range of motion (ROM). *Balance* means that the capsular ligamentous elements are pulled out to length but are not excessively stretched and certainly are not buckling or lax. It is one of the most complex and important issues in the whole operation. Soft tissue symmetry will need to be reestablished while the tibia and femur are aligned normally with one another. Proper balance must be established in every case, whether deformity coexists or not; severe deformity would call for more specialized techniques. Every attempt must be made during this process to not introduce instability, which may be a reason for early failure; instability may also lead to abnormal loading that may result in long-term failure of the implant. Imbalance can influence the ROM; ROM can be reduced, causing stiffness, or increased, leading to instability, subluxation, or dislocation.

THE CHALLENGES

Because of the presence of varying degrees of bone, cartilage damage, and ligament deficiency or excision (ACL), the implant will need a certain amount of stability or constraint. The underlying principle of TKA is to use the least constrained device and rely on the patient's soft tissue envelope so that there are reduced stresses on its fixation in bone; this will reduce the risk of revision.[15] When using an implant with the least constraint necessary, it becomes imperative to rely on a combination of the patient's soft tissue tension in the capsule and ligaments in conjunction with the articular surface geometry of the implant, matching the implant constraint to the soft tissue envelope.

The most constrained implant would be a hinge; when using this design, soft tissue balancing becomes superfluous as the entire stability is afforded by the constrained design. However, a more constrained implant would lead to more stresses on its fixation and would therefore entail additional fixation in bone with resultant bone destruction, which makes a subsequent revision more challenging. If the surgeon opts for a hinge, everything that follows is irrelevant.

Adding to the complexity of soft tissue balancing are the lack of consensus on the precise definition of and quantification of stability (and therefore what constitutes a "balanced joint"), asymmetry of native soft tissue structures, presence of varying degrees and types of deformity, wide spectrum of pathology encountered, the differential effect and efficacy of various surgical steps and devices, variations in implant positioning and design, and changes in laxity that may occur over time. All these render balancing an unresolved and difficult-to-understand subject.

Furthermore, during surgery, the active muscle envelope is relaxed, and therefore the knee is in a nonloaded paralyzed condition; judgment of laxity therefore is based on passive ligament tension. Even under these conditions, assessment of balance is based on subjective "feel," and this can be affected by the size and weight of the thigh and surgeon's ability to stabilize the knee while assessing stability. Various newer technologies to assist in this endeavor are still under evaluation. Surgical technique is further influenced by surgical experience, training, and volume. Objective data of correlation of stability with outcome measures and patient satisfaction is still emerging (and some of it is conflicting); whereas, studies focusing on revision TKA clearly identify instability as one of the main indications for revision.[16]

Thus not balancing the joint is clearly fraught with the real possibility of failure. Yet what constitutes a balanced joint and how to achieve it is akin to John Saxe's "The Blind Men and the Elephant" poem of six blind men trying to describe an elephant.[17] Everyone thinks they know what it is. I shall nevertheless attempt to examine some

of these factors in greater detail, scrutinize some evidence-based conclusions, and present a systematic and rational basis for balancing the prosthetic joint.

Laxity in Normal Knees

Before I begin our quest of balancing an arthritic knee, let us first look at the normal knee. There are various studies in normal subjects and nonarthritic cadavers using radiographs, MR scans, navigation, and robotics with different stresses applied to determine what can be defined as "envelopes of passive knee joint motion" (p. 705).[18] All these studies show that in the normal knee, medial and lateral laxity are not equal, and this difference varies with flexion. In general, the lateral gap is greater than the medial gap, and the difference increases with flexion. Even in cadaveric studies, it has been shown that there is an asymmetry of medial and lateral gaps right through from extension up to flexion; this gap is greater in flexion than in extension. There are no studies that suggest that these gaps are equal medially and laterally and that the flexion and extension gaps are equal. This is true not only of varus-valgus but also of anteroposterior and rotational laxity. Whether gaps in a prosthetic knee should mimic the normal joint or seek to establish equal gaps is a subject of debate.

With stress radiographs using a tensioner with 15 Nm torque, varus laxity of 2.8 degrees, and valgus laxity of 2.3 degrees in full extension in healthy subjects was reported.[19] (Applying elementary trigonometry, 1 degree roughly equals 1 mm over the length of a normal femur or tibia.) When knees were flexed to 90 degrees and imaged in neutral and under a varus-valgus stress in an open MRI system, the lateral joint gap opened by 6.7 mm with a varus stress, whereas the medial joint gap opened by only by 2.1 mm, indicating that the lateral joint gap is significantly lax.[20] One study has shown that the mean varus-valgus limits are smallest at 0 degrees flexion and increase nearly linearly with flexion; the varus limit increases more rapidly than the valgus limit. The ranges of the varus and valgus limits are both largest at 90 degrees flexion (2.6 and 1.1 degrees, respectively).[21] A robotic study in cadavers has shown that the native medial and lateral gaps are tightest in extension at 1.3 and 2.2 mm, respectively. These gaps increase by 3 to 4 mm with 0 to 20 degrees of flexion and then plateau. The lateral native gap is 1.3 mm larger than the medial gap throughout the range.[22] Generally, larger differences in laxity of more than 2 to 3 degrees between medial and lateral gaps over the entire range are not seen.[23]

After ACL Release

After the ACL is resected, the most cadaveric studies using tensioners show an increase in extension gaps, with the medial side increasing by 2.1 mm and the lateral gap increasing by 2.8 mm with 100 N force and increasing 2.5 and 3.1 mm, respectively, with 200 N force. Flexion gaps increase minimally after ACL resection, medially by 0.4 mm and laterally by 0.9 mm with 100 N force and increasing 0.4 mm and 0.9 mm, respectively, with 200 N force.[24]

After PCL Release

In contrast, PCL release leads to larger increases in the flexion than the extension gap. Older cadaveric studies have shown that the tibia can be distracted from the femur by 5.3 mm at rest and 6.4 mm under tension.[25] In varus knees, after PCL resection and using a tensioning device, the flexion gap increased medially by 4.8 mm and laterally by 4.5 mm. The extension gap increased by <1 mm.[26] The lateral joint gap has been shown to be 5 to 6 mm more than medial from 60 to 120 degrees of flexion.[27] Flexion gaps increase in cadavers from 30 to 120 degrees flexion by 1 to 3 mm, but increasing the force from 50 to 100 N increases the mean gap by only 0.5 mm.[28] Another study using a tensioning device with 10, 20, and 30 inch-pounds (in-lb) of distraction force found no change in extension gap after PCL resection; flexion gap distance enlarged by <2 mm.[29] PCL resection increased the mean flexion gap more than the extension gap: The gaps were 2.4 mm medially and 3.3 mm laterally in flexion versus 1.3 mm medially and 1.2 mm laterally in extension.[30] What is interesting is that the *differences* in joint center gap for 20, 40, and 60 lb and varus laxity at extension and flexion were not significantly different among different joint distraction forces.[31] With the 100 N force, the medial and lateral extension gaps increased by 0.2 mm after PCL resection and by 0.2 and 0.3 mm, respectively, with 200 N; flexion gaps increased by 2.4 mm medially, 3.4 mm laterally with 100 N, and 3.4, 2.6, and 3.7 mm, respectively, with 200 N. Thus similar proportions in gap enlargement were seen with the 200 N force.[24] In general, the extension gap increases by 1 mm and the flexion gap by 3 to 4 mm after PCL release.

It may be more technically challenging to achieve perfect balance when retaining the PCL.[6] PCL should be fully released before ligament tensioning for femoral component rotation as the medial and lateral gaps increased by 0.5 to 1 mm if complete release was performed subsequent to the gaps having been measured with only partial PCL release in a cadaveric study.[32] Similarly, in a navigational study using a 150 N tensioner force, PCL release showed no effect on the extension gap but increased the flexion gap by >3 mm in 36% of patients and >5 mm in 12% of patients, with <2 mm change in 44% of patients. Thus it is recommended to release the PCL before the femoral resections are performed, as this step determines the ratio between extension and flexion gaps.[33]

Differential Effect of Deformity on Gaps

In varus knees the lateral extension gap increases with severity of deformity; it is larger with severe varus (>20 degrees) than in mild (<10 degrees) and moderate (10 to 20 degrees) varus, whereas there are no differences in the medial joint gaps among the groups.[34] A 2020 navigational study found a much greater initial difference (4.7 mm) between lateral and medial gaps in extension in more deformed knees requiring releases than in those with no release required (1 mm).[35]

On the other hand, at 90 degrees flexion, the medial-lateral laxity difference of ≤2.5 degrees was present in 91.6% of 72 knees, implying that there is no evidence of contracture in the coronal plane tissue in end-stage arthritic knees at the time of TKA.[36] This was also seen in another study where the difference between lateral and medial gaps in flexion in more deformed knees requiring releases was 1.8 and was 0.5 mm in those with no release required.[35]

Long-term Changes in Laxity

Under spinal anesthesia, medial laxity in extension increases by 0.6 degrees and lateral laxity by 1 degree when stress is applied.[37]

Mediolateral joint laxity analyzed immediately intraoperatively and 30 minutes later showed that stress relaxation occurred in all cases; mediolateral laxity increased by an average of 1 mm on the medial and lateral sides.[38] Arthrometer stress tests with 150 N force applied with the knee in 0 to 20 degrees flexion after surgery, with the patient still under anesthesia, showed no differences in laxity measurements made under anesthesia and 6 months postoperatively with either the PS or CR design.[39]

Some studies suggest that no changes occur postoperatively in the coronal laxity that is achieved intraoperatively even up to a mean of 77 months.[40] Both extension and flexion laxity remain unchanged at 5 years in CR knees and extension gaps in PS knees as assessed by stress radiographs.[41] Another study showed that medial laxity remains constant postoperatively from immediately after surgery to 12 months. However, the mean lateral laxity that was 8.6 degrees immediately after surgery decreased to 5.1 degrees at 3 months. [42] Residual medial tightness of 1 to 2 mm improved spontaneously when laxity was measured under anesthesia at the time of the staged surgery of the contralateral knee joint. There was no change in lateral laxity.[43]

These studies suggest that about 1 mm of relaxation of gaps occurs soon after surgery and then remains unchanged. Medial tightness of 1 to 2 mm may improve, and lateral laxity may reduce by up to 3 mm over time. However, this may be influenced by the overall alignment as shown in a computer simulation study where condylar liftoff occurred in neutral coronal alignment regardless of excessive LCL laxity. Condylar liftoff occurred easily in >3 degrees varus alignment even with slight laxity in the LCL. The study also noted higher peak contact forces in the medial compartment on heel strike and lateral condylar liftoff during the single-leg stance that appeared to be influenced more by the degree of varus alignment than by the amount of LCL laxity.[44]

Effect of Stability on Patient-Reported Outcome Measures

Residual imbalance of 2.8 and 1.3 degrees varus in extension and flexion, respectively, was not associated with significant differences in early clinical results of postoperative ROM and the subscales of (symptoms, patient satisfaction, patient expectation, functional activities) of Knee Society Score (KSS) among the groups categorized according to the varus-valgus gap angle and the laxity.[45] However, excessive intraoperative medial joint laxity of ≥4 mm at 90 degrees flexion decreased patient satisfaction at 1 year.[46]

Western Ontario and McMaster Universities Arthritis Index (WOMAC) scores of patients with <3 mm gaps showed worse scores for two functional items demanding knee flexion (bending to floor and getting on/off toilet), and 3 to 4 mm laxity at 90 degrees might be necessary to carry out daily life activities.[47] Anteroposterior (AP) laxity measured with an arthrometer at 60 degrees knee flexion significantly correlated with Knee Injury and Osteoarthritis Outcome Score (KOOS) pain score.[48] AP laxity of ≥7 was significantly associated with a subjective feeling of instability in TKA patients.[49]

Similarly, it has been suggested that a controlled flexion gap increase of 2.5 mm may have a positive effect on postoperative flexion and patient satisfaction after TKA.[50] In contrast, WOMAC scores were better in TKAs

with a medial-lateral balanced (<2 mm) gap[51] as were outcomes in terms of physical functioning, bodily pain, social functioning, Oxford and Knee Society scores at 6 months, and improved social functioning scores at 2 years with flexion-extension gap differences of ≤2 mm.[52] Knees in which the difference between varus and valgus laxity was <2 degrees had greater ROM by 10 degrees whereas those with >2 mm difference had lesser ROM by 9 degrees.[53] Smaller medial gaps at 60 and 90 degrees of flexion have been shown to play an important role in achieving medial pivot motion with tibial internal rotation; moreover, tibial internal rotation provides a better flexion angle after PS-TKA.[54] Patients with medial-lateral instability <5 at 30 degrees at 2 years postoperatively had superior KSS functional knee scores and 36-item Short Form Health Survey (SF-36) scores than those with greater instability.[55]

Thus there appears to be some degree of variation in the reported optimum laxity required for superior outcomes. It would appear that the medial side is key in varus knees, especially if activities involve deep flexion. It needs to be balanced to approximately within 2 mm from 0 to 90 degrees; the lateral gap especially in flexion can be more lax but not >4 mm.

This is borne out by a cadaveric study, using calibrated extensometers sutured to the LCL and sMCL, that found that the strains in both ligaments in the replaced knee are different from those in the native knee. The MCL becomes tighter in the native knee and the LCL relaxes with flexion. Both ligaments were found to be stretched in extension; in flexion the MCL was found to be relaxed, but the LCL was tight, suggesting that measured resection techniques may overstuff the joint.[56] In another study in which transducers were attached to collateral ligaments in the native knee the MCL slackened 2 mm, whereas the LCL slackened 7 mm with flexion. Post-TKA the MCL slackened a further 3 mm and the LCL a further 4 mm during flexion. A 5 degree external rotation of the femoral component slackened the MCL by a further 2 mm and tightened the LCL by 2 mm; the opposite effect was found during 5 degrees internal rotation.[57] Others have reported that a wide range of coronal plane laxity values are associated with highly satisfied TKA subjects[58] and that a controlled flexion gap increase of 2.5 mm may have a positive effect on postoperative flexion and patient satisfaction after TKA.[50] Another study determining the tibiofemoral forces and collateral ligament strain for variations in flexion and extension gaps noted that small variations in gaps had minimal effects on the soft tissue tension between 15 and 100 degrees of flexion. However, increasing the flexion gap by as little as 2 mm may reduce tibiofemoral forces beyond 90 degrees of flexion and a looser flexion gap decreases soft tissue tension beyond 120 degrees of flexion.[59]

It is not inconceivable that it may be the postoperative kinematics of the prosthetic knee that may be responsible for patient satisfaction on patient-reported outcome measures (PROMS).[60] In fact, a 2020 study reported that during closed kinetic chain movements, patients with poor PROM scores after TKA experience more anterior translation on the medial side followed by a medial midflexion instability and less posterior translation on the lateral side in deep flexion than patients with good PROM scores.[61]

Given this background information regarding gaps, some of it conflicting and contradictory, the next sections of this chapter will consider relevant aspects of the patient's history, clinical examination, and imaging that may have a bearing on balancing gaps during TKA. The surgeon often has a proclivity to bypass these steps and head directly to surgery. The surgeon is in danger of remaining oblivious about key issues that may call for a change in the surgeon's technique to address special nuances that exist between one knee and the other, often even in the same patient[62] (Fig. 9.2).

STEPS TO ACHIEVING CORRECT ALIGNMENT AND BALANCE

Although some of these vital steps have been chronicled in earlier chapters, the ones described here are particularly relevant to balancing the knee and are perhaps worthy of repetition.

Preoperative Planning

1. Relevant history
   a. Prior soft tissue trauma, which may have led to a PCL or MCL injury that may have a bearing on implant type
   b. Prior fracture with intra- or extraarticular malunion
   c. Sudden worsening of pain above or below the knee signifying a possible stress fracture (wherein, for example, a long stem tibial component may be indicated; cutting the tibia orthogonal to its long axis would be mandated regardless of one's views on kinematic or anatomical cuts. This would therefore impact flexion and extension gaps.) (See Fig. 9.3.)

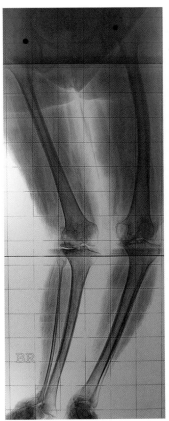

Fig. 9.2 Radiograph of a patient with windswept deformity in whom clearly the surgical technique will need to be tailored differently for the two knees. Radiograph shows valgus deformity in the right knee with a stress fracture of the ankle and varus deformity of the left knee.

   d. Prior surgery (such as high tibial ostomy [HTO], ligament reconstruction) that may be responsible for altered anatomy, kinematics, adhesions, and changes in patellar height (e.g., patella baja)
2. Preoperative clinical assessment
   • Flexion deformity (FD) is often masked by the leg lying in external rotation. The knee must be rotated internally and examined with the patella pointing upwards so that the FD manifests (Fig. 9.4).
   • Hyperextension may not be evident as the leg is lying flat on the examining couch, and it will be missed unless the leg is passively lifted with a hand supporting the ankle (Fig. 9.5). It will need a different technique of balancing than a knee with an FD.

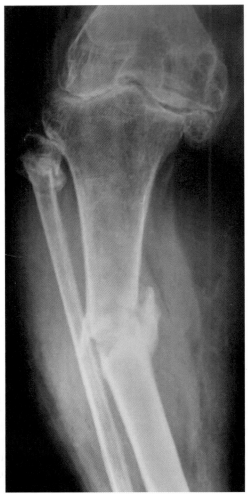

Fig. 9.3 Radiograph shows stress fracture of tibia in a patient with severe varus osteoarthritis.

- Varus-valgus stress examination with the knee flexed 10 to 20 degrees gives a very good indication if the deformity is correctable (Fig. 9.6). In full extension the posterior capsule is taut, making assessment of stability and correctability difficult; it is relaxed in slight flexion so mediolateral laxity can be better assessed.
- Patellar tracking especially in valgus knees should be assessed; maltracking will need to be addressed with appropriate releases.
- Tibial torsion is also masked in patients with a flexion and varus deformity. To detect intorsion, one needs to rotate the leg such that the patella points upward; if the foot and malleoli are internally rotated, it suggests tibial intorsion (Fig. 9.7). Incorrect tibial tray rotational placement may affect knee kinematics.[63]

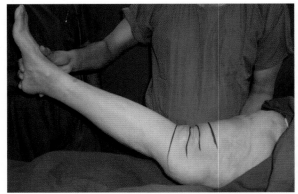

Fig. 9.5 Demonstration of the extent of hyperextension, which can often be missed, in a patient under anesthesia.

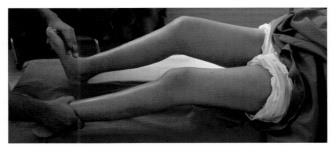

Fig. 9.4 Clinical photograph of a patient under anesthesia showing flexion deformity of left knee that appears to be lesser when the leg is in slight external rotation. In contrast, in the right knee, the true extent of flexion deformity becomes evident on internally rotating the leg such that the foot points upward.

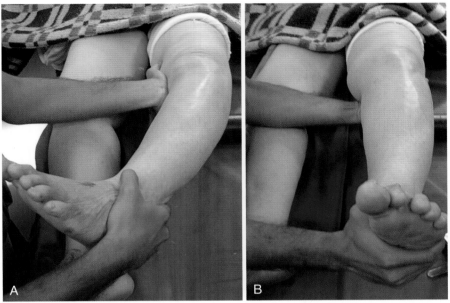

Fig. 9.6 Determining whether deformity is correctable or not: (A) the knee should be flexed slightly to ascertain whether the deformity is (B) partially or fully correctable.

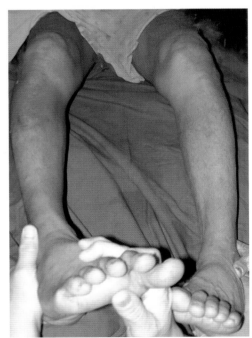

Fig. 9.7 Marked tibial intorsion that is revealed by internally rotating the legs until the patella points directly upward.

- Hip ROM has a bearing on ligament balancing; an arthritic or stiff hip or one with altered anteversion may affect orientation of the distal femur and influence femoral component orientation.
- Neurological examination: weakness of quadriceps or gastrocnemius muscle (as after a stroke) may result in hyperextension, requiring a more constrained implant. Patients with severe combined valgus and flexion deformity are at risk of developing a common peroneal nerve palsy postoperatively, and the neurological status of the lower limb needs to be documented initially.
- Flatfeet cause lateral deviation of the weight-bearing axis of the limb.[64] It is more common in patients with valgus deformity (Fig. 9.8), though it is frequently seen in patients with varus deformity. In the latter the surgeon may use this knowledge to slightly undercorrect the deformity, which would thus require a lesser release. Also the use of the second metatarsal for judging tibial jig placement may induce an error in rotational placement of the tibia tray because forefoot abduction is present in a severe flatfoot deformity.

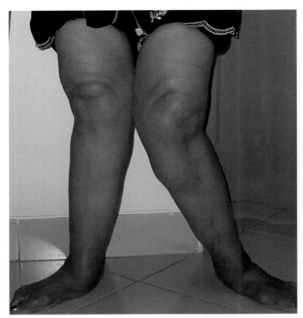

Fig. 9.8 Severe bilateral flatfeet in a patient with profound valgus deformities.

- Gait: In addition to observing for flatfeet, it is important for the surgeon to determine whether there is a major adductor thrust (Fig. 9.9) during the stance phase in varus knees. This would signify increased laxity of the lateral structures often with severe medial tibial bone loss and will need to be factored into the balancing technique.
3. Radiographic assessment

Weight-bearing long hip-to-ankle radiographs along with routine weight-bearing AP, lateral, and skyline views are valuable. A systematic assessment of radiographs should be undertaken.[65] These need to be viewed carefully for the following elements:
- Valgus correction angle (Fig. 9.10) should be noted if conventional surgery is being performed. This can often vary from 2 to 11 degrees.[66]
- Osteophyte presence, location, and size should be noted. The larger the osteophyte, the more likely that a lesser release may be required (Fig. 9.11).
- Reactive bone remodeling should be sought on the radiograph. Its presence denotes significant deformity and the possibility that reduction osteotomy may be deployed to balance gaps (Fig. 9.12).
- Bone loss or a stress fracture that may need special attention (i.e., augment, graft, sleeve, cone, stem). If a longer stem is required, this may dictate whether

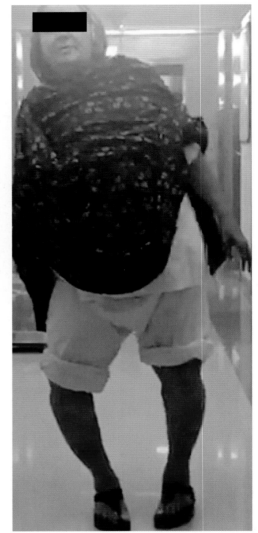

Fig. 9.9 Severe adductor thrust in the stance phase as the patient bears weight on the right leg while walking.

a classical 90 degree tibial cut should be performed over a 3 degree or more varus tibial cut to prevent stem tip abutment against the lateral tibial cortex.
- Extraarticular deformity in the femur or tibia should be identified as these knees may have to be addressed differently to align and balance them; this is discussed later. Lateral views of the length of the femur and tibia are especially mandated to determine presence and severity of extraarticular sagittal plane deformity.
- Intracapsular deformity is discussed later.

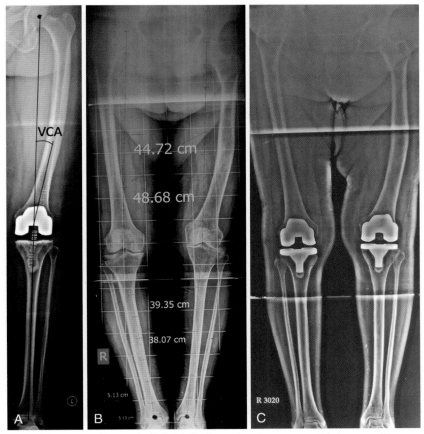

Fig. 9.10 (A) Valgus correction angle (*VCA*) is indicated and measures 11 degrees. The preoperative (B) and postoperative radiographs (C) which have taken into account the increased VCA.

- Amount of tibial subluxation and extent of lateral opening often imply severe stretching of the lateral structures (Fig. 9.13). The balancing technique will need to take this into account. By the same token, one should look for medial stretching in a valgus knee.
- Patella tracking has been alluded to above.
- Prior implant such as a staple, anchor, interference screw suggests a prior ligament reconstructive surgery and must alert the surgeon to possible ligament damage.

4. CT scan
  May be ordered if
  - there are bowing, torsional, and intracapsular deformities in the femur or tibia.
  - there is posttraumatic OA with a concern about ligament avulsion from bone, bone loss, and fracture union.

- prior HTO was performed with change in tibial slope and rotational malunion.

5. MR scan
  MR scan is useful in situations where the integrity of the MCL/PCL is in doubt.

6. Technical goals
  a. Coronal and sagittal limb alignment: the surgeon has to select and aim for classic, anatomical, kinematic, or constitutional alignment or a variant of these.
  b. Components: the surgeon should define the acceptable limits of component placement in all three planes and resection thicknesses; they should decide on the type of implant (i.e., CR, PS, constrained, hinge) that is likely to be required and the type of instruments (i.e., conventional, patient-specific instrumentation [PSI], navigation, robot) to be used for this purpose.

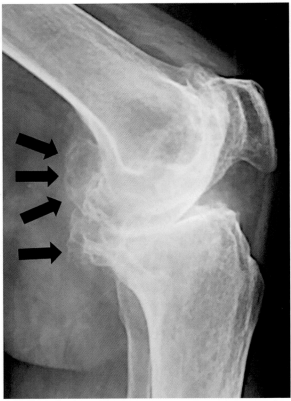

Fig. 9.11 Lateral radiograph shows large posterior femoral and tibial osteophytes.

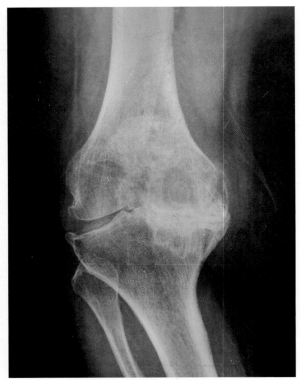

Fig. 9.12 Radiograph displays marked posteromedial reactive bone remodeling.

c. Gaps: The surgeon should also be clear regarding (1) technique of gap balancing (measured resection, gap balancing, or a variation); (2) aims in terms of acceptable flexion and extension gap differences—equal and symmetrical medially and laterally or unequal and asymmetrical and, if so, by how many mm or degrees; and (3) method of assessment of gaps and their symmetry.

Interrelationship Between Bone Cuts, Joint Line, and Stability

Each of the surgeon's decisions will have ramifications in the actual process of achieving balance. Aiming for hip-knee-ankle (HKA) axis of 177 to 180 degrees in a varus knee tight medially in flexion and extension by resecting the proximal tibia in 2 to 3 degrees varus while orienting the distal femoral cut orthogonal to its mechanical axis may result in lesser or perhaps even no

release being required to achieve balanced extension and flexion gaps (Fig. 9.14A). A rectangular extension gap can also be achieved by cutting the distal femur in varus and externally rotating the femoral component further (Fig. 9.14B) while keeping the tibial cut orthogonal. After a varus distal femoral cut and correctly rotating the femoral component, the extension gap would be balanced but the lax flexion gap would be lax laterally (Fig. 9.14C). The dashed line represents an orthogonal bone cut. By measured resection of the posterior femoral condyles (Fig. 9.14D, *dashed lines*), there will be relative internal rotation of the femoral component and a 3- to 4-mm lateral laxity at 90 degrees if no medial release is performed. To obtain a rectangular and balanced flexion gap with the component oriented parallel to the transepicondylar axis (TEA), medial release may be required to establish equivalence of medial and lateral gaps or the femoral component must be placed in excessive external rotation (Fig. 9.14E). It becomes immediately apparent that it would be expedient for the surgeon to enunciate

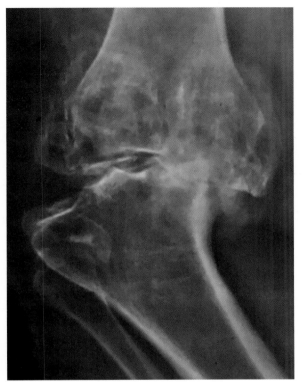

Fig. 9.13 Severe stretching of lateral structures and tibial subluxation.

their goals at the outset, rather than struggle with the various options intraoperatively. Use of PSI can help the surgeon, as will the use of navigational and robotic software.

These goals are intricately connected with the establishment of the obliquity of the articular plane of the prosthetic joint commonly referred to as *joint line.* Any cut that removes relatively more from the medial femur throws the knee into varus; a deeper medial cut on the tibia would do the same (see Fig. 9.14A). An excessively deep cut in the medial tibia might be balanced with a deep lateral cut on the femur to keep the overall tibiofemoral alignment correct. However, this combination would lead to undesirable obliquity of the joint line. In the coronal plane in normal controls the joint line is typically in 3 degrees varus, but it can vary widely,[67] with almost half being >3 degrees and even up to 10 degrees.[68] Likewise, in flexion if the axis of the posterior femoral condyles does not have a proper "neutral" rotational orientation, then as the condyles articulate with the tibial plateau in flexion, the femur goes into abnormal rotation or the tibia is positioned in abnormal varus or valgus attitude. Although properly oriented cuts from the perspective of joint line may imply normal

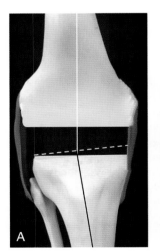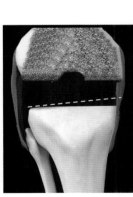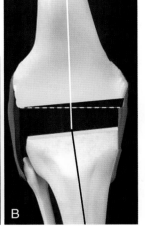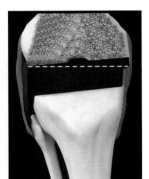

Fig. 9.14 Aiming for a hip-knee axis of 177 to 180 degrees in a varus knee tight medially in flexion and extension, by resecting the proximal tibia in 2 to 3 degrees varus while orienting the distal femoral cut orthogonal to its mechanical axis. (A) Lesser or perhaps even no release may be required for achieving balanced extension and flexion gaps. (B) A rectangular extension gap can also be achieved by cutting the distal femur in varus and externally rotating the femoral component further while keeping the tibial cut orthogonal.

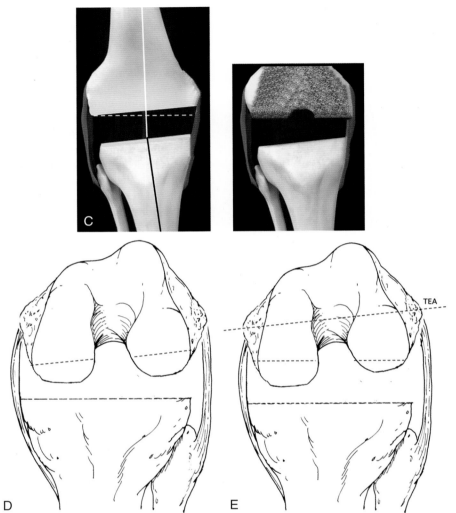

Fig. 9.14 *(Continued)* (C) After a varus distal femoral cut and correctly rotating the femoral component, the extension gap would be balanced but the lax flexion gap would be lax laterally. The *dashed line* represents an orthogonal bone cut. (D) By measured resection of the posterior femoral condyles (*dashed lines*), there will be relative internal rotation of the femoral component and a 3 to 4 mm lateral laxity at 90 degrees if no medial release is performed. (E) To obtain a rectangular and balanced flexion gap with the component oriented parallel to the transepicondylar axis (*TEA*), medial release may be required to establish equivalence of medial and lateral gaps or the femoral component must be placed in excessive external rotation.

alignment, they do not automatically recreate or maintain proper ligament balance.

Excess distal femoral resection (Fig. 9.15) draws the MCL, LCL, and PCL closer to the distal joint line. As a result, it leads to relative laxity in extension, with the same or tighter stability in flexion. Distal migration of the femoral joint line is shown in Fig. 9.16. It leads specifically to relative tightness in extension and possibly failure to achieve full extension. Anterior displacement leads to laxity in flexion (Fig. 9.17); posterior displacement leads to relatively excess tightness in flexion (Fig. 9.18).

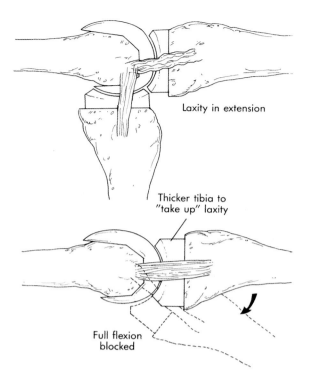

Fig. 9.15 Femoral prosthetic joint line shifted proximally. Net result is relative tendency to soft tissue collateral instability in extension. Normal or excessively tight tension presents when knee is flexed.

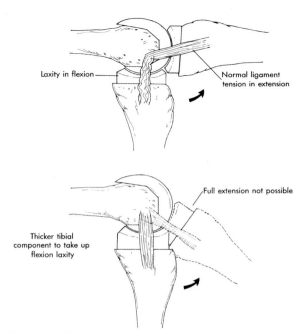

Fig. 9.17 Effect of anterior femoral component displacement. (A) Ligament attachments are closer to posterior aspect of joint and relative laxity in flexion with greater tightness in extension is seen. (B) There may be either excessive laxity in flexion or tendency to block full extension.

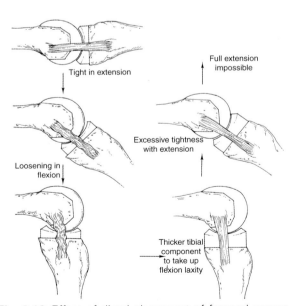

Fig. 9.16 Effect of distal placement of femoral component. (A) Ligament attachments assume positions that are proportionately farther from joint line in extension and closer in flexion. (B) Relative tightness in extension or even inability to come to full extension if knee starts with tight ligaments in flexion.

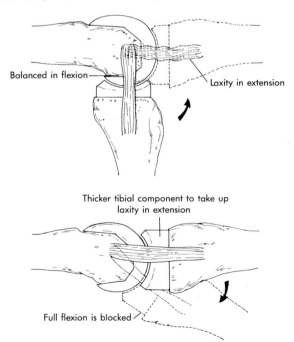

Fig. 9.18 Effect of posterior displacement of femoral component. (A) In opposite mode ligament tension is relatively tight in flexion and loose in extension. (B) Result may be block to flexion or appearance of excessive laxity toward extension.

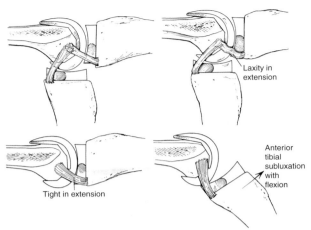

Fig. 9.19 (A) Cut-away drawing of normally positioned femoral component, demonstrating appearance in full extension and 90 degrees of flexion with essentially isometric posterior cruciate ligament. (B) Femoral component moved proximally so that origin of posterior cruciate ligament is closer to femoral joint line distally. With flexion, cruciate tightens and with extension, it appears relatively lax. (C) Femoral component has been positioned proximally and combination of tibial and femoral component thicknesses are such that posterior cruciate is tight in extension. (D) As knee is flexed, because of proximity of femoral attachment to joint line, posterior cruciate ligament tightens and draws tibia forward.

Effect of Altering the Joint Line on the PCL

A femoral joint line that is more proximal places the PCL so that it is either lax in full extension or tightens abnormally as the knee moves into flexion (Fig. 9.19). With the anterior-to-posterior vector of the PCL, the effect of its tightening should be understood. The posterior cruciate protects against abnormal posterior translation of the tibia. Its tightening pulls the tibia forward. Excessive tightening of this ligament can, in the extreme, cause the tibia to be pulled forward so that it dislocates.

Because of its somewhat anterior origin in the intercondylar notch, pathologic tightening of the PCL in extension is rarely a big problem. This is because ligaments originating more anteriorly from the femur will tend to tighten with flexion, whereas those originating more posteriorly tend to relax with flexion and tighten more with extension.

A femoral component that is too anterior would lead to relative laxity of the PCL in flexion, whereas a component that is too posterior would lead to excessive tightness in flexion.

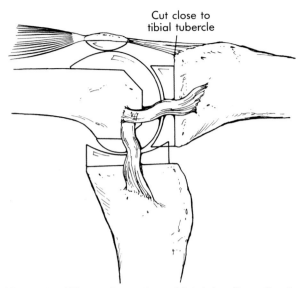

Fig. 9.20 Effect of moving tibial joint line distally. Collateral ligaments are relatively lax in both full extension and in flexion.

On the tibial side, things are simpler. Displacement of the prosthesis joint line deeper into the tibia leads to increased laxity in all aspects of motion (Fig. 9.20). Similarly, recession of ligament attachment from the tibia leads to laxity in all aspects of the motion cycle, whereas distal advancement leads to tightening throughout the ROM.

UNDERSTANDING THE PATHOANATOMY OF DEFORMITY AND IMBALANCE: A SYSTEMATIC APPROACH TO CORRECTION

It would be instructive to look separately at the two principal ingredients of deformity, the bony elements and the soft tissues, and their interaction as this will spell out the recipe to deal with deformity with the dual objective of restoring balance and reestablishing alignment. As the deformity is often in three planes, it would be convenient to address it sequentially in each plane.

The entire task can be systematized by adopting a universal classification (A. Mullaji, submitted for publication). The pathoanatomy of any knee with its specific components of deformity and instability can be precisely summarized as follows using the ELS classification system. This takes into account:

(1) the location of coronal deformity represented by the letter E followed by 0 for articular deformity, 1 for intracapsular deformity, and 2 for extraarticular deformity; thus E 0, 1, 2;

(2) soft tissue balance in the coronal plane represented by the letter L followed by 0 when flexion and extension gaps are nearly equal medially and laterally, 1 when the extension gap is asymmetrical but the flexion gap is balanced, and 2 when both extension and flexion gaps are asymmetrical and unbalanced; thus L 0, 1, 2; and

(3) soft tissue balance in the sagittal plane represented by the letter S followed by 0 when flexion and extension gaps are equal, 1 when the extension gap is less than the flexion gap, and 2 when the extension gap is greater than the flexion gap, thus S 0, 1, 2.

The Coronal Plane

The two variations in limb alignment in the coronal plane, varus and valgus deformities, can be considered as mirror images of one another. The words *concave* and *convex* are used to refer to the medial or lateral aspect of the deformed joint with varus or valgus changes. In the case of a varus deformity *concave* refers to the medial aspect and *convex* refers to the lateral aspect. The following discussion will examine more closely the overall bony contribution to deformity.

Bone Status

It is imperative to locate where the bony deformity resides, as this will have a bearing on the soft tissue sleeve and therefore on the principles of restoring both alignment and balance. Full-length radiographs are invaluable in determining the location of deformity. More recently, phenotypes of varus[69] and valgus arthritic knees[70] have been described; these may be valuable in planning and performing surgery.

Type E 0: Articular deformity. The entire arthritic process, bone loss and deformity, is confined to the articular surfaces of femur and tibia with no extraarticular deformity beyond (Fig. 9.21). The TEA (i.e., the approximate attachment of the ligament origins) is normal as is its orientation with the femoral shaft and mechanical axes.

Type E 1: Intracapsular deformity. This is perhaps the most challenging and least readily discernible deformity to the casual observer. The presence of such a deformity has vastly different implications based on whether it is located in the femur or in the tibia.

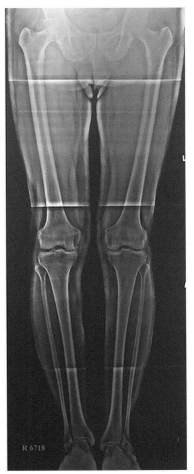

Fig. 9.21 A classical presentation of a type E 0 deformity that is confined to the articular surfaces.

On the femoral side, the deformity (Fig. 9.22) is likely to be due to congenital, developmental, or metabolic causes but rarely to traumatic causes (Fig. 9.23). In addition to the intraarticular bone loss and deformity, there is distortion of the femur between the articular joint line and the collateral-capsular attachment (as denoted by the TEA) with a sinister and subtle alteration of the angle between the distal joint line and the TEA and the mechanical and anatomical axes of the femur. Generalized bowing of the femur may also be present (see E 2 in the next section) and should be an indicator of this variation. It should be understood that a prosthetic component that comes to have proper alignment with respect to the femoral axes will not simultaneously have a proper alignment with respect to

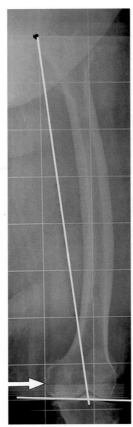

Fig. 9.22 The angle between the distal femoral joint line and the mechanical axis is decreased on the medial side such that the medial epicondylar attachment of the medial cruciate ligament (*arrow*) is closer to the joint line. There is an additional bowing of the femur which adds an element of E 2 type of deformity.

the epicondylar axis. In a typical varus case (Fig. 9.24) the medial epicondyle would be further away from the prosthetic surface and the lateral one would be much closer to the prosthetic surface. The lateral gap would be marked greater, and the gap would be substantially trapezoidal.

In a valgus knee hypoplasia of the distal femoral condyle is a common observation (Fig. 9.25). It will contribute to exacerbation of the deformity, which may be further accentuated by lateral femoral bowing. Consequently, the lateral epicondyle may be more proximal (with a lesser lateral angle between the TEA and the femoral axes) and hence further away from the prosthetic surface; the medial epicondyle would be much closer to the prosthetic

surface. The resultant medial gap would be correspondingly far greater than the lateral one.

On the tibial side, the corresponding region is between the articular joint line and the distal attachment of the sMCL. A classic example would be an overcorrected proximal tibial osteotomy (Fig. 9.26). Malunited intraarticular fractures are another cause of intracapsular deformity (Fig. 9.27). Here, the obliquity of the joint line will be markedly altered, and the soft tissue envelop would be altered either surgically or reactively over time to the osteotomized position. An orthogonal cut across the tibia will remove a great excess of medial bone; thus a disproportionately larger medial gap would ensue (Fig. 9.28). Any mild degree of varus bowing of the femur would accentuate this disparity.

Type E 2: Extraarticular deformity. Besides the intraarticular angulation, there is an extraarticular deformity away from the knee (Fig. 9.29A–E). Its effect on the putative resection levels depends on the severity of angulation (such as a malunion or prior osteotomy) and its distance from the knee joint. If the angular deformity were immediately adjacent to the hip or the ankle joint, its effect on the overall knee alignment would be minimal.

Krackow[1] has suggested, as a rule of thumb, that such shaft deformities would contribute to knee joint deformity in nearly direct proportion to the distance from the relevant hip or ankle joint in the respective case of the femur or tibia. A 10-degree shaft angulation at the midpoint of the femur, 50% along its course, would lead to approximately a 5-degree deformity at the knee, and the deformity would be with respect to the femoral joint line. A 10-degree deformity 80% of the way along the course of the femur, which is closer to the knee, would lead to approximately an 8-degree deformity at the knee; a deformity that is at the knee joint would present 100% of the 10 degrees, or a 10-degree deformity, at the knee joint and would represent type E1 (above).

More commonly, especially in Asians, there is a lateral or medial bowing of the entire femur,[71] the effect of which is computed by drawing the distal femoral resection line perpendicular to the femoral mechanical axis. When the tibial resection line is marked on the radiograph, the angle between the two resection lines (lines A and B in Fig. 9.29A) would be indicative of the magnitude of the challenge in trying to achieve a balanced gap. Likewise, metaphyseal varus bowing is often seen in Asians (Fig. 9.30). The likely effect of this can be appreciated by drawing the proximal tibial resection line

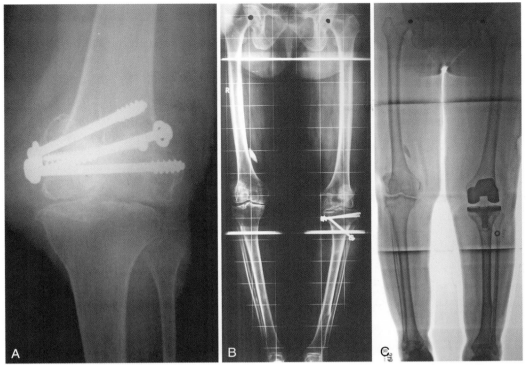

Fig. 9.23 Posttraumatic E 1 deformity: (A) distal femoral malunited fracture; (B) and (C) show preoperative and postoperative radiographs of a proximal tibial malunited fracture.

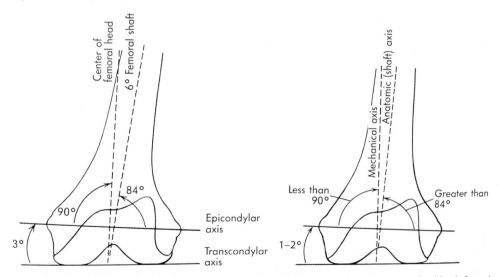

Fig. 9.24 Interrelationship of femoral joint line and epicondylar axis in normal anatomy and with deformity. (A) Normal alignment and bony structure. Epicondylar axis would be approximately perpendicular to femoral portion of mechanical axis. It would form external, lateral angle of approximately 84 degrees and medial, internal angle of approximately 96 degrees with respect to femoral shaft. Angular orientation between epicondylar axis-femoral joint axis is approximately 3 degrees. (B) Varus deformity with underlying deformed structure. Femoral joint line is rotated slightly into more varus orientation compared with normal 9-degree angle at the femoral joint. ("9-degree angle" implies 81-degree lateral angle and 99-degree medial internal angle between femoral joint line and femoral shaft.) Here it is a 84- to 85-degree lateral angle. Similarly, epicondylar axis is rotated slightly away from being perpendicular to femoral portion of mechanical axis. External angle that is formed between epicondylar axis and femoral shaft is larger and the internal angle is smaller than in a normal situation. Note differences in attitude between joint and epicondylar axis in normal versus deformed anatomy.

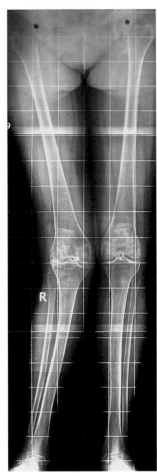

Fig. 9.25 Radiograph representative of a valgus E 1 femoral deformity with hypoplasia and wear of distal lateral femoral condyle.

perpendicular to the distal tibial axis. In similar manner, when the femoral resection line is marked on the radiograph, the angle between the two resection lines would be indicative of the likely difficulty in trying to achieve a balanced gap.

Osteophytes

As the disease progresses in each of the previously discussed types, osteophytes develop on the concave side of the deformity on the femur and tibia (also in the intercondylar notch and posteriorly, which will be alluded to later). Over time, they enlarge and do not contribute to increasing the coronal deformity, but they have

important implications on the soft tissues. Their excision alone can result in deformity correction and gap balancing in many cases.[35]

Soft tissue status

After the evaluation of the bony aspect of the lower extremity from hip to ankle, this section hones in on the soft tissues within the knee. Typically, arthritis begins in one compartment, more commonly the medial one. In the initial stages with cartilage and bone loss in one compartment, articular deformity arises because one bony surface approximates the opposite surface in that compartment, which leads to an angular deformity with concavity on side of the affected compartment. If bone loss occurred only on the tibia, the deformity would be evident in both extension and flexion. Loss distally on the femoral side would appear principally as deformity in extension; if present on the posterior condyle, it would manifest in flexion.

In the initial stage the soft issues are normal; the deformity would manifest on weight-bearing. It would appear to show collateral instability, but it would be passively correctable to neutral alignment with a stress in the opposite direction and would correct until the soft tissue structures on the concave side would be out to length. (This is best done in 10 to 20 degrees flexion to relax the posterior joint capsule.)

As the unicompartmental bone loss advances, the deformity progresses and the convex structures stretch out, further increasing the angular deformity. As this knee is examined, a sense of obvious ligament instability is present on varus-valgus testing. Assuming there is no contracture of ligaments at the concave side, the knee should passively correct to neutral alignment and not overcorrect. It will not be immediately apparent that the convex side structures are lax unless a stress is applied in the same direction as the deformity and a lack of resistance is felt until the slack is taken up.

As the wear increases, the deformity progresses on weight-bearing. The convex structures may be normal or elongated. However, the concave side structures are no longer normal, but they start to undergo contracture such that attempts to passively correct the deformity with stress in the opposite direction will have partial or no success. If the contracture of the concave structures were total, there would be no sense of correction. If it were not, then there would be a partial correction.

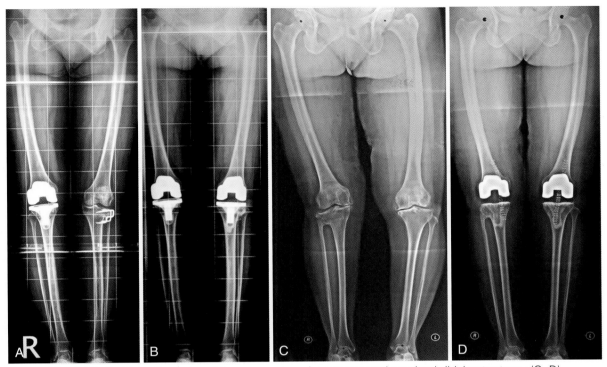

Fig. 9.26 (A, B) Radiographs of two examples of overcorrected proximal tibial osteotomy (C, D) that also show significant femoral bowing.

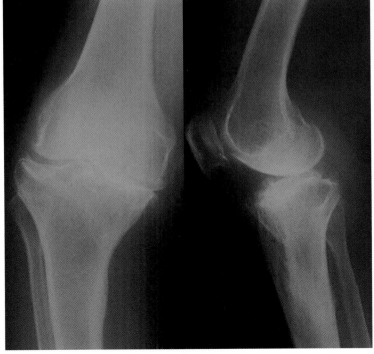

Fig. 9.27 Malunited intraarticular proximal tibial fracture.

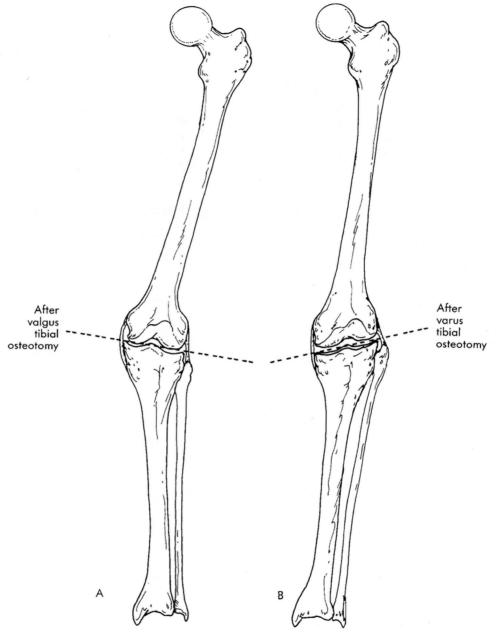

Fig. 9.28 Abnormal joint line orientations after valgus and varus proximal tibial osteotomies. (A) Arrangement after valgus proximal tibial osteotomy. Femoral joint line is drawn to show relative varus orientation. That is, external angle between femoral shaft and femoral joint line here is 86 degrees and internal medial angle is 94 degrees. This femur has approximately 5 degrees varus deformity. Resulting tibiofemoral angle for this drawing is 10 degrees valgus, which represents a 4-degree overcorrection beyond normal. Tibial joint angle itself is in substantial valgus orientation. (B) Situation with postoperative varus proximal tibial osteotomy performed for valgus deformity. Original valgus deformity is implied partly by femoral joint angle here taken to be 12 degrees. That is, external lateral angle is 78 degrees (normal would be 81 degrees), and internal or medial angle at femur is supplementary 102 degrees. Overall tibiofemoral angle is 4 degrees varus. There is obvious obliquity of resulting joint line. Medial ligamentous complex is positioned relatively distally, while lateral complex is proximal or cephalad.

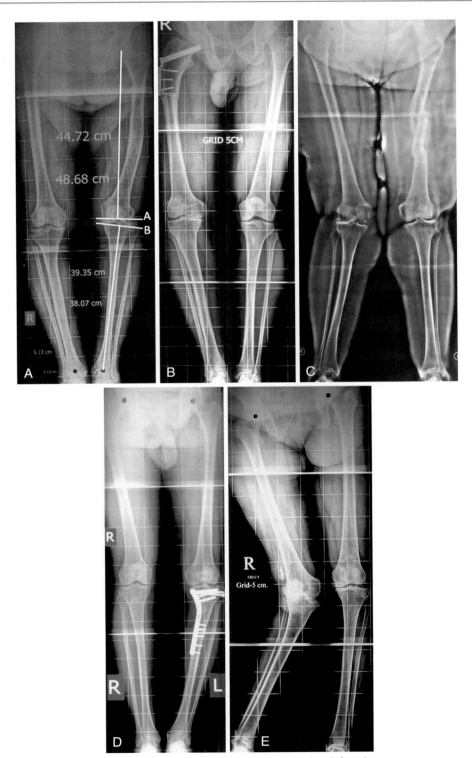

Fig. 9.29 (A–E) Examples of extraarticular deformity.

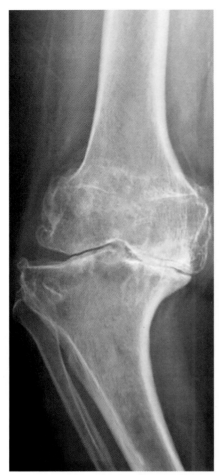

Fig. 9.30 Radiograph showing marked metaphyseal tibia vara.

Thus there are four possible combinations of soft tissue status:

- Concave and convex structures are normal (Fig. 9.31).
- Concave structures are normal, and convex structures are lax (Fig. 9.32).
- Concave structures are contracted, and convex structures are normal (Fig. 9.33).
- Concave structures are contracted, and convex structures are lax (Fig. 9.34).

In practical terms three possibilities have a direct bearing on the structures that need to be released to balance the gaps.

- Type L 0 is when flexion and extension gaps are nearly equal medially and laterally (Fig. 9.35A).
- Type L 1 is when the extension gap is asymmetrical (reduced on the concave side) but the flexion gap is balanced (Fig. 9.35B).
- Type L 2 is when both extension and flexion gaps are asymmetrical (reduced on the concave side) and unbalanced (Fig. 9.35C).

The surgeon can specify the outer limits of the range of stability that they find acceptable. For example, they may consider a difference in extension gaps of more than 2 mm as asymmetrical, and that in flexion gap exceeding 4 mm.

Which Soft Tissue Structures Undergo Contracture?

The answer to this pivotal question is key to the surgical exercise of balancing the prosthetic joint. Intuitively, one may conclude, as has been done in the past, that the MCL undergoes contracture in a varus deformity as it lies on the concave side, and the LCL does so in case of a valgus deformity. A variety of release sequences have been described as a fallout of this premise, often with deleterious effects on stability and ligament strength, culminating in the need for more constrained implants. It has become increasingly evident that the MCL and LCL do not undergo contracture. The MR scan (Fig. 9.36) depicts in no uncertain terms that the MCL, in this example of a 30-degree varus deformity, is tented substantially over the medial osteophyte rather than being contracted. I have examined over 1000 MR scans in patients undergoing arthroplasty and have yet to see a single case of contracture of the MCL. If the surgeon releases the MCL, they will compromise stability by enlarging the medial gap, thereby possibly generating an unnecessary need for a constrained implant to balance the knee. A similar fate will befall the surgeon attempting to release the LCL in a valgus knee; this will have deleterious effects particularly on the flexion gap.

The structures that undergo contracture in a varus knee are the POL, posteromedial capsule, and possibly the posterior-most fibers of the sMCL that are in close proximity to the former. In a valgus knee the analogous counterparts are the posterolateral capsule and PFL. Release of the semimembranosus and popliteus tendons have been described by some authors, but it is more

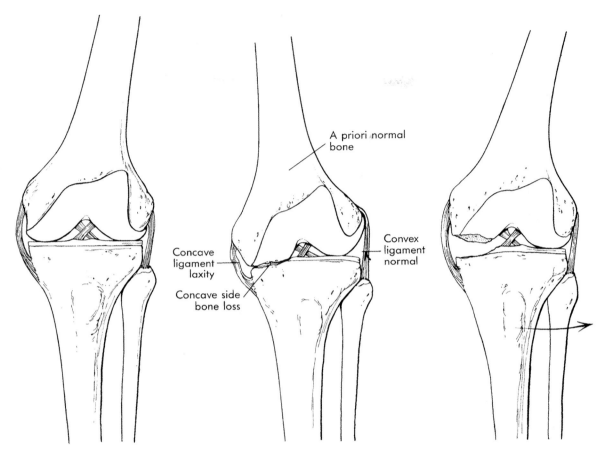

Fig. 9.31 Concave and convex structures are normal. (A) Normal knee with collateral ligaments, cruciate ligaments, and normal orientation of respective femoral and tibial joint angles. (B) Weight-bearing arrangement. Articular cartilage and bone attrition are shown. Axial deformity and ligamentous laxity on concave aspect are present. (C) Passive correction. With distraction and rotation to correct deformity, a normal tibiofemoral angle can be achieved, and collateral ligaments are simultaneously tight. There is gapping of the compartment of concave side and sensation of ligamentous laxity.

likely that it is the effect of release of the adjacent structures mentioned previously rather than these structures.

Osteophytes cause tenting of the soft tissues on the concave side and diminish or eliminate passive correctability. They would also diminish the pseudoligamentous laxity, such that stresses in the opposite direction would demonstrate only limited or no correctability. However, their excision plays a pivotal role in restoration of both alignment and balance.[35] Closely related

to osteophytes is the reactive bone formation on the posteromedial tibia often indistinguishable from the osteophytes that produces a posteromedial flare of bone that furthers tents the soft tissues. Reduction osteotomy[72–74] and removal of this bony protrusion after the osteophytes have been excised can provide additional assistance in equalizing gaps.

This analysis of bony deformity has been in the coronal plane with consideration of the medial and

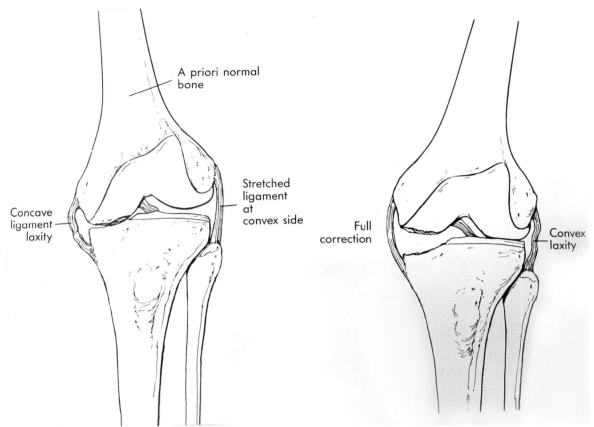

Fig. 9.32 Concave structures are normal, convex are lax. (A) Weight-bearing arrangement. Loss of cartilage and bone on concave side of deformity is seen. There is laxity of collateral ligament on same side. Collateral ligament on convex side is stretched, and there is distraction of joint. (B) Passive correction. With tension across the joint or other forces to attempt to correct deformity, it is seen that there is full correction. There is distraction of joint surfaces at the originally concave side. The ligament on that side comes out to full length. Previously stretched ligament on the convex side is lax. There is a sensation of ligamentous laxity if back and forth varus-valgus examination maneuver is undertaken.

lateral soft tissues. Next, the deformity in the sagittal plane will be discussed, with a focus on the posterior capsule.

The Sagittal Plane
Flexion and Hyperextension

The two deformities possible in the sagittal plane are FD and hyperextension. Analogous to the concave and convex sides in the coronal plane, the posterior aspect

is considered as being the concave side and the anterior aspect as the convex side. Likewise, bony and soft tissue components must be assessed.

Bone Status

In similar fashion to coronal plane deformity the locus of deformity in the sagittal plane should be sought, articular, extraarticular, or intracapsular, though these are much rarer. Articular causes of FD would be posterior tibial bone loss exceeding anterior bone deficiency;

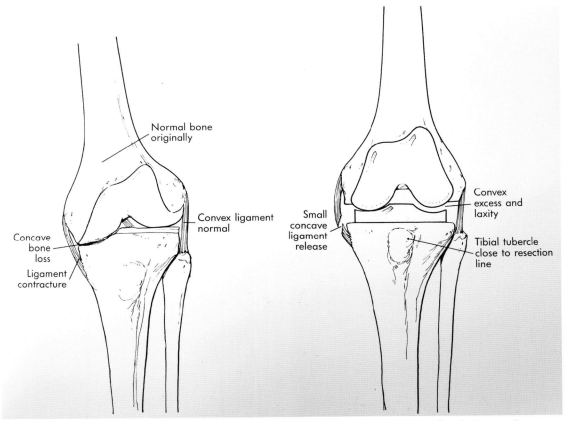

Fig. 9.33 Concave structures are contracted, convex are normal. (A) Loss of articular cartilage and bone on concave side of deformity and ligament complex has become contracted. (B) Effect of managing this situation with minimal medial release and removal of enough bone to implant the prosthetic components. Femoral component assumes normal relationship to epicondyles and original joint line. There is a small amount of concave ligament release. This was necessary to make enough space for component. However, convex ligament has not been "balanced." Relative excess of soft tissue still is on the convex side, and convex laxity may be present.

in hyperextension, the reverse is discernible more markedly on the distal femoral condyles. Extraarticular elements contributing to these deformities (hyperextension is rare, but FD is more common in the femur; in the tibia, FD is more likely) would be excessive anterior bowing of the femur or a prior fracture or osteotomy. More subtle changes in the sagittal joint line, such as from excessive or reduced posterior tibial slope (Fig. 9.37) and "molding" or hypoplasia of the femoral condyles, would exemplify intracapsular causes. Trauma and proximal tibial osteotomy are the common causes for alterations in the proximal tibia. The surgeon

would be well advised to look carefully at lateral and full-length lateral radiographs (Fig. 9.38) so as not to miss these findings.

Soft Tissue Status

Flexion contracture is not an alignment aberration, but it is a ROM abnormality. Although the exact sequence of development of FD from soft tissue causes remains unclear, congenital causes are most uncommon; hence FD is obviously a consequence of arthritis. Pain relief is often experienced by patients when the knee is flexed over a pillow; this may be an etiological agent (cases

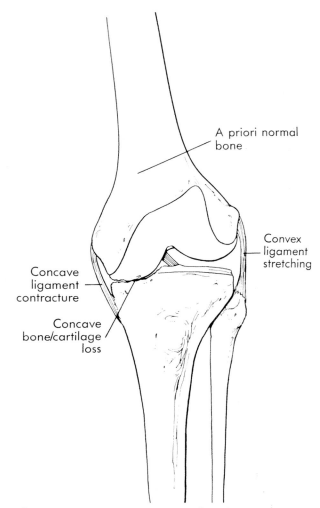

A priori normal bone

Convex ligament stretching

Concave ligament contracture

Concave bone/cartilage loss

Fig. 9.34 Concave structures are contracted, and convex structures are lax.

of functional FD get completely corrected under anesthesia). FD usually begins to manifest after the ACL is disrupted and as wear progresses further posteriorly on the tibia. Ensuing contracture of the posterior capsule, in conjunction with spasm or contracture of hamstrings and gastrocnemius muscle, aggravates the situation further. Release and management of FD must not only straighten but must also lead to increased motion toward the extension side of the ROM arc. Long-standing FD can engender weakness in the extensor mechanism. Despite full passive correction of FD, there may be relapse unless the quadriceps power also recovers.

No correlation has been seen between soft tissue tension in 90-degree flexion and postoperative flexion angle, however soft tissue tension in extension affects postoperative extension angle and stability in extension and 30 degrees flexion. In fact, high tension of the soft tissue in extension intraoperatively may result in FD.[75,76]

The role of the PCL as a major causative factor in a flexion contracture situation can be questioned. A lax PCL, by itself, would have no way of causing a flexion contracture, and a tight PCL pulls the tibia into a relatively anterior position. Whether this would occur with the knee in flexion, mild flexion, or extension would not appear to contribute to a flexion contracture.

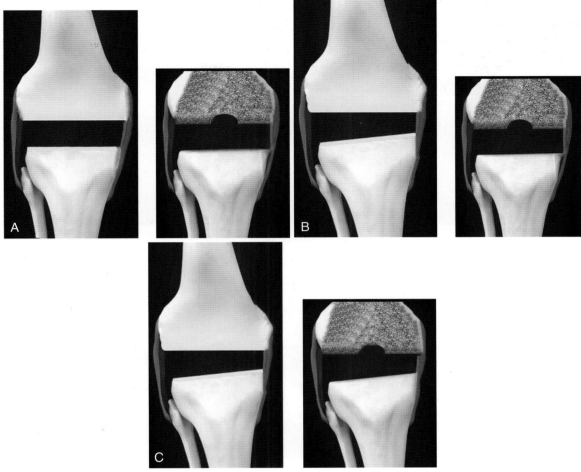

Fig. 9.35 Three possible situations in terms of mediolateral gap balance: (A) L 0: flexion and extension gaps are nearly equal medially and laterally; (B) L 1: extension gap is asymmetrical (reduced on the concave side) but the flexion gap is balanced; (C) L 2: both extension and flexion gaps are asymmetrical.

Hyperextension is much less commonly seen, but it also can be more easily missed. Often it manifests only under anesthesia and if the surgeon lifts the leg up while it is unsupported except at the heel. It is imperative to have excluded a possible neurological etiology. Typically, this deformity is caused by excessive stretching of the posterior capsule and oblique popliteal ligament and possibly by attenuation of the ACL and PCL. The posterior elongated structures are relaxed in flexion, so flexion remains unaffected. The collateral ligaments are also neither elongated nor contracted; hence the flexion gap would be balanced unless other contracted structures are affected by concomitant varus or valgus deformity. As the knee extends, tension in the normal collaterals and the camming effect of the femoral component prevents hyperextension.

Based on the relative extension and flexion gaps, the combinations of soft tissue balance can be reduced to three variants:

- Type S 0 when flexion and extension gaps are equal (Fig. 9.39A)
- Type S 1when the extension gap is less than the flexion gap, which is typically seen with FD (Fig. 9.39B)

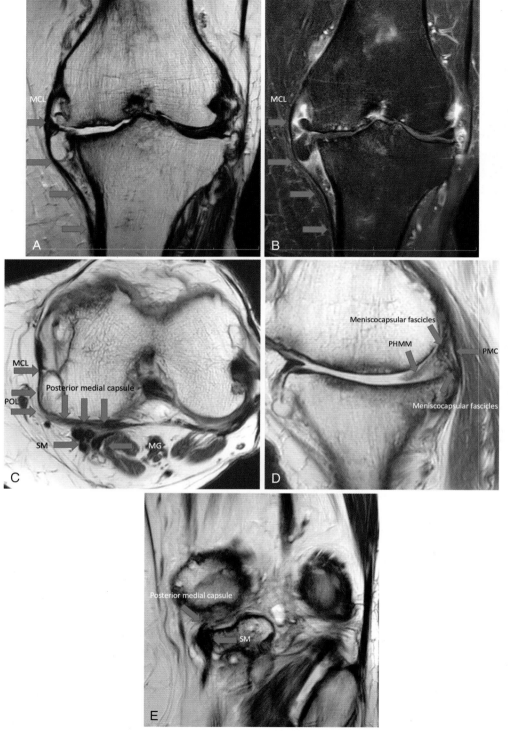

Fig. 9.36 (A–E) MR scans) of a patient with a 30-degree varus deformity to depict the medial cruciate ligament (*MCL*) tented over the medial osteophyte and the thickened posterior oblique ligament (*POL*) and posteromedial capsule (*PMC*). Note the location of the semimembranosus (*SM*) and gastrocnemius (*MG*). *PHMM* is the posterior horn of the medial meniscus.

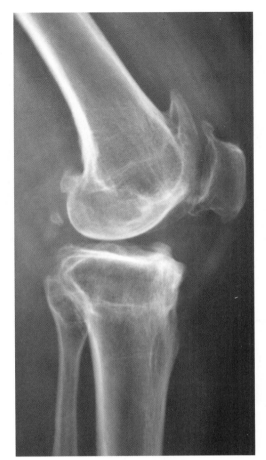

Fig. 9.37 Reversal of tibial slope after high tibial ostomy.

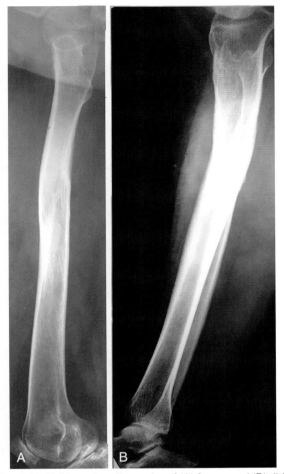

Fig. 9.38 Full-length radiographs of (A) femur and (B) tibia depicting extraarticular deformity in the sagittal plane.

- Type S 2 when the extension gap is greater than the flexion gap, which is typically seen with HE deformity (Fig. 9.39C)

Just as for coronal deformity, the surgeon can specify the outer limits of the range of stability that they find acceptable. For example, they may consider a difference in gaps of >3 mm as asymmetrical.

Osteophytes

As the disease advances, osteophytes enlarge, and those on the posterior aspect of the femur and tibia do not accentuate flexion deformity but merely limit its correctability by tenting the posterior capsule. However, an anvil osteophyte and intercondylar osteophytes anteriorly in the midline can create a limitation to terminal extension. Osteophytes are seldom seen posteriorly in hyperextending knees.

The Transverse Plane

Transverse plane aberrations can be even more difficult to discern. These are most likely to be extraarticular or intracapsular from fracture or osteotomy. However, a more challenging variety is caused by congenital or developmental torsional deformity in the femur or more commonly in the tibia. On the femoral side, alterations in anteversion of the proximal femur with respect to the TEA would have little bearing on gait and positioning of TKA components if the hip joint has normal rotations. An arthritic or stiff hip with restricted internal rotation and altered anteversion would affect the orientation of the distal femur when the knee is flexed to assess rotation of the femoral component.

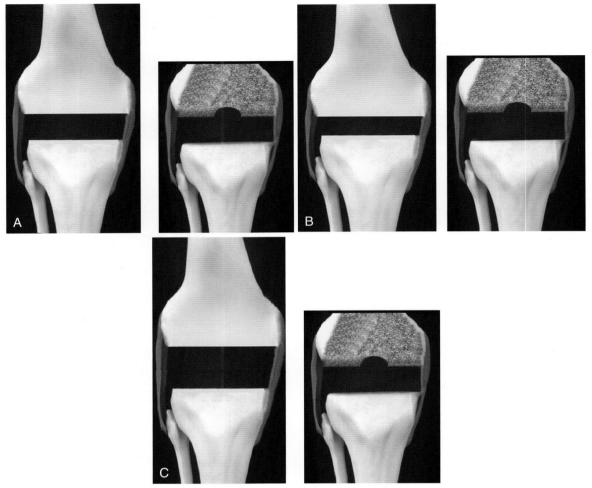

Fig. 9.39 Three possible situations in terms of flexion-extension gap balance: (A) S 0: flexion and extension gaps are equal; (B) S 1: extension gap is less than the flexion gap; (C) S 2: extension gap is greater than the flexion gap.

On the tibial side, it is often seen that internal torsional deformity occurs in varus cases and external torsion in the valgus cases. However, with a normal hip joint, these patients may not walk with in-toeing (or out-toeing) as there is compensatory rotation of the whole leg such that the foot points forward, and the knee may appear to be in varus (or valgus) and somewhat flexed. It is important to conduct the examination with the patella pointing forward, when internal torsion manifests itself in the form of the foot pointing inward (Fig. 9.40) often with an associated flexion contracture.

An analogous internal rotation would present a valgus deformity.

The previous analysis is extremely comprehensive and may appear daunting at first. But it is important to not lump all varus knees together, just as it is incorrect to regard all valgus knees as the same. By adopting this classification, each possible combination and permutation of malalignment and imbalance can be assigned a unique category. Thus a valgus deformity with an extraarticular tibial malunited fracture with laterally tight gaps in extension and flexion and a flexion

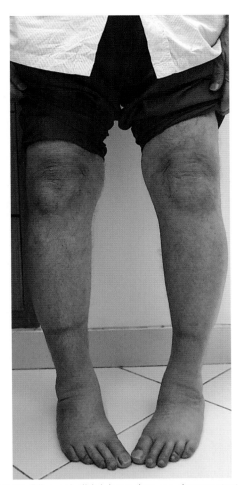

Fig. 9.40 Bilateral tibial intorsion as demonstrated by in-toeing when the patient is asked to stand with the patellae facing forward.

knees. However, to balance the knee, attention to the soft tissue envelop is the key step. For this, it behooves the surgeon to be able to discern normal from stretched and contracted structures before they embark upon the task of achieving soft tissue balance.

The first step in this assessment involves the *tension stress technique* (Fig. 9.41). In particular, the surgeon must seek to balance the soft tissues by providing tension in the opposite direction to the deformity (i.e., a valgus stress for a varus deformity) across the joint during examination and then inspecting to see how much actual deformity is still present. All of the initial deformity may be present, or some, possibly all of it, may have been corrected. The greater the deformity that persists, the greater the concave contracture and soft tissue balancing that is required. The tension stress analysis is important in the preoperative and intraoperative stages.

The second step is the *reverse tension stress*. I is performed at a later stage during the operation when the extension gap has already been created by bone cuts and distraction or reverse stress is applied with a spacer block or trial components in place. Thus in a varus deformity, a *varus* stress is applied to uncover excess laxity on the convex side.

It is pertinent to emphasize the point that these tests when performed to assess the extension gap equality should be done with the knee slightly flexed to relax the posterior capsule, which may obscure any mediolateral imbalance that may exist. Performance of this with the knee flexed to 90 degrees requires a little more attention to grasping the thigh firmly while giving varus and valgus stresses to the leg.

deformity would be a valgus type E 2 L 2 S 1 knee. The usefulness of this system will be seen not only in distinguishing each subtype for diagnostic and comparative purposes but also from a surgical perspective in addressing each subtype.

Assessment of Deformity and Balance

It is of paramount importance to appreciate the fact that alignment restoration essentially involves bony surgery (i.e., the bone cuts to position the prosthetic components in the correct relationship the various axes of the long bones). This does not automatically confer balance and stability to the joint. It may do so in less arthritic

TECHNIQUE OF BALANCING: GAP BALANCING VERSUS MEASURED RESECTION

After the knee joint is exposed, the menisci and ACL (and PCL in PS knees) are excised. Further steps may include preparation of the tibia first or femur first. This would depend on which of the two general techniques is adopted for establishing balance with regard to extension and flexion: the "classical" gap-balancing technique proposed by Freeman, Insall, Ranawat, and others, or the measured resection technique suggested by Hungerford and Krackow.

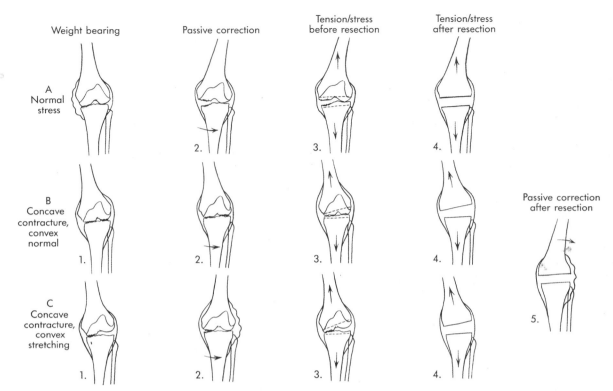

Fig. 9.41 Analysis of soft tissue sleeve element in axial deformity. (A) Deformity present with weight-bearing without deformity in soft tissue sleeve. In *1* maximum deformity is present with laxity of soft tissues at concave aspect. In *2* with passive correction, deformity disappears and disappears also with tension stress (*3*). With tension stress or reverse stress after bone cuts (*4*), deformity is corrected and rectangular extension space is seen, assuming cuts were made properly. (B) Same amount of deformity in weight-bearing posture as in A. No laxity present on either side of soft tissue sleeve. Soft tissue sleeve asymmetry and deformity going right with overall apparent deformity on weight-bearing. *2*, With attempted passive correction, no change in position. *3*, With tension stress, no change in position. *4*, After properly oriented bone cuts have been made, the tibiofemoral angle remains at the same abnormal relationship, and the extension space remains trapezoidal with tension or reverse stress. *5*, With attempted passive correction after removing joint surfaces, normal tibiofemoral orientation can be achieved with cut bone surfaces now describing rectangular form. Originally the concave ligament is tight, while the convex side is lax. (C) Soft tissue sleeve deformity with stretching on convex side. *1*, Weight-bearing and deformed attitude. Deformity is present, and soft tissues are essentially out to length. *2*, With attempted passive correction, deformity diminishes. Soft tissue sleeve is lax on one aspect. *3*, With tension stress, there is the same alignment as in *1*. Deformity is present, and soft tissue sleeve is out to tension. *4*, After properly oriented bone cuts have been made, deformity is still present if joint is tension stressed or reverse stress is applied. *5*, It is possible to passively correct and bring joint surfaces to rectangular parallel orientation. However soft tissues are not balanced.

In the gap-balancing technique a 90-degree tibial cut is first performed and any releases are carried out; this is followed by distracting the femur from the tibia at 90 degrees and performing the posterior femoral cut parallel to the tibial cut. The femoral component is thus rotated in a manner that will create a symmetrical flexion gap. The knee is then extended, similarly distracted, and the distal femoral cut is performed at a level such that the extension gap equals the flexion gap.

In the measured resection technique the distal and posterior femoral bone is resected by an amount equal to the distal and posterior thicknesses of the femoral component so that the femoral component is spatially correctly oriented in relation to the PCL and collateral ligament attachments on the femur. Specific anatomical landmarks may be used to determine femoral rotation. The tibia is resected independently to allow the thinnest component to be seated. Soft tissue deformity is corrected to achieve proper flexion-extension balance.

These two techniques can be combined: the posterior condyles can be cut in a measured fashion and the femoral component size and rotation established. The flexion gap created is then measured and an equal extension gap created in a balanced fashion.

Most metaanalyses and randomized controlled trials comparing these techniques have revealed very little difference between the two methods.[77,78] Some studies have shown that gap-balancing techniques resulted in statistically significant improvements in the restoration of mechanical and rotational alignment and mean KSS and KSS functional knee scores 2 years postoperatively, but they resulted in greater elevation of the position of the joint line.[79,80] Other studies have suggested that measured resection can lead to lateral femoral condylar liftoff.[81,82] In general, both techniques work well except in the presence of excess contracture or bone loss.[83] Nevertheless, the surgeon should be familiar with the ramifications of the complications that may ensue in both methods.

To illustrate the susceptibility of both techniques to create problems, look at a knee with a substantial flexion contracture. Assume that it has not been fully corrected by soft tissue release (Fig. 9.42). In the gap-balancing technique the flexion gap is prepared, and this will be unaffected as the contracted posterior capsule is relaxed. As the knee is extended and the femur distracted to perform the distal cut, the extension gap is narrowed by the

incompletely released posterior capsule, and the collaterals have not been taken to their full length. The cut that is made will therefore resect more distal femur and raise the joint line. The knee will be stable in full extension as the posterior capsule is taut. However, in midflexion, the posterior capsule is relaxed and the collaterals, which are relatively lax, cannot provide varus-valgus stability.

In measured resection for the same scenario resecting the distal femur accurately will lead to a residual flexion contracture as the extension gap is relatively tight. If the surgeon chooses to resect more of the distal femur to correct the FD, a similar outcome of a raised joint line and midflexion instability will occur. The distal femoral cut thus principally affects the extension gap.

In a cadaveric study recutting the distal femur not only increases the maximum knee extension achieved but also increases coronal plane laxity in midflexion. For a 10-degree flexion contracture, resecting 2 mm more of the distal femur increased overall coronal plane laxity by 4 degrees at 30 degrees of flexion and by 2 degrees at 60 degrees of flexion. A further 2-mm recut increased midflexion laxity by 6 degrees at 30 degrees of flexion and by 4 degrees at 60 degrees of flexion.[84]

In gap balancing if the distal femoral cut were made more distally, it would lead to extension tightness and relative flexion laxity. Movement of the femoral component posteriorly because of decreased bone resection would lead to flexion tightness and extension laxity; moving it anteriorly would cause flexion laxity and extension tightness. The posterior femoral cut thus principally affects the flexion gap.

In both techniques changing the posterior tibial slope would result in similar effects on the flexion gap: A reduced slope would narrow it and limit knee flexion, and an increased slope would enlarge it. In a CT scan study in cadavers with virtual bone cuts incrementally increasing the posterior slope by 1 degree led to the extension gap both medially and laterally and the flexion gap medially increasing by 0.5 to 0.6 mm; the lateral flexion gap increased by 0.9 mm.[85]

A varus tibial cut would increase the medial gap in both flexion and extension, and a valgus cut would do the same to the lateral gap. The tibial cut thus affects both flexion and extension gaps. Awareness of these consequences can be used to advantage in balancing gaps as will be discussed later.

If there is a marked, uncorrected contracture laterally, as may occur in a valgus deformity, and the femur

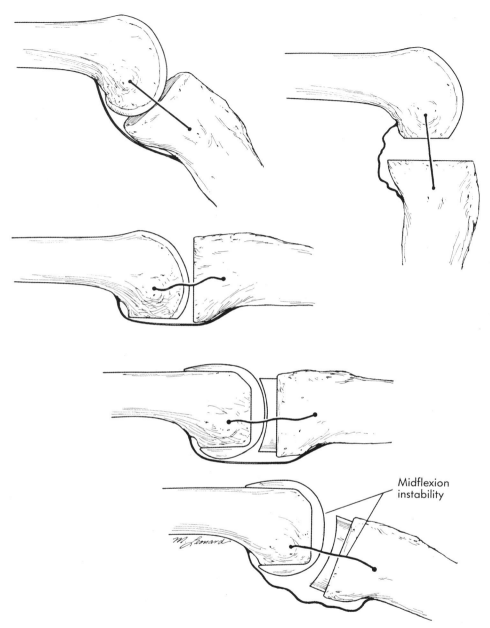

Fig. 9.42 Unreleased posterior contracture in flexion deformity causing midflexion instability. Flexion contracture and flexion-extension gap-balancing technique. (A) Flexion contracture present at 45 degrees with joint surfaces, posterior capsule, and collateral ligaments shown. (B) Proximal tibial and posterior femoral cuts are made. Flexion gap is created, and collateral ligaments are tense. (C) Knee is brought to essentially full extension, made possible by combination of proximal tibial resection and posterior femoral resection. Collateral structures are typically lax at this point. (D) Distal femoral cut has been made at level sufficient to permit implantation of femoral and tibial components. Posterior structures are still tight. However, collateral structures are still relatively lax. (E) As knee is brought into flexion, posterior soft tissue relaxation in combination with collateral laxity, which is still present at gentle flexion, permits either distraction of tibia or general sensation of global instability. This sequence of events may be tolerable. Situation may provide adequate stability; however, stability probably will not be perfect and *may* not even be adequate.

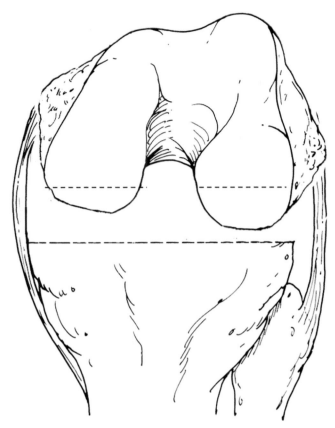

Fig. 9.43 An uncorrected contracture laterally in flexion in a valgus deformity may lead to excessive internal rotation of the femoral component in a balanced gap technique.

is distracted in flexion and cut parallel to the tibia, it is likely to be cut in excessive internal rotation (Fig. 9.43). The reverse would occur with a tight medial flexion gap (Fig. 9.44). This may lead to deleterious effects on stability and patellar tracking. An accurate tibial cut is a prerequisite, or else both gaps and positions of both components could be affected.

In measured resection if releases are performed after the implants are positioned, they may lead to instability as some releases may increase the flexion gap more than the extension gap. Conventional anatomical landmarks for femoral rotation determination have not been found to be reliable and accurate.[86] In a study of 1000 consecutive CT scans on patients who had been evaluated for TKA marked imbalances were created using a mechanically aligned measured resection technique. In this study ≥3 mm extension gap imbalances were

created in 25% of varus and 54% of valgus knees, and ≥5 mm imbalances were created in up to 8% of varus and 19% of valgus knees. Higher flexion gap imbalances were created using TEA compared with posterior condylar axis.[87]

As discussed in the earlier chapter on alignment, there are some variations of limb and component alignment (i.e., constitutional, kinematic, and restricted kinematic) that are available to the surgeon. Similar early clinical outcomes have been reported with both mechanical alignment and restricted kinematic alignment, with subsequent knee balancing accomplished using sensor technology.[88] The surgeon can apply the concepts and techniques that follow to any alignment they choose to pursue, and they can define the limits of laxity that are acceptable. The etiopathology of deformity remains the same. The surgeon can perform

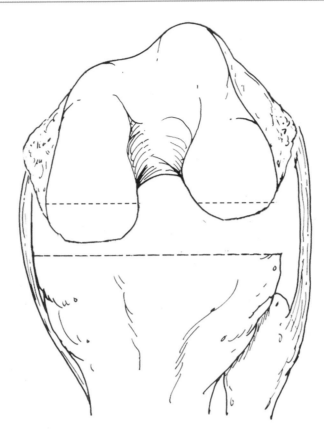

Fig. 9.44 An uncorrected contracture medially in flexion in a varus deformity may lead to excessive external rotation of the femoral component in a balanced gap technique.

the same analysis to determine the manner in which and the extent to which alignment and balancing are affected in a given instance.

Distraction Methods, Forces, and Pitfalls

A key question is how much force should be used to distract the gaps. Various studies have used a large range of forces, and this adds to the difficulty in interpreting the data. Again, it would appear that as the force increases, there is a proportional increase in the gaps, especially in flexion. Additionally, there are large patient-to-patient variations in these values as well. What is of surgical importance is the gap difference both between medial and lateral gaps from extension to flexion and the difference between the extension and flexion gaps.

A variety of distraction devices have been used, ranging from manual torque or stressing to laminar

spreaders and tensioners with forces ranging from 50 to 178 N; most have used lower forces in flexion than in extension. If the joint is considered as a mechanism with 2 degrees of freedom of motion (flexion-tibial rotation), then the motion pathways measured (using a roentgen stereophotogrammetric system) along these limits are defined as the envelopes of passive knee joint motion.[18] These pathways are consistent and are not greatly influenced by axial forces up to 300 N and AP forces of 30 N.

Distraction and manual torque to stress the ligaments have been shown in cadaveric studies to produce small differences but similar trends in gap values after soft tissue releases.[89] Similar results have been found with spring-loaded distractors versus manual tensioners.[90]

The use of laminar spreaders can result in extension and flexion gaps that are oversized and asymmetrical compared with the same gaps when specific forces are applied with a tensioner (100 N in extension and 80 N in flexion).[91]

When less tension is applied to the soft tissues (via the tensioner), the soft tissues are less stiff and will therefore permit more joint instability; conversely, if the tissues are greatly tensed (with the tensioner), the tissues become stiffer, less pliable, and so permit a lesser range of motion.[3]

The surgeon should be aware when using some tensioners that have an upper seesaw plate that as the distraction force increases, the lateral gaps can increase more than medial gaps in flexion and extension. This is because the medial tissues have greater stiffness than the lateral ones. Thus the gaps are trapezoidal.[92] The femoral component may then be placed in excessive external rotation.

In cadaveric knees there was a <2 mm difference in the flexion gap across four ligament-tensioning devices (LTD). Some of the largest differences exceeded 3 degrees, which might affect condylar liftoff and patellofemoral tracking; the differences were possibly a result of the stronger distraction force with some LTDs.[93]

Newer navigational software is available that permits accurate and reproducible values of gaps[94] to be seen in real-time while manual stressing into varus and valgus is performed through the entire ROM. Advantageously, this assessment can be performed with the patella reduced. Similar software is used in robotic systems.

While assessing the flexion gap, the surgeon should be aware that there can be posterior tibial translation with overestimation of the flexion gap[95] and internal rotation of the tibia.[96] Hence the thigh should be supported, and the flexed knee should be drawn forwards while the flexion gap is measured.

Another important detail for the surgeon to note when gaps are measured is whether the posterior condyle is intact, resected, or replaced with the trial prosthesis. This is because the posterior capsule follows the contour of the posterior condyle or prosthesis instead of taking a straighter path once the condyles are resected. When the extension gap is assessed with spacer blocks or tensioners, the gaps are therefore different before and after the posterior condyle is cut. The extension gap increases medially and laterally by 3 mm if it is measured after the posterior condyles are cut.[97] The extension gap reduces by 5 mm[98] with a trial femoral component in place and by 2 to 4 mm if the posterior condylar offset is increased by 4 mm.[99]

It would therefore be preferable to measure the extension gap before the posterior condyles are resected, in other words addressing the extension gap before preparing the flexion gap. Once the posterior condyles have been resected, the gaps should not be measured unless the trials are in place.

A nice method of assessing balance with the trials in place is to introduce plastic spatulas or spacers from the unicompartmental instrument set of thicknesses from 2 mm upward into the concave side gap between the femoral trial and insert or between the femur and spacer block to elicit laxity. Such use of monocompartmental spatulas has been found to be very reliable.[100]

Patellar eversion increases the intraoperative load of the lateral compartment at knee flexion angles of 10, 45, and 90 degrees.[101] The flexion gap is slightly larger with the patella *in situ* than when it is everted; this difference may be too small to be considered clinically relevant.[102] One study found the lateral gap to be 1.56 mm larger with a gap angle greater by 0.9 degrees if it were *in situ* rather than everted.[103]

Sensor-Guided Technology

Pressure sensors incorporated into tibial trial inserts are available that indicate compartmental loads, which indirectly reflect the soft tissue tension. These are being used to quantify the balance in the medial and lateral compartments through the full ROM.

Surgeon-defined assessment of knee balance has a lower accuracy of around 60% compared with pressure sensor data; the capacity to determine an unbalanced knee worsens as flexion increases.[104] In a cadaveric study similar laxity patterns were noted with use of a tensioner and a sensor device; however, use of sensors improved load distribution in the arc of motion.[105] Second-generation electronic balancing devices have been shown to be more accurate than mechanical distraction devices in cadaver testing.[106]

Patients with postoperative liftoff on fluoroscopic analysis were found to have a pressure imbalance as noted intraoperatively with sensors in the same compartment and at the same flexion angle. Also, if there were similar pressures and distributions in both compartments throughout the ROM, condylar liftoff greater than 1.0 mm was not seen.[107]

A study comparing mechanical alignment with restricted kinematic alignment showed that both alignment strategies with subsequent knee balancing using sensor technology produced similar early clinical outcomes.[88]

Assessment of knee balance using sensors is dependent on the validity of the sensors and on the limb position. The high precision of sensors in quantifying balance may lead to releases that may not translate into clinically meaningful changes. Sensors record compartmental loads, which are a surrogate measure of soft tissue tension; the clinical and biomechanical correlation between these two variables remains to be elucidated. Also, equality of compartmental loads may have little relationship to the loading that occurs in the weight-bearing situation, particularly on the implant-bone interface, and this has been found to correlate with alignment. A deviation of 1 degree varus from neutral alignment increases the medial load share by 5%.[108] This again underlines the importance of alignment *and* balance. These technology-driven assessments are covered more in depth in Chapter 9.

Is There a Single Technique of Release for Balancing TKA?

Even though medial release is the standard intraoperative mode of balancing for a varus knee, there is a lack of evidence to support current methods. The correct method for defining intraoperatively the sequence, extent, and magnitude of releases required for a varus deformity remains ill-defined[109]; this perhaps is more true for the less common valgus knees. The spectrum of releases for a varus knee ranges from not performing any releases at all and using bone cuts alone to performing extensive releases that strip the sMCL off the proximal tibia!

In a study in which no soft tissue releases were performed and with bone cuts alone flexion-extension and medial-lateral gaps within 2 mm of each other were achieved in 782 knees. Ninety-three percent of the patients were satisfied with lower pain scores. There were 14% "outliers" with regard to coronal mechanical axis >±3 degrees, and two patients with aseptic mechanical loosening.[110] The kinematic alignment technique also espouses bony cuts and abstinence from soft tissue releases.[111] At the other extreme, there was no difference in vivo tibiofemoral contact kinematics using radiostereometric analysis and patient-reported outcomes between patients who received minimal medial soft tissue releases intraoperatively and those who received extensive releases.[112]

As a middle path, selective soft tissue release for gap balancing in primary TKA has been shown to be a safe and effective technique associated with excellent clinical and radiographic results. Compared with the more global release of tight concave structures advocated in the early TKA experience, selective soft tissue release may avoid subsequent flexion instability and the need for increased levels of prosthetic constraint.[113]

A SYSTEMATIC APPROACH TO KNEE BALANCING

A systematic approach to knee balancing is based on my preference of performing a PS-TKA by preparing the tibia first and using a gap-balancing technique. However, the principles could be applied to any sequence the surgeon chooses and with their acceptable goals of alignment and laxity; these need not always be a condition of "perfect" ligamentous balance but frequently one of "acceptable" instability. In all cases the surgeon needs to assess the degree of deformity and imbalance not only at the outset of the case but also after each corrective move or series of moves has been made intraoperatively. Only in this way can the surgeon know when to continue with deformity and instability management maneuvers and not overdo it (i.e., overcorrecting or creating new unwanted instability problems). Each cut or release in knees with varus deformity results in increases in the medial gap from 1.2 to 3.8 mm on average.[114]

When there is instability and one compartment is tighter than the other in extension, the solution is not to insert a thicker insert. It will either not be possible to get the insert in position, or there will be a block to extension. A similar imbalance in flexion would block the knee from flexing suitably. The solution would be to balance the gaps.

The exposure in a varus knee should be limited initially to resect the ACL (and PCL if a PS knee is being used) and menisci. Thus only the deep collateral ligament will be released if the dissection is restricted to the proximal 1 cm of the medial tibial plateau (Fig. 9.45) in a varus knee. In a valgus knee no release should be performed medially whatsoever. After the tibial cut, the tension medially and laterally in extension gap is checked with a tensioner (or manual stress) using equal distraction (or force) medially and laterally (with the knee slightly flexed). This gives a sense of the extension gap

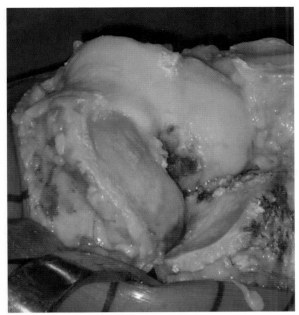

Fig. 9.45 Limited medial exposure in a varus knee, sufficient to excise medial osteophytes.

balance. Alignment of the limb is assessed. Any medial tibial and femoral osteophytes present are excised after dissection just below the medial joint line to free the deep MCL from the osteophytes.

There are three balancing scenarios with corresponding specific releases that need to be performed.

Scenario 1. L 0: Extension gap symmetrical, flexion gap symmetrical, alignment acceptable (Fig. 9.46)

- If the alignment is acceptable and the tension medially and laterally is balanced in extension, no releases are called for. I have yet to see a knee balanced in extension but not in flexion.
- The distal femoral resection is performed. The shape of the resulting gap should be inspected when the soft tissues are tensed. A rectangular space implies that the soft tissues are balanced. Tension stress and reverse tension stress is applied using the thickest possible spacer block that can be inserted in the gap (Fig. 9.47). The flexion gap is assessed and found symmetrical by evaluating it as follows. The knee is flexed to 90 degrees; with the thigh supported and the tibia drawn anteriorly, the flexion space is distracted with a manual tensioner (that can individually distract medial and lateral compartments), with slightly less force

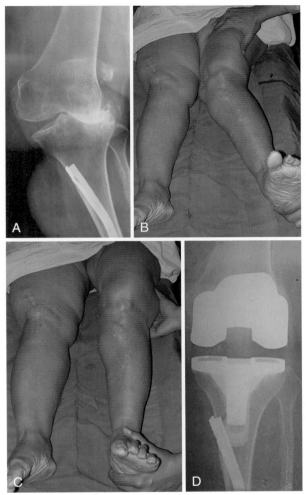

Fig. 9.46 A valgus knee with L 0 type of coronal balance. (A) Preoperative radiograph; the patient had undergone nailing for a prior tibial shaft fracture. (B) Demonstration of maximum valgus deformity with the application of valgus stress under anaesthesia. (C) Correctibility of deformity with varus stress. (D) Postoperative radiograph.

being applied laterally than medially. A nonslotted AP cutting block of the estimated femoral component size is mounted on the distal femur and rotated in position using all available landmarks but principally the tibial cut surface. An anterior stylus or "angel wing" excludes anterior notching (Fig. 9.48). The block is then securely pinned in place, and the last spacer block used to measure the extension space is placed between the tibial

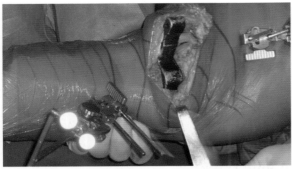

Fig. 9.47 Assessing the extension gap with varus and valgus stress with a spacer block in the gap.

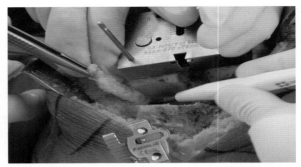

Fig. 9.49 Excision of the thickened posteromedial capsule.

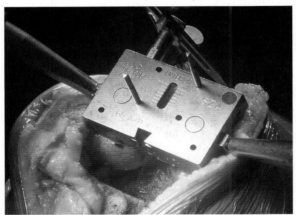

Fig. 9.48 View of the "putative" flexion gap with a non-slotted anteroposterior cutting block pinned in place. A stylus anteriorly mitigates against the possibility of anterior notching.

surface and the cutting block. Varus and valgus stress is applied again to ascertain balance.

- The remaining cuts and final implantation are done.

Scenario 2. L 1: Extension gap tight on the concave side, flexion gap symmetrical

After the distal femoral cut is made, if the extension space is trapezoidal when the soft tissues are tensed and while stress testing with a spacer block in place, then this implies soft tissue imbalance. With reverse stressing in extension, the surgeon can assess alignment and measure the distance (say "x" mm) between the spacer block and the distal femoral cut surface on the convex side. This is noted and the surgeon moves on to assess the flexion gap. If this is rectangular and balanced in

varus knees, the contracture is in the posteromedial structures (POL, posteromedial capsule) or is due to posterior osteophytes. Posterior femoral osteophytes are excised with a curved osteotome. This may suffice to balance the extension gap (i.e., an "x" mm thicker spacer block is snug). If an imbalance is seen, transverse capsulotomy is performed just posterior and lateral to the MCL but much short of the midline neurovascular structures while the knee is flexed with the thigh supported or a segment of capsule can be excised[115] (Fig. 9.49). A finger placed along the capsule will identify the taut part of the capsule. A vertical capsulotomy has also been described and selectively increases the extension gap by 2.7 mm.[116] Fig. 9.50 depicts the clinical and radiographic appearances before and after correction with these techniques.

In valgus knees the IT band may be tight and can be released in a Z format to provide some insurance against overrelease and subsequent lateral instability. The Z, or step cut, is arranged to leave anterior fibers intact distally and posterolateral ones intact proximally. Alternatively it can be dissected off Gerdy tubercle. However, the posterolateral capsule contracture is the main culprit. This is released from its tibial attachment from the posterolateral corner (Fig. 9.51) moving medially toward the popliteal tendon, while the surgeon remains cognizant of the fact that the peroneal nerve is near. Often there are posterolateral tibial osteophytes that can be excised with an narrow osteotome. Posterior femoral osteophytes are excised with a curved osteotome inserted in the space superior to the popliteal tendon coursing obliquely across the posterolateral space. Fig. 9.52 depicts the radiographic appearances before and after correction with these techniques.

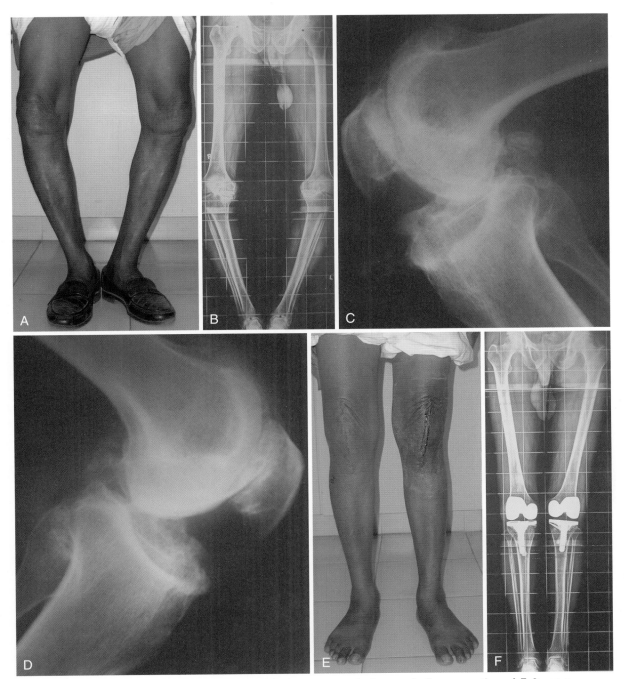

Fig. 9.50 (A) Clinical and (B) radiographic appearances before and after correction of E 0 varus deformity. Note the tibial defects in C and D. Posterior cartilage is intact, and thus the collateral ligaments remain at their normal lengths in flexion. (E) Postoperative clinical appearance. (F) Full-length postoperative scanogram. (G–J) Depict the postoperative anteroposterior and lateral radiographs.

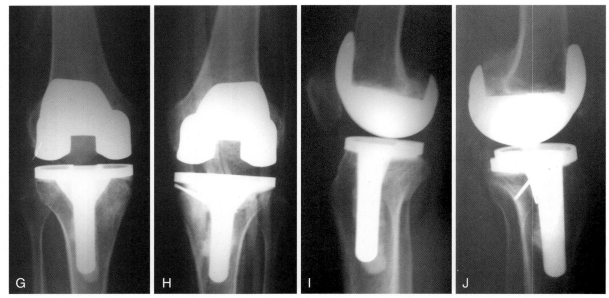

Fig. 9.50 *(Continued)*

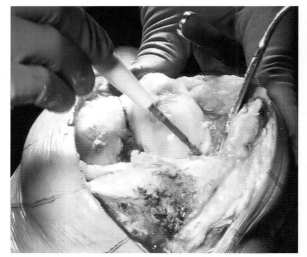

Fig. 9.51 Release of posterolateral corner in a valgus knee.

After these have been addressed, persisting asymmetry and malalignment imply that there is an extraarticular or intracapsular bony deformity, and further intervention may be required. Stability is then checked with the trials in place, with the patella reduced, through the entire range while giving varus-valgus stresses. Patella tracking is observed, and the rotational position of the tibial tray is marked on the tibia.

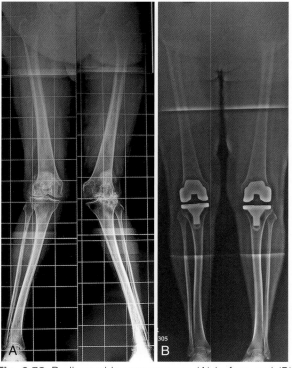

Fig. 9.52 Radiographic appearances (A) before and (B) after correction of E 0 valgus deformity.

Scenario 3. L 2: Concave side extension and flexion gaps both tight

If after tibial and distal femoral cuts, the extension gap is tight on the concave side and so is the flexion gap (assessed with the cutting block positioned but before the anterior and posterior femoral cuts), the surgeon can intervene in the following ways.

- In varus knees reduction osteotomy of the postero-medial tibial flare is then performed. Fig. 9.53 depicts the clinical and radiographic appearances before and after correction with these techniques. The reduction osteotomy helps to achieve correction by reducing the tenting of the MCL[72–74,117] (Fig. 9.54).

- Rarely is release required of the semimembrano-sus,[118] sMCL, or pes anserinus from their tibial attachment along the posteromedial surface of the upper tibia.
- Severe subluxation of the tibia laterally is often a very daunting situation (Fig. 9.55). Examination under anesthesia may reveal that it is fairly correctable deformity. Any medial release of the MCL is only going to make matters worse by making the knee more unstable in the transverse plane. The sMCL therefore should be maintained intact. If there is difficulty in restoring the tibia back to its correct position beneath the femur, the problem may lie with the PFL, which

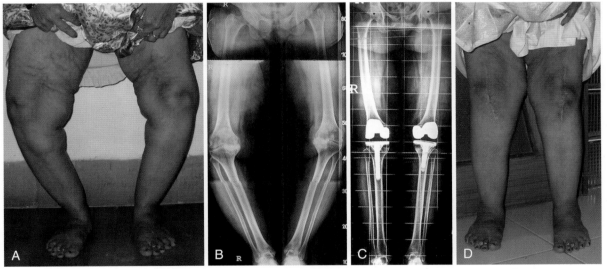

Fig. 9.53 (A–D) Reduction osteotomy facilitates restoration of alignment and balance in these severe varus deformities.

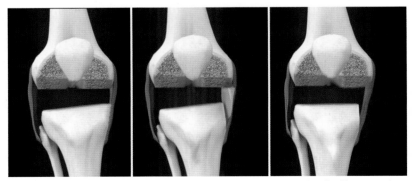

Fig. 9.54 By removing the posteromedial flare of tibia, its "bowstring" effect on the medial collateral ligament is taken away.

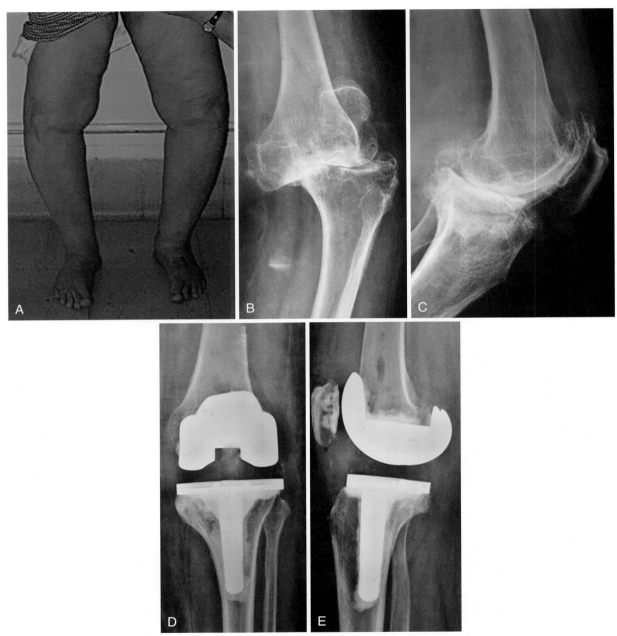

Fig. 9.55 (A–E) An example of severe stretching of the lateral collateral ligament and lateral sub-luxation of tibia, amenable to a posterior-stabilizing implant. (D and E) The stem is used in view of the medial tibial defect.

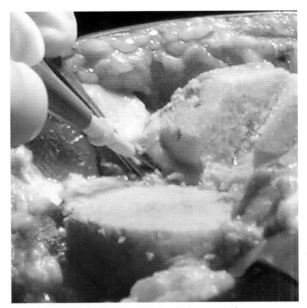

Fig. 9.56 Popliteofibular ligament release.

may have a contracture. In most instances the tibia is externally rotated. By releasing the PFL transversely lateral and inferior to the popliteal tendon traversing the posterolateral compartment obliquely, the tibia can be translated back to center beneath the femur

(Fig. 9.56). Occasionally, the laxity is such that the flexion gap exceeds the jump height of the PS post. In these rare circumstances a more constrained implant may be used (Fig. 9.57).

- If imbalance and deformity persist, it implies that there is a tibial extra-articular deformity (EAD).[119,120] This should have been detected and anticipated in the planning stage. The extension gap may be rectangular, but the overall alignment is still in varus. If the gap is trapezoidal, then the surgeon can obtain a rectangular extension gap by recutting proximal tibia. Any residual varus deformity is corrected by closed-wedge osteotomy at the apex of deformity usually in the tibial metaphysis.

- In valgus knees (Fig. 9.58) the flexion gap may be tighter laterally[121] and further release may be required of the posterolateral corner and PFL, which is divided with cautery in the interval between the popliteal tendon and posterior margin of the lateral tibial plateau. It is useful to insert a laminar spreader to distract the lateral femur from the tibia while the thigh is supported and the knee flexed. The surgeon should take note of the proximity of the common peroneal nerve. As the PFL is released with the laminar spreader in place, a sudden "pop" may be felt, and the laminar spreader can be opened up by a few more ratchets (Fig. 9.58).

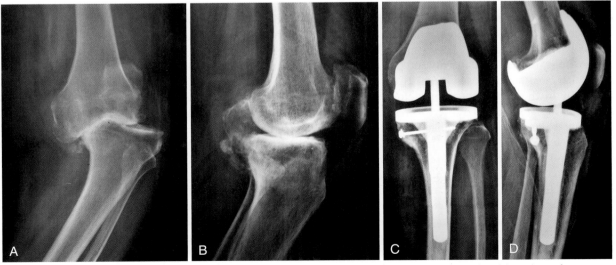

Fig. 9.57 (A–D) Marked stretching of the lateral collateral ligament and lateral subluxation of tibia, with an unbalanced flexion gap, not amenable to a posterior-stabilized implant. A more constrained implant was used.

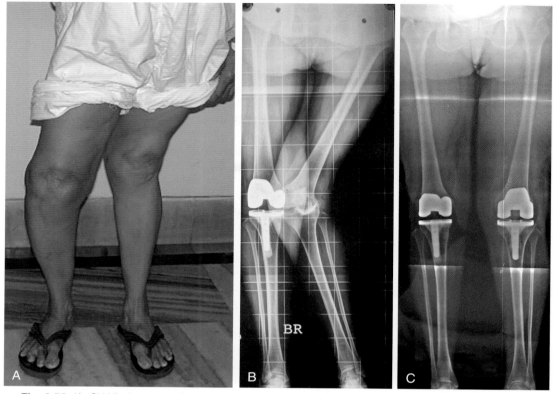

Fig. 9.58 (A–C) Windswept deformity with staged surgery. The left knee had E 0 valgus deformity, which was aligned and balanced without releasing the lateral collateral ligament and popliteal tendon.

- If residual valgus persists despite these releases, then it suggests a hypoplastic posterior lateral femoral condyle, which requires a lateral epicondylar sliding osteotomy (condyle slid distally and posteriorly).

In the most severe cases of varus deformity and especially in those cases of varus deformity wherein stretching of lateral collateral structures has occurred adequate balancing of the collateral soft tissues by medial release may be exceptionally difficult or virtually impossible. However, in several thousand consecutive cases of varus deformity, I have not been compelled to release the sMCL or pes and have been able to balance the gaps satisfactorily while achieving mechanical alignment. Some degree of lateral laxity is acceptable provided the limb is not in excess varus. If there is excess stretching of the lateral ligament, reconstructive procedures can be found in Appendix A to this chapter for the rare occasion that the surgeon may be called upon to perform them. Alternatively, the surgeon may consider the use of a more varus-valgus constrained implant (Fig. 9.59).

Although some lateral laxity may be accepted in varus knees, the same is not true of medial laxity in valgus knees. Even if well aligned, there is every possibility of continued painful stretching of the medial structures with weight-bearing over time. A plano-valgus deformity of the foot and mild valgus alignment will exacerbate the problem and also overload the lateral compartment. In low-demand, elderly patients in whom the previously described releases have failed and for whom sliding osteotomy may be too substantial a procedure a more constrained implant may be a compromise solution. Reconstructive procedures to perform medial advancement can be found in Appendix B.

In a valgus deformity there is an added issue that may need to be addressed, that of patellar maltracking. As the initial exposure is being completed and before an attempt to flex the knee, the patella should

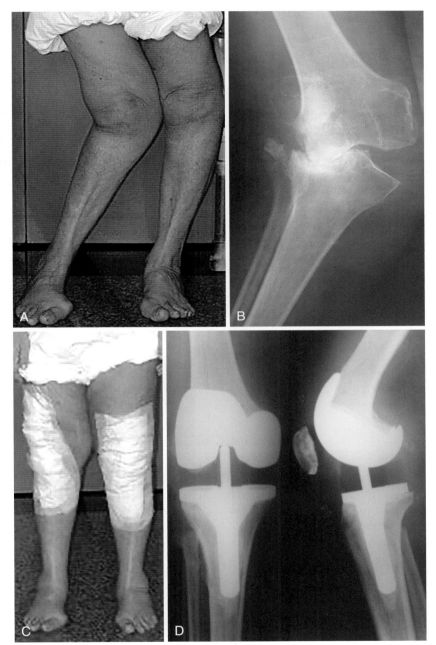

Fig. 9.59 (A–D) Use of a more varus-valgus constrained implant in a valgus knee with excess stretching of the medial soft tissue complex. Note the fibular head resection (discussed later).

be grasped by the surgeon's nondominant hand and lifted in an anterior and very slightly lateral direction to assess its mobility and the possible need for lateral patellar release.

If lateral patellar release is necessary, most retraction can be performed by the surgeon. The synovial plica divided longitudinally, and the deeper retinacular fibers are divided from within the joint to give the desired

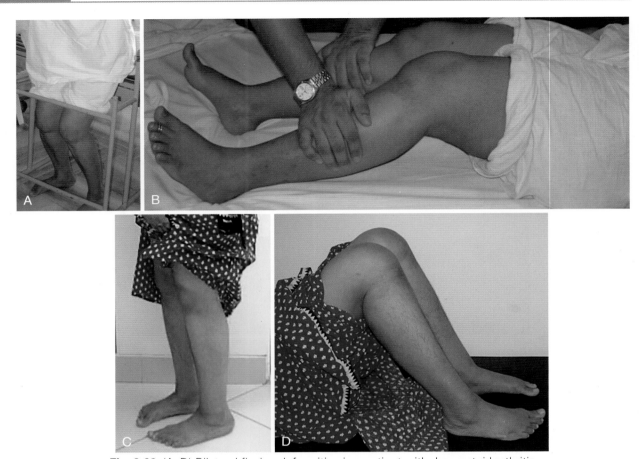

Fig. 9.60 (A–D) Bilateral flexion deformities in a patient with rheumatoid arthritis.

amount of patellar mobility. The same can be performed from the outer side of the retinaculum, taking care of the superior lateral genicular artery.

In terms of sagittal deformity, this chapter presents two corresponding scenarios: first for FD then for hyperextension. The techniques are described in sequence for convenience, but intraoperatively they need to be considered concurrently with the previous scenarios.

Scenario 1. S 0: Extension gap equals flexion gap

- The spacer block thickness used in extension is noted. In flexion the same thickness is used to check the gap. If this provides balance while the AP cutting block of the estimated femoral size is used and the anterior and posterior resections are of an acceptable thickness, it implies that the flexion gap is equal to the extension gap. No releases are required. The surgeon can proceed with final implantation.

Scenario 2. S 1: Extension gap is narrower than flexion gap

This scenario would be likely in patients with a flexion contracture (Fig. 9.60). The surgeon can follow this sequence of steps to correct the FD.

- Posterior tibial and femoral osteophytes must be meticulously resected. An accompanying varus (Fig. 9.61) or valgus deformity must be treated as described in Scenario 2. L 1. If this step does not suffice to balance gaps, then the following steps are carried out sequentially till the gaps are equalized, while inspecting repeatedly the relative size of the flexion and extension gaps and, at the same time, devoting attention to the relative position of the epicondyles to the femoral joint lines: (1) transverse posterior capsulotomy on either side of and avoiding posterior midline neurovascular structures (Fig. 9.62); (2) detachment of gastrocnemius from the femoral

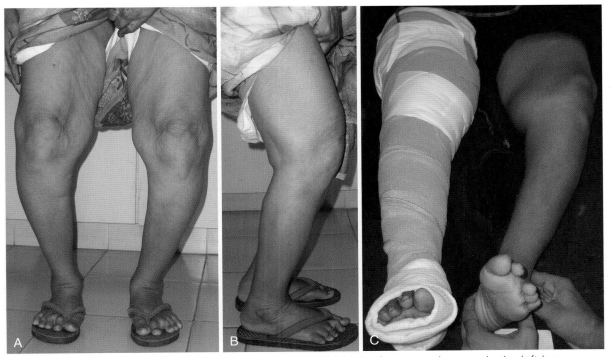

Fig. 9.61 (A, B) Bilateral flexion contractures with tibial intorsion as can be seen in the left leg, where the patella is pointing externally when the foot is pointing upwards. (C) On the right side, a plaster slab has been applied immediately after surgery and is kept overnight to maintain the correction of a rigid flexion deformity.

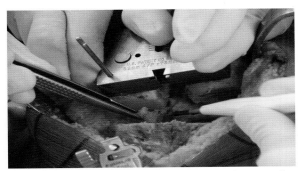

Fig. 9.62 Posteromedial release from tibia in varus flexion contracture cases helps management of both varus components of deformity and flexion contracture.

condyle by stripping it using a broad gouge wrapped in a sponge (Fig. 9.63); (3) upsizing and posteriorizing the femoral component in order to balance the larger flexion gap. This ploy has the least negative impact on postoperative knee kinematics and

kinetics with PS-TKA compared to flexing the component or resecting more distal femoral bone.[122] In fact, flexing the femoral component >3.5 degrees is itself associated with a higher risk for a postoperative flexion contracture.[123] The mean femoral component flexion was 7.3 degrees in patients with a postoperative contracture >10 degrees;[124] (4) resection of 2–4 mm more of distal femur as the last resort; (5) occasionally percutaneous or open tenotomy of hamstrings may be required.

- Rarely, preoperative splinting, even serial casting for profound deformities for a period of 1 to 2 weeks may be warranted. Rarely, would there arise a need to perform a posterior surgical release as a preliminary operation.
- Postoperative splinting or bracing is often required but rarely does a cast need to be applied to maintain the correction achieved (Fig. 9.61C).

Most authors have used some or all these methods with minor variations in the sequence of the steps.[125–127]

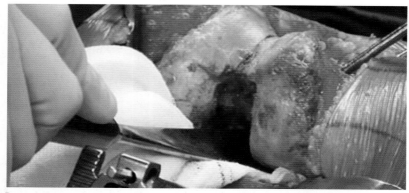

Fig. 9.63 Detachment of gastrocnemius from the femoral condyle by stripping it using a broad gouge wrapped in a sponge.

In patients with flexion deformity >15 degrees progressive improvement of 2 to 5 degrees in the FD angle occurred with each step of release: after medial release, 5.2 degrees; after PCL release, another 2.5 degrees; after routine bone cutting, 3.1 degrees; after trial insertion and posterior clearance, 2.7 degrees; after additional femoral bone cutting, 4.8 degrees.[128] Posterior capsular release from its femoral attachment is not detrimental to overall AP stability as it causes only a small change in AP laxity (1.4 mm).[129]

Somewhat surprisingly, studies have shown only a minor effect of excision of posterior osteophytes on FD correction. After posterior condylar osteophytes are removed, the gaps in extension increased by 1.8 mm, whereas flexion gap increased by 2 mm.[130] However, a 2019 study in which the resected posterior osteophyte thickness was nearly 8 mm found that both extension and flexion gaps changed <1 mm.[131]

The Common Peroneal Nerve in Valgus Deformity

In valgus knees there is the additional concern regarding possible damage to and elongation of the peroneal nerve. It must be borne in mind that the nerve is about 6 to 18 mm from the posterolateral corner of the tibia.[132,133] The nerve travels along the posterior margin of the biceps femoris muscle and wraps around the fibular head laterally to dive deep to the peroneus longus anteriorly and other anterior compartment muscles. With lateral collateral release, stretching of the lateral aspect of the knee, and movement of the tibia into a more varus attitude, it would appear that the nerve is simply being stretched and also "bowstrung" at the fibular head and neck. It would not appear to be entrapped by any fibroosseous or fibrous tunnel. Therefore release of the peroneus longus muscle and any fibromuscular "roof" would seem to be of dubious efficacy, though it has been lately reported as a "prerelease" through a separate incision before commencing the TKA.[134]

Subperiosteal Fibular Head Resection

Another option recommended in cases in which there is severe and long-standing flexion deformity with valgus is to subperiosteally resect the fibular head[135,136] at the level of the fibular neck to "decompress" the nerve and prevent its bowstringing across the fibular head. The lateral tibial dissection is continued with a cautery, and the fibular head is exposed in subperiosteal fashion such that the LCL and biceps tendon attachment is in continuity with the intact soft tissue sleeve. The dissection proceeds to the neck of the fibula, which is then osteotomized and excised (Fig. 9.64). A precaution is to keep the knee slightly flexed in the postoperative period until the effects of anesthesia have worn off and the neurological status of the foot has been ascertained.

Scenario 3. S 2: Extension gap is larger than flexion gap
- The initial assessment under anesthesia and the tension assessment of the extension gap after the tibial cut is key to detecting hyperextension (Fig. 9.65).
- Less initial resection of distal femur and proximal tibia needs to be performed. Instead of the routine

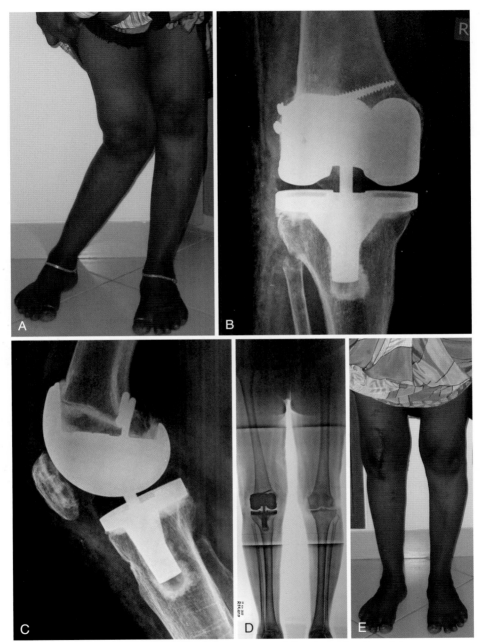

Fig. 9.64 (A–E) Rigid valgus and flexion deformity. A sliding lateral epicondylar osteotomy was performed, along with subperiosteal fibular head resection to prevent bowstringing of the peroneal nerve on the fibular head when the deformity was corrected.

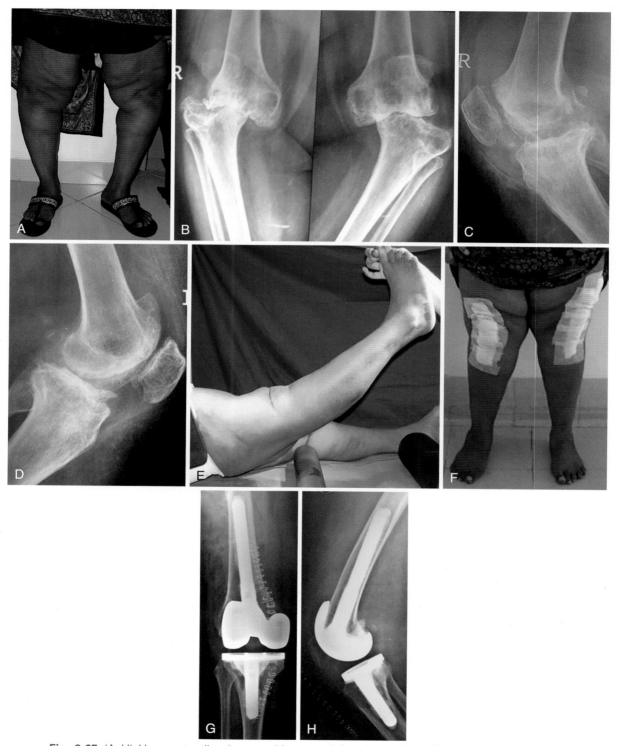

Fig. 9.65 (A–H) Hyperextending knees with varus deformity and significant bone loss on the distal right femur for which a long stem was used.

8- to 9-mm resection thickness, 5 to 6 mm may be initially resected.[137] Otherwise, the gaps that result may be much larger than the available thicknesses of inserts. Because of the increasing radius of curvature of the femoral component as the surgeon moves anteriorly on the femoral condyles, a "camming" action takes place. The increasing radius of curvature leads to progressive tightening of the collateral ligaments to a point at which further extension is blocked.

- No release whatsoever must be attempted posteriorly.
- A thicker tibial insert may be needed to balance the extension gap.
- A smaller femoral component size may be required to accommodate the thicker tibial insert.

Once again, it is stressed that balancing pertains to establishing flexion-extension soft tissue stability. Alignment must be restored by appropriate bony surgery. Irrespective of whether the coronal deformity is type E 0, 1, or 2, one of the previously described scenarios is likely to be present in each of the coronal and sagittal planes and will need to be addressed as outlined (Fig. 9.66). If it is a purely articular deformity (E 0) then the described steps would restore both alignment and balance. An extraarticular deformity (E 1) closer to the hip joint would have negligible effect on the surgical cadence. The closer the EAD and the greater the angulation, the more likely that a corrective osteotomy would be essential at the same or prior sitting to restore alignment; however, the balancing scenarios would be the same.[119] Type E 2 with a substantially altered epicondylar position with respect to the femoral cuts would call for a sliding epicondylar osteotomy; both alignment and balance would be restored. Management of the more severe deformity states may require acceptance of certain compromises and evaluation of the pros and cons of doing additional procedures versus using a more constrained implant to restore balance.

Traditional Collateral Ligament Release

Until a few years ago, it was de rigueur to perform extensive posteromedial releases to correct severe varus deformities and release the LCL in severe valgus deformities.[1,138] In fact, there is little evidence to support the various methods of releases described for varus deformity.[109] Several studies have suggested that collateral ligaments need not be released as they are not contracted.[115]

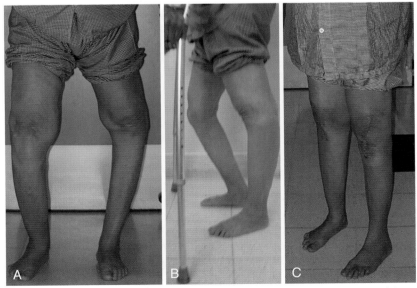

Fig. 9.66 (A) Flexion deformity in the right knee, (B) hyperextension in the left knee and (C) the corrected knees

In a large series of nearly 500 varus deformities the MCL did not require release even in one knee, and satisfactory balancing of gaps was achieved in two-thirds of cases with no release or merely excision of osteophytes.[35] Collateral release may in fact precipitate instability and increase the need for thicker inserts[139] and constrained implants.[140]

Extensive release can markedly and differentially enlarge the medial flexion gap in varus knees and the lateral flexion gap in valgus knees. As most deformities do not create flexion asymmetry, releasing the collaterals leads to a disproportionate and unwanted flexion gap imbalance. After release of the anteromedial sleeve 8 cm from the medial joint line in a medial release sequence, there was a 10-degree increase in valgus laxity in flexion, and almost the same increase when the LCL was released.[141] Release of the anterior portion of the sMCL was found to affect the flexion gap, whereas release of the POL was found to mainly affect the extension gap. Release of more posterior structures (the posterior aspect of the capsule, PCL, POL, and posterolateral corner) on either side of the joint had a greater effect on the extension gap than on the flexion gap.[89] Hence it would be preferable to release the posteromedial structures selectively to achieve balance in extension.

Another reason to desist from releasing even the anterior fibers of the MCL is to avoid midflexion instability. In a study using mobile videofluoroscopy to capture radiographic images of the knee in six patients, the anterior fibers of the MCL showed highest elongation at 50 to 60 degrees of knee flexion, therefore excessive release of these fibers should be avoided to reduce the risk of midflexion instability.[142] Release of the anteromedial tibial sleeve in cadaveric knees 4 cm below the joint line weakened the ligament complex by approximately 13%, and release 6 cm below the joint line reduced stiffness and stability by 15% to 20% over the entire ROM. After detachment of the MCL, stability was only about 60% of its initial value.[7] Distal release of the sMCL leads to a higher risk for increased mediolateral laxity because of overrelease.[143]

In valgus knees a variety of extensive lateral releases[138,144,145] have been described, many with satisfactory results and others with serious unwanted consequences such as instability[146] (because of the release of the LCL as part of the technique.[147] Hence some authors

have recommended desisting from LCL release by only releasing the iliotibial band, posterolateral capsule, and PFL and resorting occasionally to lateral sliding osteotomy.[115,148] One study has suggested performing only a posterolateral capsular release and then resecting the distal femur in as much valgus as is required to achieve a balanced gap with residual valgus alignment up to 16 degrees.[149]

Both medial approaches and lateral approaches (Fig. 9.67) for valgus deformity have been described, the latter with and without tibial tubercle osteotomy and a proximal quadriceps snip.[150,151] A systematic review has suggested that the lateral approach (combined with a tibial tubercle osteotomy or proximal quadriceps snip) is more useful and safer than the medial approach for severe uncorrectable valgus knee deformity provided that the surgeon is familiar with the pathological anatomy of the valgus knee.[152]

The use of constrained devices is reserved for valgus knees when it is not possible to obtain final satisfactory balance, which is <5 degrees of residual frontal laxity in extension and a tibiofemoral gap difference not in excess of 3 mm between flexion and extension.[153]

Pie Crusting and Multiple Needle Puncturing

Perhaps because of disenchantment with traditional collateral ligament release, two fairly analogous techniques have been proposed and deployed. One is pie crusting (PC), and the other is multiple needle puncturing (MNP). Multiple needle punctures with 16-, 18-, and 19-gauge needles and PC with 11 or 15 blade of the anterior, posterior fibers, and entire sMCL have been described in an attempt to avoid traditional release of the sMCL from its tibial attachment. Cadaveric and clinical studies suggest that lengthening of the MCL by 4 to 8 mm can be achieved with an increase of medial gap in flexion and a slightly less increase in extension. Releasing anterior fibers has a greater effect on the flexion gap, and releasing posterior fibers has a greater effect on the extension gap.

A cadaveric study has shown that PC of anterior fibers of MCL results in a 1-degree increase in extension and flexion laxity; PC of posterior fibers results in a 3-degree increase in extension and flexion; complete PC results in a 4- to 5-degree increase in extension and flexion; and complete open release leads to 4-degree laxity in extension and 7-degree laxity in flexion. PC of

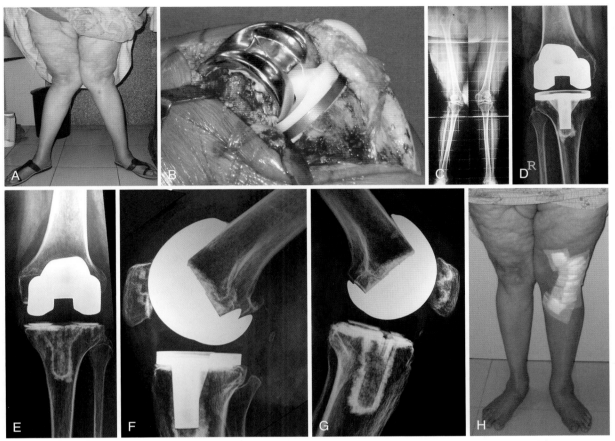

Fig. 9.67 (A–H) Lateral approach was used for this patient with severe bilateral valgus deformities.

anterior fibers increases internal and external rotational laxity by nearly 3 degrees at 90 degrees of flexion.[154]

The effect of PC may vary based on whether it is performed with the knee flexed or extended, and PC can lead to unpredictable gap increments and to frequent overrelease.[155] PC has been shown in a study to not be a reproducible technique, with variability in the number of punctures required, regardless of needle size (16 or 18), to elongate or lead to failure of the MCL.[156] The stiffness, force, and stress required to cause ligament elongation have been shown to be less in the PC group compared with a control group but not statistically different from a traditional release group; further, PC is likely to be technique-dependent because failure occurs within the ligament itself. The authors conclude that "caution should be used before employing the pie-crusting technique." (p. 1309)[157]

In a clinical study a 2- to 4-mm maximal mediolateral joint line opening was obtained in extension and a 2- to 6-mm opening in flexion with a 19-gauge needle while stressing the knee in valgus; 5% overreleases occurred.[158] Another study concluded that PC with an 11 blade lengthened the MCL by 6 to 8 mm both in flexion and extension. A selective release of the anterior and/or posterior fibers of the MCL could be done: releasing anterior fibers if they were tight in flexion, and posterior fibers if they were tight in extension. Traditional release of the superficial MCL from the tibia was advocated only in severe varus knees.[143]

Stress radiographs in extension and outcomes at 6 months and 1 year after MNP was performed with 11-gauge needle selectively (anteriorly or posteriorly or both) were not markedly different compared with those knees where MNP was not required.[159] The use of constrained inserts was significantly lower in patients who underwent PC than in patients with "classic" subperiosteal release of the medial soft tissue sleeve.[140]

It would appear that both these methods, which seem attractively simple, are somewhat technique-dependent and unpredictable, with a possibility of ligament damage because of the narrowness of the sMCL. If the ligament fails, repair of the pie-crusted or needle-punctured structure may be close to impossible.

PC has been described in valgus deformity.[160,161] Cadaveric dissections have revealed that PC without the effective release of the LCL can result in only a small amount of correction (depending on the number of pie-crust stabs made). It is only once the LCL is effectively released that substantial correction can be obtained, which in turn causes a disparity in the flexion and extension gaps.[25]

Combinations of Techniques

Several authors have reported combinations of releases involving MNP with other maneuvers such as reduction osteotomy, a thicker insert,[162] and semimembranosus release.[118,163]

Reduction Osteotomy

The purpose of the reduction osteotomy is to remove the tenting effect of the medial flare of the proximal tibial bone on medial and posteromedial soft tissue structures. Reduction osteotomy[72-74] is performed by removing the posteromedial tibial bony flare by using a tibial trial component as a reference to mark the eventual position of the tibial tray. This delineates the excess bone that is to be excised. Care must be taken to note the sizes of the femoral and tibial components and to ensure that the tibial tray being used as a guide is of a size compatible with that of the femoral component. An osteotome is directed almost vertically downward, or an oscillating saw is used to execute the osteotomy (while protecting the MCL). It can attain deformity correction in a predictable manner (approximately 1 degree of correction per 2 mm of osteotomy).[73] Knees treated with reduction osteotomy were associated with greater improvements in pain and function than knees treated with conventional extensive medial soft tissue release.[117] I have not experienced any adverse effect of this maneuver either in the short or long term (Fig. 9.68).

Corrective Osteotomy for Femoral Extraarticular Deformity

Mild deformities in the proximal femur may not call for any major intervention (Fig. 9.69). For extraarticular coronal angulation that is severe and closer to the knee, the surgeon should assess on preoperative radiographs whether a standard femoral resection is likely to produce an extremely trapezoidal gap. Often, it is possible to achieve reasonable balance and alignment with reduction osteotomy alone (Fig. 9.70). If such a resection may be difficult to balance or is likely to disrupt the collateral ligament attachment to the epicondyle, a corrective osteotomy in the femur may be indicated (Fig. 9.71). This may be performed as a prior procedure where a closed-wedge osteotomy is carried out at the apex of the deformity (Fig. 9.72). The osteotomy is fixed with an intramedullary locked nail or a plate and screws in the proximal two-thirds of the femur. TKA can be performed at the same stage; if an intramedullary (IM) nail is used or a plate and screws, navigation would be helpful as the IM guide would not be usable.

In the lower one-third of the femur use of a long stem or sleeve may dispense with the need for an IM nail or plate, and it can be part of the TKA construct. In the latter scenario tibial preparation is completed first. The distal femur is resected at an angle of 5 to 7 degrees to the anatomical femoral axis distal to the angulation. The remaining cuts are completed to balance gaps. A closed-wedge osteotomy is performed at the apex of the deformity after making two vertical marks with a pen on either side of the osteotomy to avoid rotational malalignment. The osteotomy can be stabilized with a plate and bone clamps while preparation is made for a stem or sleeve to stabilize the osteotomy. If the trial stem is unable to confer rotational stability, a derotation plate may be additionally used (Fig. 9.73). Alternatively, the TKA could be performed after consolidation of the osteotomy, usually after 6 months.

A bowing of the femoral diaphysis is more likely than a sharp angular deformity. In varus knees there is typically lateral bowing, and in valgus knees it is medial bowing. If this bowing is significant, it adds to the difficulty in restoring alignment and balance. The surgeon could compromise by performing the distal femoral cut in 3 to 4 degrees of varus to reduce the mediolateral extension gap difference. If the convex side extension gap was greater by 5 to 10 mm, I would resort to a sliding

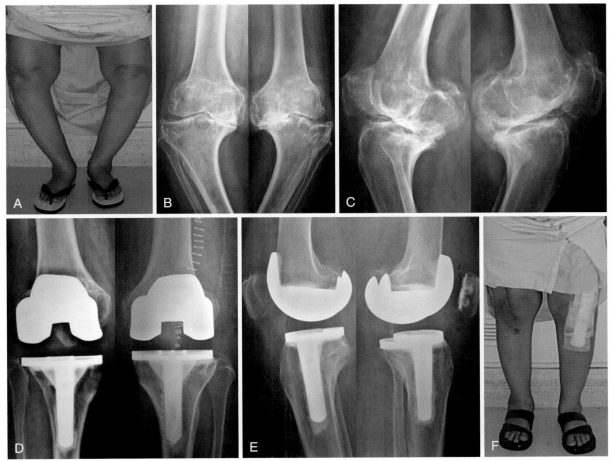

Fig. 9.68 (A–F) Flexion deformity with marked varus bilaterally with severe metaphyseal tibia vara. Reduction osteotomy permitted excellent restoration of stability and alignment.

epicondylar osteotomy (see later discussion). For large angular deformities resulting in the likelihood of >10-mm disparity in gaps, an extraarticular closed-wedge osteotomy would be appropriate.

Corrective Osteotomy for Tibial Extraarticular Deformity

Lesser degrees of deformity can be tackled intraarticularly and occasionally by sliding epicondylar osteotomy (see later discussion). Larger deformities may be treated by a corrective osteotomy that is performed as a prior procedure where a closed-wedge osteotomy is carried out at the apex of the deformity (Fig. 9.74). The osteotomy is fixed with a plate and screws. After consolidation

of the osteotomy (usually after 6 months), TKA can be performed.

Alternatively, to obviate the need for two procedures, the osteotomy can be performed during the TKA as follows.[119] After performing the releases described previously, the amount of residual limb deformity and the shape of extension gap are noted. The distal femoral cut is first performed. The proximal tibial cut is then performed at an angle equal to the amount of residual deformity such that the extension space is rectangular. Using a spacer block, the surgeon determines the flexion gap and femoral size so extension and flexion gaps are balanced. They complete the anteroposterior, notch, and chamfer cuts. Through a separate incision

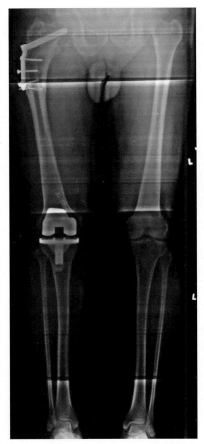

Fig. 9.69 Malunited fracture in the proximal femur has a negligible effect on limb alignment.

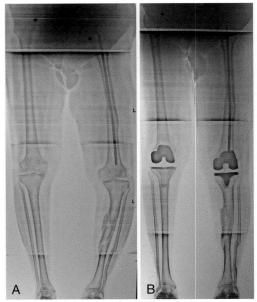

Fig. 9.70 (A, B) Diaphyseal fracture malunions in femur and tibia create an additive effect on limb alignment. This was however amenable to restoration of alignment and balance with reduction osteotomy.

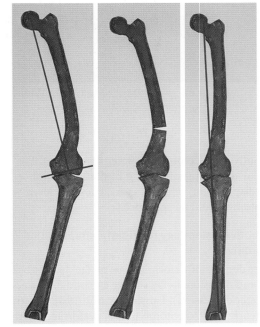

Fig. 9.71 Diagrammatic representation of correction of distal femoral deformity by a preliminary closed wedge osteotomy.

over the apex of the tibial deformity, the surgeon performs a closed-wedge osteotomy at the metaphyseal-diaphyseal junction. The angle of the wedge equals the angle of residual deformity. The osteotomy is then closed with a valgus force. It may be stabilized with a plate and screws if the apex of the deformity is in the lower two-thirds of the tibia; if it is in the upper third of the tibia, it is stabilized with a long tibial stem extension. For the latter, the canal is reamed using progressively larger reamers. A tibial tray and long cementless stem of a length enough to stabilize the osteotomy is inserted, and adjustments to the level of tibial resection and soft tissue balance are done if needed. The tibial base plate and the proximal part of the stem engaging the metaphysis are cemented, taking care that no

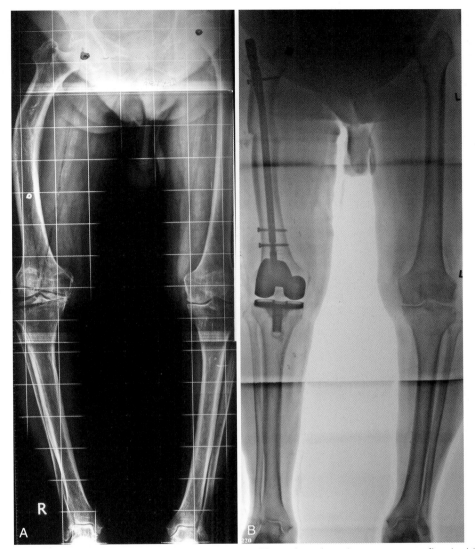

Fig. 9.72 (A, B) Proximal femoral deformity corrected by a closed wedge osteotomy, fixed with an intramedullary nail, followed by navigated total knee arthroscopy in the same sitting.

cement extruded into the osteotomy site (see Figs. 9.75 and 9.76). With stress fractures in the lower half of the tibia, I have, on a few occasions, done a closed reduction of the fracture and immobilized it in a plaster cast. Partial weight-bearing ambulation in a long-leg knee brace for 4 to 6 weeks is advised. With satisfactory healing, patients are allowed full weight-bearing ambulation with a stick for 3 months.

Medial Condylar Sliding Osteotomy

The medial condylar sliding osteotomy (Fig. 9.77) is useful in selected cases in which there is a severe varus deformity[164,165] that is intracapsular and in some cases of severe femoral bowing causing extraarticular deformity. Here the relationship of the TEA and joint line is affected with respect to the femoral axes, usually associated with lateral femoral bowing (i.e., type E 2 deformity).

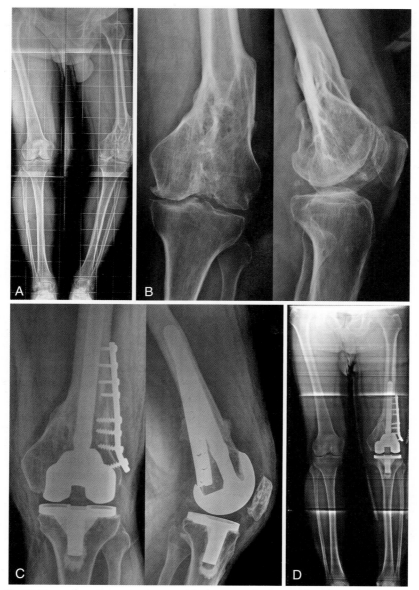

Fig. 9.73 (A–D) Closed wedge osteotomy with the use of a femoral stem and derotation plate for a distal femoral malunion.

Tibial and distal femoral cuts are performed and the extension gap asymmetry noted. Flexion gap is measured and component size and rotation selected such that the posterior medial condyle resection thickness would be approximately 9 to 10 mm. The spacer block thickness is checked to balance the flexion gap (say

12 mm). Then the thinnest spacer block (say 8 mm) that can be inserted is placed such that the medial collateral is taut with the knee fully extended. The surgeon gives a varus stress to assess the laxity laterally. If the lateral gap opens by 6 mm, then a final insert of 8 + 6 mm (= 14 mm) will be required to balance

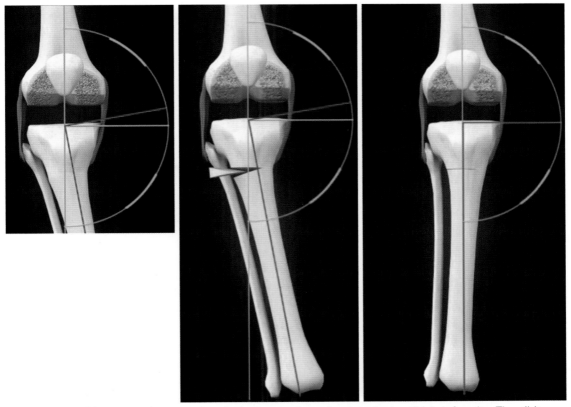

Fig. 9.74 Diagrammatic representation of correction of extraarticular tibial deformity. The tibia is cut after a preliminary medial release such that the extension gap is rectangular, ignoring the distal tibia for the moment. This is followed by a closed wedge osteotomy, the angle of the wedge equal to the residual deformity.

the extension gap, and the fragment will need to slide 6 mm distally. However, the flexion gap will need to be enlarged by 2 mm. Options for accomplishing this are anteriorizing or downsizing the femoral component and increasing the tibial slope slightly. The remaining cuts are completed.

The medial margin of the trial femoral component is marked with a pen on bone and then removed. A mark 6 mm proximal to the marking along the distal margin is made on the fragment to be osteotomized. The osteotomy is made with the knee in 90 degrees of flexion. It is performed in the sagittal plane using a reciprocating saw, angled proximally and slightly medially, so that the epicondylar block is 10- to 15-mm thick. The cut is started around 1 to

2 mm lateral to the marking of the outer margin of the femoral component. The fragment is shaped by resecting 6 mm from the distal edge and the chamfer edges. With the trials in place (and a 14-mm insert), the knee is carefully extended, using a flat periosteal elevator to ease the epicondylar fragment into position within the outer margin of the femoral component. Once stability, patellar tracking, and alignment are confirmed, the components are cemented in place. The fragment is held with a towel clip in its new distal position with the knee in extension. With the fixed knee flexed to 45 degrees, the fragment is fixed with two to three cannulated cancellous screws with washers and is angled laterally and lightly proximally (Fig. 9.78).

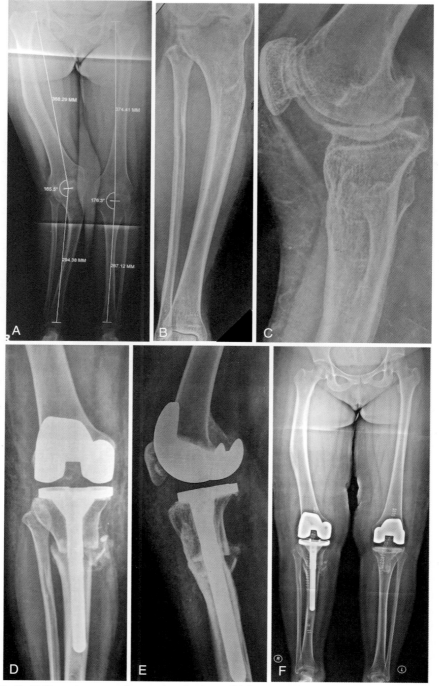

Fig. 9.75 (A–F) Complex varus femoral and valgus tibial extraarticular deformities. The tibial deformity was corrected by a closed wedge osteotomy and stabilized by a long tibial stem. The femoral deformity did not require an osteotomy.

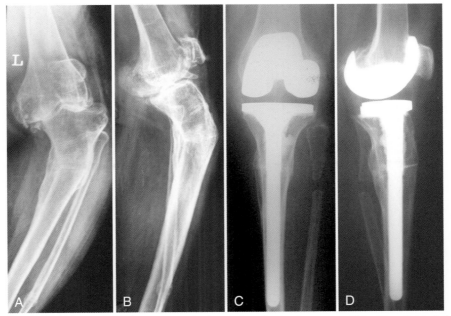

Fig. 9.76 (A–D) Varus and flexion extraarticular deformity in the upper tibia. The tibial deformity was corrected by a closed wedge osteotomy and stabilized by a long tibial stem.

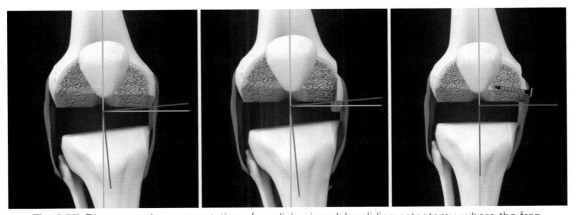

Fig. 9.77 Diagrammatic representation of medial epicondylar sliding osteotomy, where the fragment about 10- to 15-mm thick is slid distally to attain a rectangular extension gap. The fragment is then fixed with cancellous screws.

This facilitates equalization of medial and lateral gaps, thereby ensuring a stable well-aligned knee without using constrained implants. Postoperatively, full weight-bearing is permitted but knee flexion is restricted by using a long leg brace for 2 to 3 weeks.

Lateral Sliding Epicondylar Osteotomy

The lateral sliding epicondylar osteotomy is useful in selected cases where there is a fixed valgus deformity that is intracapsular. Here the relationship of the TEA and joint line are both affected with respect to the

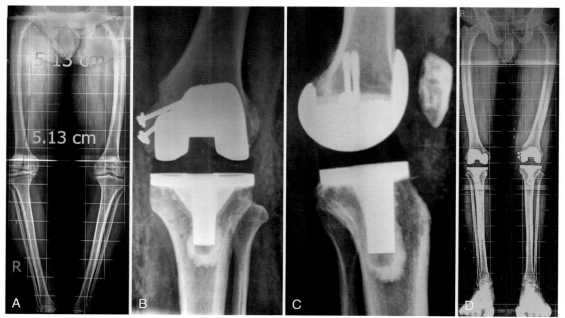

Fig. 9.78 (A–D) Combined E 1 and E 2 varus deformity requiring a medial epicondylar sliding osteotomy.

femoral axes, usually associated with lateral femoral condylar hypoplasia (i.e., type E 1 deformity) (Fig. 9.79). Occasionally severe medial bowing causing extraarticular deformity may also be an indication (Figs. 9.80–9.82). The osteotomy may be done via a lateral approach[148] or a standard medial approach.[166]

Tibial and distal femoral cuts are performed, and the extension gap asymmetry is noted. Flexion gap is measured, and component size and rotation are selected such that the posterior medial condyle resection thickness would be approximately 9 to 10 mm. The spacer block thickness is checked to balance the flexion gap (say 12 mm). Then the thinnest spacer block (say 8 mm) that can be inserted is placed such that the LCL is taut with the knee fully extended. The surgeon gives a valgus stress to see the laxity medially. If the medial gap opens by 6 mm, then a final insert of 8 + 6 mm (= 14 mm) will be required to balance the extension gap, and the fragment will need to slide 6 mm distally. However, the flexion gap will need to be enlarged by 2 mm. Options for accomplishing this are anteriorizing or downsizing the femoral component and increasing the tibial slope slightly. The remaining cuts are completed.

The lateral margin of the trial femoral component is marked with a pen on bone and then removed. A mark that is 6 mm proximal to the marking along the distal margin is made on the fragment to be osteotomized. The osteotomy is made with the knee in 90 degrees flexion. It is performed in the sagittal plane using a reciprocating saw, angled proximally and slightly laterally, so that the epicondylar block is 10- to 15-mm thick. The cut is started around 1 to 2 mm medial to the marking of the outer margin of the femoral component. The fragment is shaped by resecting 6 mm from the distal edge and the chamfer edges. With the trials in place (and a 14-mm insert), the knee is carefully extended, using a flat periosteal elevator to ease the epicondylar fragment into position within the outer margin of the femoral component. Once stability, patellar tracking, and alignment are confirmed, the components are cemented in place. The fragment is held with a towel clip in its new distal position with the knee in extension. With the fixed knee flexed to 45 degrees, the fragment is fixed with two to three cannulated cancellous screws with washers and is angled medially and lightly proximally (Fig. 9.83). Postoperatively, full weight-bearing is permitted but knee flexion is restricted by using a long leg brace for 2 to 3 weeks.

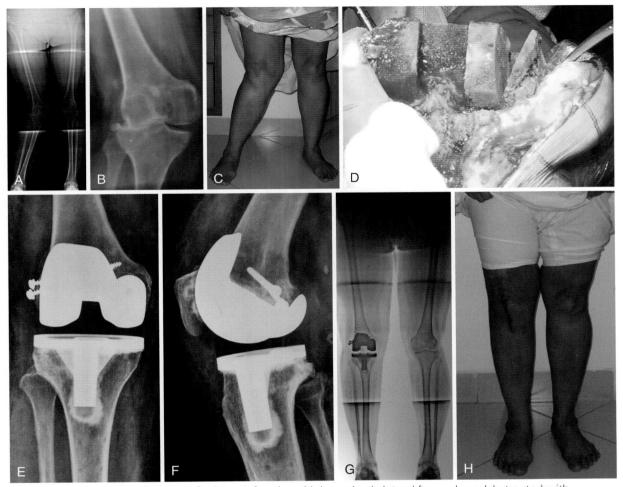

Fig. 9.79 (A–H) E 1 type of valgus deformity with hypoplastic lateral femoral condyle treated with a lateral epicondylar sliding osteotomy.

A variation of this technique can be performed when there is considerable hypoplasia of the posterior lateral femoral condyle and marked flexion gap asymmetry (L 2) that continues despite posterolateral capsular and PFL releases and excision of posterior osteophytes. Here the fragment is slid posteriorly by the amount required to achieve balanced medial and lateral flexion gaps (Fig. 9.84).

SUMMARY

Balancing pertains to establishing flexion-extension soft tissue stability. Alignment must be restored by appropriate bony surgery. How one chooses to align the limb and prosthesis will affect the flexion and extension gaps. Laxity in the normal knee varies in individuals, between medial and lateral sides, and with flexion. The gaps are differentially affected by pathology, by cruciate resection, and by how and what soft tissues are released. Restoring balance and not increasing instability is an avowed aim of arthroplasty. Lack of balance may lead to instability, which is a known and important cause of revision surgery. However, what is the optimal stability and balance in a prosthetic knee for optimum function and durability is only slowly being uncovered. In the future it is possible that there may be convergent attempts to influence kinematics of the knee with a combination of implant alignment and

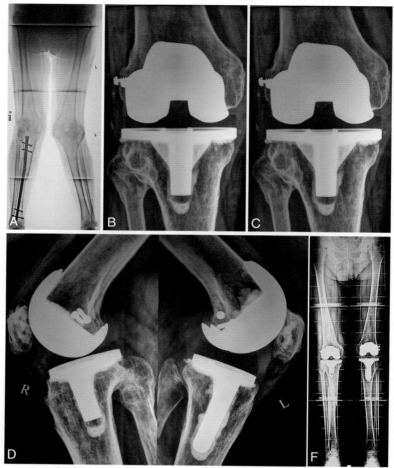

Fig. 9.80 (A–E) E 1 and E 2 valgus deformity with bilateral valgus deformities in a rheumatoid patient. Bilateral staged lateral epicondylar sliding osteotomies were performed.

design, appropriate soft tissue balancing, and targeted physiotherapy to attain the holy grail of TKA, namely, enhanced patient satisfaction.

APPENDIX A LATERAL COLLATERAL TIGHTENING

In the most severe cases of varus deformity and especially in those cases of varus deformity wherein stretching of lateral collateral structures has occurred adequate balancing of the collateral soft tissues by medial release may be exceptionally difficult or virtually impossible.

"Adequate" balancing here implies not only that straightening of the knee has been accomplished but also that satisfactory ligamentous stability has been established. The just mentioned potential problem with lateral subluxation of the tibia in cases with extensive medial stripping is an example of this type of problem.

If recreating and reconstructing ligamentous function by means of soft tissue techniques and not by prosthetic constraint is important, then such cases invite the consideration of lateral ligament reconstructive and tightening procedures. On the lateral aspect of the knee, when instability is present in the management for specific varus cases, two different techniques

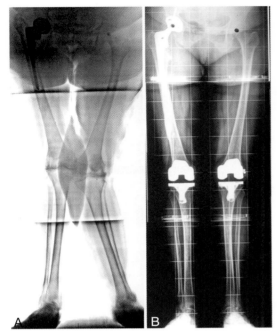

Fig. 9.81 (A, B) Bilateral severe valgus deformities with a failed loose left hip hemiarthroplasty. Lateral epicondylar sliding osteotomy was required on the left side.

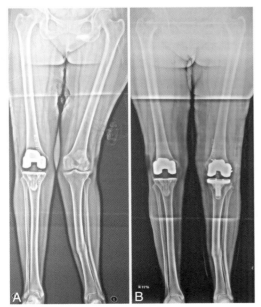

Fig. 9.82 (A, B) Marked E 1 and E 2 valgus deformity of the left knee exacerbated by an extraarticular deformity of the tibia. Lateral epicondylar sliding osteotomy was needed on the left side.

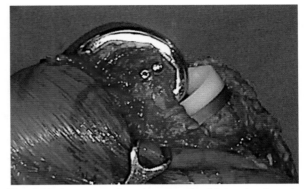

Fig. 9.83 Intraoperative photograph of lateral epicondylar sliding osteotomy, fixed with two screws.

for reconstitution of lateral ligament stability have been used.

DISTAL COLLATERAL ADVANCEMENT

Distal advancement can be performed as shown in Fig. 8.54. An auxiliary incision is made straight and longitudinally over the lateral collateral ligament and proximal fibula. The peroneal nerve is identified, mobilized, and protected. The fibular head is predrilled for later internal fixation and is then osteotomized and separated from the proximal tibial metaphysis by means of dissection and division across the capsule of the proximal tibiofibular joint. The fibular head is mobilized to the extent that the distal traction on it is resisted only by the lateral collateral and biceps femoris insertions and not by any soft tissue attachment to the tibia itself. After final implantation of prosthetic components, the knee is held in about 10 degrees of flexion, the fibular head is pulled distally, the overlapping fibular shaft is resected while the peroneal nerve is protected, and the fibular head is fixed to the remaining shaft by a longitudinal intermedullary lag screw. This procedure results in a distal advancement of the lateral collateral and biceps femoris structures to reestablish lateral soft tissue stability. Under the assumption that the lateral collateral ligament on the femur has retained a proper relationship to the lateral femoral condylar surface in regard to centers of rotation and epicondylar anatomy, this distal advancement will behave appropriately in terms of flexion-versus-extension ligament tension (see Fig. 8.55). Postoperatively, patients are protected from

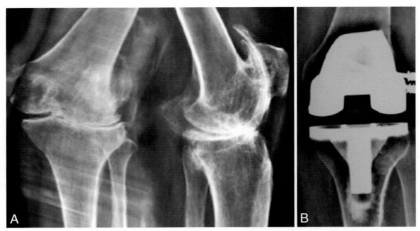

Fig. 9.84 (A, B) Extremely hypoplastic lateral femoral condyle distally and posteriorly, with a rigid valgus and flexion deformity. This required sliding lateral epicondylar osteotomy where the fragment was slid posteriorly and distally.

unwanted varus deformation by braces. However, they are allowed to continue with range-of-motion exercise work at physical therapy. Protection is provided by a hinged immobilizer type of brace. During specific episodes of physical exercise, the patients are allowed to mobilize the knee into flexion without wearing any form of brace or splint.

A general caution concerning fixation of this reconstruction is in order. In particular, such fixation difficulties are compounded by the fact that these patients typically have osteoporotic bone on the aspects of the knees involved with such reconstructions. These are the convex sides of their deformities—those aspects of the knees that have borne less weight as the concave, here medial, aspects of the knees have undergone excess strain and wear. This differential osteoporosis in response to the differential loading secondary to deformity makes fixation of such reconstructive elements more tenuous.

A particular caution with respect to the distal advancement of the fibular head is in order, owing to a unique characteristic of this form of ligament reconstruction. The caution is simply to recognize the interrelationship of flexion and stress on the fibular head because a lateral knee flexor, biceps femoris, is attached to the fibular fragment. On one hand, active flexion exercise can be expected to stress the ligament repair and may even lead to failure of the repair. On the other hand, passive knee flexion work would not seem to be

any different from any other for this type of ligament advancement.

PROXIMAL LATERAL COLLATERAL ADVANCEMENT

In some cases the posterolateral aspect of the knee is amenable to proximal advancement of the lateral collateral, popliteus complex. In this way the desired lateral stability can be achieved without an accessory incision, without any dissection around the peroneal nerve, and without any concern for direct muscle pull against the reconstructive elements.

The essentials of this reconstruction are shown in Fig. 8.56. The entire reconstruction is typically performed through the main knee incision. The extensor mechanism has been retracted sufficiently laterally to allow blunt and sharp dissection in the region of the posterolateral capsule and to define the posterolateral corner adequately. One needs to develop an exposure of the posterolateral capsule analogous to that necessary for an Ellison procedure, a sling and reef, or a Rowe-Zarins procedure—all of which are ligament operations that have an extraarticular component.[3,8,12] They involve exposure of the posterolateral capsule and lateral isolation of the lateral collateral ligament.

The lateral collateral is not dissected separately for the proximal advancement being done during the total knee arthroplasty. Rather, it, the popliteus, and some of the posterolateral capsule are removed from the femur and freed as the distally based capsular ligamentous flap, which will be advanced proximally.

Recognizing the importance of establishing ligament attachment at the proper physical point in relation to joint surface and centers of rotation, one must reapply this soft tissue element at such a location. That is, the elevated tissue is pulled tight in typically a proximal and anterior direction. It is, however, reapplied to the bone at the proper epicondylar or instant center relationship to the femoral component. This focal soft tissue application is achieved by a soft tissue staple or washer-screw arrangement. The excess tissue present proximally is simply left adjacent to femoral bone at this more proximal site. Strength of repair is achieved by use of a special ligament suture technique and by securing the tails of this ligament suture to more proximally located hardware, such as screws or staples (see Fig. 8.57).

Just as with the distal advancement technique previously described, patients are protected postoperatively from varus deformation, which may be expected to disrupt the ligament repair. They are permitted gentle active and passive range-of-motion work at physical therapy, with conscious effort to protect the reconstruction while the brace is off. Otherwise, they wear an elaborate hinge brace to minimize varus or valgus protection for at least 6 weeks.

LIGAMENT RECONSTRUCTION IN TOTAL KNEE ARTHROPLASTY

Ligament-tightening procedures as part of the management of fixed deformity are only infrequently indicated and would certainly not be indicated if one wanted to move to a higher degree of prosthetic constraint. In the case of lateral ligament tightening for varus deformities the frequency of use of such a technique is minimal. It has been undertaken in approximately 3% to 5% of patients having significant varus deformity or only 1% to 2% of all total knee arthroplasties. The frequency with which I perform medial ligament tightening for specific cases of valgus deformity is slightly higher; it is described below.

Such ligament reconstruction techniques are difficult but clearly can be done and can provide excellent success, yielding good stability and satisfactory range of motion, together with insertion of a minimally constrained

prosthesis. To those who fear that postoperative ligamentous stability may not be "normal" if patients are allowed early range of motion after such reconstructions, I can only say: (1) many of these patients demonstrate normal or essentially normal ligament stability, and (2) others are certainly comparable to the differential stability that may be expected if large concave release alone were undertaken (see Fig. 8.58). That is, in the type of severe deformities being considered one's ability to release the tight concave side to the point of achieving the appearance of full, normal, collateral ligament stability is typically limited. After all, significant soft tissue asymmetry was the reason for undertaking the collateral tightening procedure in the first place.

The discussion of ligament-tightening procedures in this text is not offered as a strong inducement to perform these procedures rather than focus greater attention on concave release or change tack and use a prosthesis of increased constraint. Rather, it is offered as a workable alternative to be considered and perhaps tried by the brave and careful.

APPENDIX B DISTAL ADVANCEMENT ON THE TIBIA

This technique has been described elsewhere.[5] It involves extension of the skin incision 1 to 2 inch further distally and performance of a corresponding proximal-to-distal incision at the pes insertion, as well as an oblique incision along the proximal border of the sartorius to allow its retraction peripherally, medially, and distally while the insertion edge of the pes group is incised (see Fig. 8.62).

The original longitudinal capsular periosteal incision just proximal to the proximal margin of the pes group is addressed. The medial edge of this tissue is grasped and the medial periosteal-capsular-ligamentous flap is dissected free from the entire anteromedial, midmedial, and posteromedial aspect of the proximal tibia as necessary. Again, the pes tendons are held in a retracted peripheral, anteromedial, and distal position. The aforementioned elevation includes the entire superficial medial collateral ligament, which has been attached just under the pes group.

At the final placement of all total knee components and with the knee held in a position of approximately 10 to 20 degrees of flexion, this entire capsular-ligamentous-periosteal sleeve is pulled distally and reattached to bone, using a combination of staples, sutures, and/or ligament soft tissue washers and screws.

For this technique to provide adequate medial stability, dissection and freeing of tibial soft tissue must be complete so that distal pull and displacement cause traction on the femoral attachments and recreate medial stability. Incomplete release from the proximal margin of the tibia will imply that distal advancement is totally or partially pulling on more proximal remaining tibial attachment and not providing a tension transmitted up to the femur, which is necessary for recreation of medial stability.

To the degree that the origin of the medial ligamentous complex remains properly placed with respect to the distal femoral prosthetic joint surface (i.e., in a "natural epicondylar" relationship), one can expect the flexion-versus-extension ligament balance of this reconstruction to be proper. To the extent that the mobilization of the tibial sleeve has been complete and has included the posteromedial corner, such a technique should also provide suitable posteromedial corner stability.

The technique outlined requires some distal extension of the skin incision. Furthermore, it involves a takedown and repair of the pes mechanism and disruption of the entire soft tissue sleeve from the proximal medial tibia, including the posteromedial corner. Because of this extensive dissection and the extensive release and potential instability that could result because of inadequacy of reattachment, my preference has been for the alternative procedure described in the next section.

PROXIMAL ADVANCEMENT ON THE FEMUR

An alternative technique of ligament advancement, which uses tightening at the femoral aspect, has been developed. If the option of tightening the medial soft tissue structures is planned for at the outset, then the skin incision is moved slightly medially to facilitate development of the exposure of the medial femoral capsular plane to the level of the posteromedial corner. The dissection required is analogous to that described for the Nicholas 5-1 procedure.[9] Once the decision for this form of medial tightening has been made, the medial ligamentous complex is elevated from the medial epicondyle as shown (see Fig. 8.63). The elevated tissue includes the superior and deep medial collateral ligament and the posterior oblique complex. It represents

a triangular or trapezoidal flap of capsular ligamentous, even synovial, tissue, which has an apex coming from the epicondylar origin and whose distal aspect spans to include the soft tissue elements for the entire midmedial and posteromedial aspect of the knee.

After final implantation of total knee components, the medial soft tissue flap is pulled tight in typically a proximal, slightly anterior direction. The proper reinsertion point is located in relation to the condylar surface geometry of the femoral component, and bony reattachment of the ligament sleeve is planned to be centered at this point. Specific ligament sutures are placed in the tissue. The femoral, attachment point is freshened, and the tissue is applied to this point with a staple or ligament washer and screw. The tails of the ligament sutures are fixed farther proximally, by tying over the washer of an ancillary screw placed just for this purpose.

To the extent that the tissue is properly "reoriginated" (i.e., in proper relationship to the neighborhood of centers of rotation for the condylar geometry), the flexion-extension ligament balance behavior of this correct reconstruction is quite good. Note that the technique is not performed simply as a straight proximal advancement of the medial ligament origin. Such ought to lead to adequate stability in extension but excess laxity in flexion. Instead, the technique described is a proximal advancement with *reapplication* of the tissue at the proper center of rotation.

The amount of extra soft tissue dissection is not that great, and the amount of soft tissue elevation and release from bone is minimal. The resulting flap of tissue is substantial and takes sutures and staple fixation well. Its proximal advancement provides at once both straight medial and posteromedial restabilization.

Management of the lateral side and corner of the knee in these type II cases (Fig. 9.32A) can be considered in several different ways. In cases where medial tightening has been undertaken after maximum lateral release has been performed nothing further needs to be considered with respect to the lateral side. In the second class of type II patients in whom the performance of a medial ligament tightening is planned from the outset the surgeon has the option of omitting any lateral collateral, capsular, or iliotibial band release. The goal is simply to remove enough distal femur and proximal tibia to get both the femoral and tibial components in place with good lateral stability and then to provide all necessary medial stability by ligament tightening.

GENERAL COMMENTS

Admittedly, the medial and lateral ligament-tightening procedures are fraught with limitations and difficulties as described later. However, with careful planning, the medial advancement on the femur can be performed with less soft tissue cutting and dissection and in less operative time than the otherwise necessary extensive lateral, possibly posterior, release that would be undertaken and might be insufficient in the end. The point is simply that some of this ligament advancement work need not be as complex and time consuming as it might seem to be at first. It certainly is not so grandiose if the alternative extreme and extensive release work are kept clearly in mind.

Maximum fixation of ligament reconstructive elements for these complex total knee procedures is of paramount consideration for at least two reasons. First is the desire, even requirement, to be able to allow the patient range of motion in the postoperative period in nearly the same fashion as any other total knee replacement patient. Second is the soft tissue fixation problem inherent in these particular types of deformed total knee arthroplasty cases. In particular, I am referring again to the differential bone density issue. Tightening occurs on the originally convex side of the deformity, which was also the side bearing less weight and hence was typically quite osteoporotic. For this reason the elaborate ligament fixation suturing techniques were developed[6,7] (see Fig. 8.64).

Advancement of either the medial collateral distally or proximally with a bone wafer is not recommended in these cases. The soft bone wafer does not provide significant additional stability of fixation, and its creation weakens the substrate bone at the condyle or metaphysis from which it was removed.

These considerations can well explain surgeons' disenchantment with ligament reconstruction procedures in combination with total knee arthroplasty. Unless the special soft tissue fixation techniques are used to maintain position of the reconstructive elements and unless the frailty of the situation is appreciated, then as patients carry out postoperative motion exercises, the chance of reconstruction failure is excessive.

Management of patients with medial ligament reconstruction is the same as that for the smaller number of patients with lateral procedures. Excessive valgus displacement is at all times guarded by use of a knee immobilizer, a hinged long brace, or by specific patient and therapist attention during range-of-motion exercise at home or in the physical therapy department. With the exception of these specific exercise periods, in which all bracing is removed to facilitate range of motion, the knee and its ligament reconstruction elements are in a brace for at least 6 weeks.

SURGICAL PROCEDURE FOR OVERCORRECTED PROXIMAL TIBIAL OSTEOTOMIES

Preoperative planning in type III cases usually reveals a relatively varus distal femoral joint line and a severely valgus proximal tibial joint line. For this and other reasons, I recommend adoption of classical alignment considerations in the planning of the resection cuts.

That is to say, the distal femoral cut will be made, on the average, at 5 to 7 degrees of valgus, and the proximal tibial cut will be made at 0 degrees or perpendicular to the tibial shaft. The alternative anatomical cuts (distal femoral cut at approximately 9 degrees of valgus and proximal tibial cut at 2 to 3 degrees of varus) involve greater asymmetry of bone resection on both the femoral and the tibial sides.

In rough outline a complex soft tissue reconstruction is done on the entire midmedial, posteromedial, and central posterior aspect of the tibia, bringing all soft tissue elements distally along with their original, attached tibial cortical bone.

The technique is illustrated in Fig. 8.67. A longer, otherwise standard median parapatellar exposure is performed with a standard quadriceps and medial capsular exposure of the joint. The pes anserinus tendon group is incised longitudinally adjacent to its bony insertion. The upper cephalad border of the sartorius is incised in the direction of the overlying fascia, running in the direction of the sartorius tendon itself so that the pes group can be retracted peripherally, anteromedially, and distally. The anteromedial capsulotomy is performed in standard fashion, and the midanterior and anterolateral aspects of the tibia are freed of soft tissue in the usual fashion for total knee arthroplasty exposure. However, no similar stripping of medial soft tissue is performed at the posterior tibia. The more superficial capsular plane is exposed by subcutaneous undermining over the medial aspect of the knee. This aspect of the exposure requires a generous skin incision both distally and proximally. In other words, a medial capsular plane is developed analogous to what one would do before performing an extensive medial ligament reconstruction.

The superficial medial collateral ligament is located visually and by palpation and by applying valgus tension stressing of the joint. Longitudinal, definitive incisions straight to bone are made at the anterior and posterior margins of the superficial medial collateral ligament, running from just distal to the medial femoral epicondyle to the region of the tibial insertion of the medial collateral ligament, again, at the anterior and posterior margins of the superficial medial collateral ligament. Recall that, at this point, the pes group overlying the tibial insertion of the medial collateral ligament is being retracted out of the way. Dissection is performed at and below the tibial joint line to free the deep and superficial medial collateral ligament from the tibia everywhere except at the specific bony insertion under the pes group.

The entire discrete bony insertion of the superficial medial collateral ligament is ascertained, and its center is drilled with a 3.2-mm or ⅛-inch drill bit. The bony insertion location is then elevated from the tibia as a piece measuring approximately 1×1 to 1.5 cm (width by length) preferably by using a very fine, end- and side-cutting bit. The bone is typically too hard for easy use of even a sharp osteotome. After elevation of this centrally perforated bone rectangle at the distal end of the superficial medial collateral ligament, tension on the end of the medial collateral should be transmitted totally to the femoral side of the joint; the deep attachments of this soft tissue strip to the underlying tibia should have been divided.

Later, when the tibial resection cut is made, it is made as a minimum-thickness resection from the lateral plateau, which leads to a relatively large amount of bone resection from the medial plateau. No subperiosteal freeing at the posteromedial and posterior aspect of the tibia is to be performed. Thus the cut and freed wafer of proximal tibial bone is thin laterally, thick medially, and devoid of soft tissue attachments anterolaterally, anteriorly, and anteromedially, but it is fully attached to soft tissue posteromedially and at the midposterior aspect where the posterior cruciate ligament inserts. The anterior cruciate ligament has been released earlier as would ordinarily be the case.

After mobilization and preliminary freeing of the tibial wafer, this bone is drawn forward, and working either from the joint surface aspect or from the cancellous undersurface, a sharp end- and side-cutting high-speed burr is used to separate the majority of this tibial wafer from a portion of its peripheral rim, particularly that portion at the central and the medioposterior aspect, which still has attached to it the posterior cruciate ligament, the posteromedial capsule, and the posterior oblique medial ligament.

After final preparation of the femur and tibial cuts, anterior-to-posterior drill holes of approximately $^3/_{32}$-inch diameter are placed across the top of the tibia, and heavy ligament sutures are positioned through the posterior cruciate ligament, posteromedial capsule, and posterior oblique. Wire suture passers are used (26 gauge), and the respective peripheral bone shells are drawn down to the remaining cortical-tibial rim. Care is taken to free soft tissue from the peripheral aspect of the proximal tibia just below the resection cut at the location of the posterior cruciate, posteromedial capsule, and posterior oblique so that the attached cortical bone will fit snugly immediately adjacent to the tibia.

On final implantation of all components, the knee is held in approximately 10 degrees of flexion; the sutures are drawn tight and tied, effecting a distal advancement of the posterior cruciate ligament, the posteromedial capsule, and the posterior oblique structures. The bony insertion of the superficial medial collateral ligament is drawn distally until it is tight, and the underlying bone is drilled with a 3.2-mm bit. The superficial medial collateral ligament is then fixed with an AO screw, conveniently, the 4.5-mm malleolar type, which obviates tapping and automatically lags the fragment into position. Also, this particular screw, because of the shape of its tip, very easily locates the far cortex. A ligament suture may be placed in the superficial medial collateral ligament and tied over either this screw or an additional, distal screw.

Despite the relatively large amount of medial tibial bone that has been removed (i.e., the depth of the tibial cut), so far no problem has occurred with significant violation of the tibial tubercle to accomplish this cut. With all of the steps planned carefully, the procedure progresses quite smoothly. The fixation achieved is excellent, and postoperative stability has uniformly been superb, even too good in one patient, who was iatrogenically driven into a 5- to 10-degree flexion contracture because the superficial medial collateral ligament was drawn too tightly (see Fig. 8.68).

Ligamentous soft tissue fixation here is different from such fixation in the average valgus or varus deformity case, where differential bone density in association with convex underloading is typically seen. These type III patients, who were initially medially overloaded, typically maintain good medial bone density, which facilitates the strength of fixation of soft tissue reattachment.

Alternative consideration of proximal femoral advancement of medial soft tissues has not been used in these patients, because the asymmetrical tibial cut judged necessary to achieve a reasonable tibial bone surface is sufficiently deep to disrupt the posterior and the posteromedial soft tissue attachments. No provision for this fact would exist if the soft tissues were simply advanced proximally on the femur.

The bone island advancement technique has been sustained in these type III cases but abandoned in the type II cases, which are handled with distal medial soft tissue advancement. It was found that in these other type II patients with such differential bone density, the creation of this bone plug can dangerously weaken bone adjacent to the joint line and lead to fracture. Postoperative management of the type III patients is the same as for any of the medial or lateral ligament reconstruction cases.

REFERENCES

1. Krackow KA. *The Technique of Total Knee Arthroplasty.* : The C. V. Mosby Company; 1990.
2. Fitzpatrick CK, Clary CW, Rullkoetter PJ. The role of patient, surgical, and implant design variation in total knee replacement performance. *J Biomech.* 2012;45(12):2092–2102. https://doi.org/10.1016/j.jbiomech.2012.05.035.
3. Asano H, Muneta T, Hoshino A. Stiffness of soft tissue complex in total knee arthroplasty. *Knee Surg, Sports Traumatol, Arthrosc.* 2008;16(1):51–55. https://doi.org/10.1007/s00167-007-0387-8.
4. Robinson JR, Bull AMJ, Amis AA. Structural properties of the medial collateral ligament complex of the human knee. *J Biomech.* 2005;38(5):1067–1074. https://doi.org/10.1016/j.jbiomech.2004.05.034.
5. Sugita T, Amis AA. Anatomic and biomechanical study of the lateral collateral and popliteofibular ligaments. *Am J Sports Med.* 2001;29(4):466–472. https://doi.org/10.1177/03635465010290041501.
6. Zalzal P, Papini M, Petruccelli D, De Beer J, Winemaker MJ. An in vivo biomechanical analysis of the soft-tissue envelope of osteoarthritic knees. *J Arthroplasty.* 2004;19(2):217–223. https://doi.org/10.1016/j.arth.2003.09.008.
7. Völlner F, Fischer J, Weber M, Greimel F, Benditz A, Renkawitz T, Grifka J, Craiovan B. Weakening of the knee ligament complex due to sequential medial release in total knee Arthroplasty. *Arch Orthop Trauma Surg.* 2019;139(7):999–1006. https://doi.org/10.1007/s00402-019-03181-z.
8. Iwaki H, Pinskerova V, Freeman MAR. Tibiofemoral Movement 1: The shape and relative movements of the femur and tibia in the unloaded cadaver knee. *J Bone Joint Surg Br.* 2000;82(8):1189–1195. https://doi.org/10.1302/0301-620X.82B8.10717.
9. Grood ES, Stowers SF, Noyes FR. Limits of movement in the human knee. Effect of sectioning the posterior cruciate ligament and posterolateral structures. *JBJS.* 1988;70(1):88–97. https://journals.lww.com/jbjsjournal/Fulltext/1988/70010/Limits_of_movement_in_the_human_knee-Effect_of.14.aspx.
10. Vincent JP, Magnussen RA, Gezmez F, Uguen A, Jacobi M, Weppe F, Al-Saati M'ad F, et al. The anterolateral ligament of the human knee: An anatomic and histologic study. *Knee Surg, Sports Traumatol, Arthrosc.* 2012;20(1):147–152. https://doi.org/10.1007/s00167-011-1580-3.
11. Neri T, Dalcol P, Palpacuer F, Bergandi F, Michel PJ, Farizon F, Philippot R, Peoc'h M. The anterolateral ligament is a distinct ligamentous structure: A histological explanation. *Knee.* 2018;25(3):360–366. https://doi.org/10.1016/j.knee.2018.03.012.
12. Zens M, Feucht MJ, Ruhhammer J, Bernstein A, Mayr HO, Südkamp NP, Woias P, Niemeyer P. Mechanical tensile properties of the anterolateral ligament. *J Exp Orthop.* 2015;2(1):1–7. https://doi.org/10.1186/s40634-015-0023-3.
13. Siston RA, Giori NJ, Goodman SB, Delp S. Intraoperative passive kinematics of osteoarthritic knees before and after total knee arthroplasty. *J Orthop Res. September, no. August.* 2006;24(8):1607–1614. https://doi.org/10.1002/jor.
14. Sasaki K, Neptune R. Individual muscle contributions to the axial knee joint contact force during normal walking. *J Biomech.* 2010;43(14):2780–2784. https://doi.org/10.1016/j.jbiomech.2010.06.011.Individual.
15. Avino RJ, King CA, Landy DC, Martell JM. Varus-valgus constraint in primary total knee arthroplasty: A short-term solution but will it last? *J Arthroplasty.* 2020;35(3):741–746. https://doi.org/10.1016/j.arth.2019.09.048. e2.
16. Dyrhovden GS, Lygre SHL, Badawy M, Gøthesen Ø, Furnes O. Have the causes of revision for total and unicompartmental knee arthroplasties changed

during the past two decades? *Clin Orthop Relat Res.* 2017;475(7):1874–1886. https://doi.org/10.1007/s11999-017-5316-7.

17. Martin G. *Famous Poems From Bygone Days.* New York: Courier Dover Publications; 1995.

18. Blankevoort L, Huiskes R, De Lange A. The envelope of passive knee joint motion. *J Biomech.* 1988;21(9):705–720.

19. Heesterbeek PJC, Verdonschot N, Wymenga AB. In vivo knee laxity in flexion and extension: A radiographic study in 30 older healthy subjects. *Knee.* 2008;15:45–49. https://doi.org/10.1016/j.knee.2007.09.007.

20. Tokuhara Y, Kadoya Y, Nakagawa S, Kobayashi A, Takaoka K. The flexion gap in normal knees. *J Bone Jt Surg [Br].* 2004;86B(8):1133–1136. https://doi.org/10.1302/0301-620X.86B8.15246.

21. Roth JD, Howell SM, Hull ML. Native knee laxities at 0°, 45°, and 90° of flexion and their relationship to the goal of the gap-balancing alignment method of total knee arthroplasty. *J Bone Jt Surg Am.* 2015;97:1678–1684.

22. Sami S, Moschetti WE, Dabuzhsky L, Jevsevar DS, Keggi JM, Plaskos C. Laxity profiles in the native and replaced knee—application to robotic-assisted gap-balancing total knee arthroplasty. *J Arthroplasty.* 2018;33(9):3043–3048. https://doi.org/10.1016/j.arth.2018.05.012.

23. Gladnick BP, Boorman-padgett J, Stone K, Kent RN, Cross MB, Mayman DJ, Pearle AD, Imhauser CW. Primary and coupled motions of the native knee in response to applied varus and valgus load. *Knee.* 2016;23(3):387–392. https://doi.org/10.1016/j.knee.2016.01.006.

24. Nowakowski AM, Majewski M, Muller-Gerbl M, Valderrabano V. Measurement of knee joint gaps without bone resection: Physiologic extension and flexion gaps in total knee arthroplasty are asymmetric and unequal and anterior and posterior cruciate ligament resections produce different gap changes. *J Orthop Res.* 2012;30(April):522–527. https://doi.org/10.1002/jor.21564.

25. Mihalko WM, Krackow KA. Posterior cruciate ligament effects on the flexion space in total knee arthroplasty. *Clin Orthop Relat Res.* 1999;no. 360:243–250. https://doi.org/10.1097/00003086-199903000-00029.

26. Kadoya Y, Kobayashi A, Komatsu T, Nakagawa S, Yamano Y. Effects of posterior cruciate ligament resection on the tibiofemoral joint gap. *Clin Orthop Relat Res.* 2001;no. 391:210–217. https://doi.org/10.1097/00003086-200110000-00023.

27. Tanaka K, Muratsu H, Mizuno K, Kuroda R, Yoshiya S, Kurosaka M. Soft tissue balance measurement in anterior cruciate ligament-resected knee joint: Cadaveric study as a model for cruciate-retaining total knee arthroplasty.

J Ortho Sci. 2007;12:149–153. https://doi.org/10.1007/s00776-006-1108-8.

28. Mayman D, Plaskos C, Kendoff D, Wernecke G, Pearle AD, Laskin R. Ligament tension in the ACL-deficient knee: Assessment of medial and lateral gaps. *Clin Orthop Relat Res.* 2009;467:1621–1628. https://doi.org/10.1007/s11999-009-0748-3.

29. Ma Y, Jia Chen W, Nagamine R. Comparative evaluation of posterior cruciate ligament in total knee arthroplasty: An in vivo study. *J Orthopaedic Surg.* 2017;25(1):1–6. https://doi.org/10.1177/2309499017690976.

30. Kayani B, Konan S, Horriat S, Ibrahim MS, Haddad FS. Posterior cruciate ligament resection in total knee arthroplasty: The effect on flexion-extension gaps, mediolateral laxity, and fixed flexion deformity. *Bone Jt J.* 2019;101-B(10):1230–1237. https://doi.org/10.1302/0301-620X.101B10.BJJ-2018-1428.R2.

31. Nagai K, Muratsu H, Takeoka Y. The influence of joint distraction force on the soft-tissue balance using modified gap-balancing technique in posterior-stabilized total knee arthroplasty. *J Arthroplasty.* 2017;32(10):2995–2999. https://doi.org/10.1016/j.arth.2017.04.058.

32. Foge DA, Baldini TH, Hellwinkel JE, Hogan CA, Dayton MR. The role of complete posterior cruciate ligament release in flexion gap balancing for total knee arthroplasty. *J Arthroplasty.* 2019;34(7S):S361–S365. https://doi.org/10.1016/j.arth.2019.03.017.

33. Schnurr C, Eysel P, König DP. Is the effect of a posterior cruciate ligament resection in total knee arthroplasty predictable? *Int Orthop.* 2012;36(1):83–88. https://doi.org/10.1007/s00264-011-1295-6.

34. Okamoto S, Okazaki K, Mitsuyasu H, Matsuda S, Iwamoto Y. Lateral soft tissue laxity increases but medial laxity does not contract with varus deformity in total knee arthroplasty. *Clin Orthop Relat Res.* 2013;471:1334–1342. https://doi.org/10.1007/s11999-012-2745-1.

35. Mullaji A. Can isolated removal of osteophytes achieve correction of varus deformity and gap-balance in computer-assisted total knee arthroplasty? An analysis of navigation data. *Bone Jt J.* 2020;102-B(6 Suppl A):49–58. https://doi.org/10.1302/0301-620X.102B6.BJJ-2019-1597.R1.

36. McAuliffe MJ, Roe J, Garg G, Whitehouse SL, Crawford R. The varus osteoarthritic knee has no coronal contractures in 90 degrees of flexion. *J Knee Surg.* 2016;30(4):297–303.

37. Tsukeoka T, Tsuneizumi Y. Varus and valgus stress tests after total knee arthroplasty with and without anesthesia. *Arch Ortho Trauma Surg.* 2016;136(3):407–411. https://doi.org/10.1007/s00402-015-2405-5.

38. Bellemans J, D'Hooghe P, Vandenneucker H, Van Damme G, Victor J. Soft tissue balance in total knee arthroplasty: does stress relaxation occur perioperatively?

Clin Orthop Relat Res. 2006;no. 452:49–52. https://doi. org/10.1097/01.blo.0000238790.29102.95.

39. Ishii Y, Matsuda Y, Noguchi H, Hiroshi K. Effect of soft tissue tension on measurements of coronal laxity in mobile-bearing total knee arthroplasty. *J Ortho Sci.* 2005;10:496–500. https://doi.org/10.1007/s00776-005-0935-3.

40. Takeda M, Ishii Y, Noguchi H, Matsuda Y, Sato J. Changes in varus – valgus laxity after total knee arthroplasty over time. *Knee Surg Sports Traumatol Arthrosc.* 2012;20:1988–1993. https://doi.org/10.1007/s00167-011-1783-7.

41. Matsumoto T, Muratsu H, Kubo S, Matsushita T, Kurosaka M, Kuroda R. Intraoperative soft tissue balance reflects minimum 5-year midterm outcomes in cruciate-retaining and posterior-stabilized total knee arthroplasty. *J Arthro.* 2012;27(9):1723–1730. https://doi.org/10.1016/j.arth.2012.02.020.

42. Sekiya H, Takatoku K, Takada H, Sasanuma H, Sugimota N. Postoperative lateral ligamentous laxity diminishes with time after TKA in the varus knee. *Clin Orthop Relat Res.* 2009;467(6):1582–1586. https://doi.org/10.1007/s11999-008-0588-6.

43. Tsukeoka T, Tsuneizumi Y. Residual medial tightness in extension is corrected spontaneously after total knee arthroplasty in varus knees. *Knee Surgery, Sports Traumatol, Arthrosc.* 2018;7(3):692–697. https://doi.org/10.1007/s00167-018-4967-6.

44. Kuriyama S, Ishikawa M, $nichiro Nakamura S, Furu M, Ito H, Matsuda S. No condylar lift—off occurs because of excessive lateral soft tissue laxity in neutrally aligned total knee arthroplasty: A computer simulation study. *Knee Surg, Sports Traumatol, Arthrosc.* 2015;24(8):2517–2524. https://doi.org/10.1007/s00167-015-3687-4.

45. Tanaka Y, Nakamura S, Kuriyama S, Nishitani K, Ito H, Lyman S, Matsuda S. Intraoperative physiological lateral laxity in extension and flexion for varus knees did not affect short—Term clinical outcomes and patient satisfaction. *Knee Surg, Sports Traumatol, Arthrosc.* 2020;28(12):3888–3898. https://doi.org/10.1007/s00167-020-05862-4.

46. Azukizawa M, Kuriyama S, Nakamura S, Nishitani K, Lyman S, Morita Y, Furu M, Ito H, Matsuda S. Intraoperative medial joint laxity in flexion decreases patient satisfaction after total knee arthroplasty. *Arch Ortho Trauma Surg.* 2018;138(8):1143–1150. https://doi.org/10.1007/s00402-018-2965-2.

47. Fujimoto E, Sasashige Y, Tomita T, Sasaki H, Touten Y, Fujiwara Y, Ochi M. Intra-operative gaps affect outcome and postoperative kinematics in vivo following cruciate-retaining total knee arthroplasty. *Int Orthop (SICOT).* 2015;40(1):41–49. https://doi.org/10.1007/s00264-015-2847-y.

48. Matsumoto K, Ogawa H, Yoshioka H, Akiyama H. Postoperative anteroposterior laxity influences subjective outcome after total knee arthroplasty. *J Arthro.* 2017;32(6):1845–1849. https://doi.org/10.1016/j.arth.2016.12.043.

49. Mochizuki T, Tanifuji O, Sato T, Hijikata H, Koga H, Watanabe S, Higano Y, et al. Association between anteroposterior laxity in mid-range flexion and subjective healing of instability after total knee arthroplasty. *Knee Surg, Sports Traumatol, Arthrosc.* 2017;25(11):3543–3548. https://doi.org/10.1007/s00167-016-4375-8.

50. Ismailidis P, Kuster MS, Jost B, Giesinger K, Behrend H. Clinical outcome of increased flexion gap after total knee arthroplasty. Can controlled gap imbalance improve knee flexion? *Knee Surg, Sports Traumatol, Arthrosc.* 2016;25(6):1705–1711. https://doi.org/10.1007/s00167-016-4009-1.

51. Jawhar A, Hutter K, Scharf HP. Outcome in total knee arthroplasty with a medial-lateral balanced versus unbalanced gap. *J Ortho Surg.* 2016;24(3):298–301.

52. Chia Z-Y, Pang H-N, Tan M-H, Yeo S-J. Gap difference in navigated TKA: A measure of the imbalanced flexion-extension gap. *SICOT-J.* 2018;4(30):1–5.

53. Matsuda Y, Ishii Y, Noguchi H, Ishii R. Varus-valgus balance and range of movement after total knee arthroplasty. *J Bone Jt Surg Br.* 2005;87B(6):804–808. https://doi.org/10.1302/0301-620X.87B6.15256.

54. Kamenaga T, Takayama K, Ishida K, Muratsu H, Hayashi S, Hashimoto S, Kuroda Y, et al. Medial knee stability at flexion increases tibial internal rotation and knee flexion angle after posterior-stabilized total knee arthroplasty. *Clin Biomech.* 2019;68:16–22. https://doi.org/10.1016/j.clinbiomech.2019.05.029.

55. Seah RB, Jin YS, Lin CP, Yew AKS, Chi CH, Nung LN. Evaluation of medial-lateral stability and functional outcome following total knee arthroplasty: Results of a single hospital joint registry. *J Arthro.* 2014;29(12):2276–2279. https://doi.org/10.1016/j.arth.2014.04.015.

56. Delport H, Labey L, De Corte R, Innocenti B, Vander J, Bellemans J. Collateral ligament strains during knee joint laxity evaluation before and after TKA. *Clin Biomech.* 2013;28(7):777–782. https://doi.org/10.1016/j.clinbiomech.2013.06.006.

57. Ghosh KM, Merican AM, Iranpour F, Deehan DJ, Amis AA. Length-change patterns of the collateral ligaments after total knee arthroplasty. *Knee Surg, Sports Traumatol, Arthrosc.* 2012;20(7):1349–1356. https://doi.org/10.1007/s00167-011-1824-2.

58. McAuliffe MJ, Connor PBO, Garg G, Whitehouse SL, Crawford RW, Phty B. Highly satisfied total knee arthroplasty patients display a wide range of soft tissue balance. *J Knee Surg.* 2018;33(3):247–254.

59. Jeffcote B, Nicholls R, Schirm A, Kuster MS. The Variation in medial and lateral collateral ligament strain and tibiofemoral forces following changes in the flexion and extension gaps in total knee replacement. *J Bone Jt Surg [Br]*. 2007;89(11):1528–1533. https://doi.org/10.1302/0301-620X.89B11.18834.

60. D'Lima DD. CORR Insights®: Are TKA kinematics during closed kinetic chain exercises associated with patient-reported outcomes? A preliminary analysis. *Clin Orthop Relat Res*. 2020;478(2):264–265. https://doi.org/10.1097/CORR.0000000000001061.

61. Onsem SV, Verstraete M, Van Eenoo W, Van Der Straeten C, Victor J. Are TKA kinematics during closed kinetic chain exercises associated with patient-reported outcomes? A preliminary analysis. *Clin Orthop Relat Res*. 2020;478(2):255–263. https://doi.org/10.1097/CORR.0000000000000991.

62. Shetty GM, Mullaji A, Khalifa AA, Ray A. Windswept deformities—An indication to individualise valgus correction angle during total knee arthroplasty. *J Orthop*. 2017;14(1):70–72. https://doi.org/10.1016/j.jor.2016.10.007.

63. Mihalko WM, Williams JL. Computer modeling to predict effects of implant malpositioning during TKA. *Orthopedics*. 2010;33(10):71–75. https://doi.org/10.3928/01477447-20100510-57.

64. Mullaji A, Shetty GM. Persistent hindfoot valgus causes lateral deviation of weightbearing axis after total knee arthroplasty. *Clin Orthop Relat Res*. 2011;469(4):1154–1160. https://doi.org/10.1007/s11999-010-1703-z.

65. Khalifa A, Mullaji AB, Mostafa AM, Farouk OA. A protocol to systematic radiographic assessment of primary total knee arthroplasty. *Orthop Res and Rev*. 2021;13:95–106.

66. Mullaji AB, Shetty GM, Kanna R, Vadapalli RC. The Influence of preoperative deformity on valgus correction angle: An analysis of 503 total knee arthroplasties. *J Arthrop*. 2013;28(1):20–27. https://doi.org/10.1016/j.arth.2012.04.014.

67. Bellemans J, Colyn W, Vandenneucker H, Victor J. Is neutral mechanical alignment normal for all patients? The concept of constitutional varus. *Clin Orthop Relat Res*. 2012;470(1):45–53. https://doi.org/10.1007/s11999-011-1936-5.

68. Shetty GM, Mullaji A, Bhayde S, Wook NK, Keun OH. Factors contributing to inherent varus alignment of lower limb in normal asian adults: Role of tibial plateau inclination. *Knee*. 2014;21(2):544–548. https://doi.org/10.1016/j.knee.2013.09.008.

69. Mullaji AB, Shah R, Bhoskar R, Singh A, Haidermota M, Thakur H. Seven phenotypes of varus osteoarthritic knees can be identified in the coronal plane. *Knee*

Surgery. *Sports Traumatol, Arthrosc*. 2021 https://doi.org/10.1007/s00167-021-06676-8.

70. Mullaji AB, Bhoskar R, Singh A, Haidermota M. Valgus arthritic knees can be classified into nine phenotypes. *Knee Surg. Sports Traumatol, Arthrosc*. 2021 https://doi.org/10.1007/s00167-021-06796-1.

71. Mullaji AB, Marawar SV, Mittal V. A comparison of coronal plane axial femoral relationships in asian patients with varus osteoarthritic knees and healthy knees. *J Arthropl*. 2009;24(6). https://doi.org/10.1016/j.arth.2008.05.025.

72. Mullaji AB, Padmanabhan V, Jindal G. Total knee arthroplasty for profound varus deformity: Technique and radiological results in 173 knees with varus of more than 20°. *J Arthropl*. 2005;20(5):550–561. https://doi.org/10.1016/j.arth.2005.04.009.

73. Mullaji AB, Shetty GM. Correction of varus deformity during TKA with reduction osteotomy knee. *Clin Orthop Relat Res*. 2014;472(1):126–132. https://doi.org/10.1007/s11999-013-3077-5.

74. Tang Q, Yu HC, Shang P, Tang Skun, Xu HZ, Liu HX, Zhang Y. Selective medial soft tissue release combined with tibial reduction osteotomy in total knee arthroplasty. *J Orthop Surg Res*. 2017;12(1):1–7. https://doi.org/10.1186/s13018-017-0681-1.

75. Asano H, Hoshino A, Wilton TJ. Soft-tissue tension total knee arthroplasty. *J Arthropl*. 2004;19(5):558–561. https://doi.org/10.1016/j.arth.2004.01.003.

76. Asano H, Muneta T, Sekiya I. Soft tissue tension in extension in total knee arthroplasty affects postoperative knee extension and stability. *Knee Surg, Sports Traumatol, Arthrosc*. 2008;16(11):999–1003. https://doi.org/10.1007/s00167-008-0591-1.

77. Li S, Luo X, Wang P, Sun H, Wang K, Sun X. Clinical outcomes of gap balancing vs measured resection in total knee arthroplasty: A systematic review and meta-analysis involving 2259 subjects. *J Arthrop*. 2018;33(8):2684–2693. https://doi.org/10.1016/j.arth.2018.03.015.

78. Moon YW, Kim HJ, Ahn HS, Park CD, Lee DH. Comparison of soft tissue balancing, femoral component rotation, and joint line change between the gap balancing and measured resection techniques in primary total knee arthroplasty: A meta-analysis. *Med (Baltim)*. 2016;95(39):1–7.

79. Sina B, Dowsey MM, Stoney JD, Choong PFM. Gap balancing sacrifices joint-line maintenance to improve gap symmetry: A randomized controlled trial comparing gap balancing and measured resection. *J Arthrop*. 2014;29(5):950–954. https://doi.org/10.1016/j.arth.2013.09.036.

80. Huang T, Long Y, George D, Wang W. Meta-analysis of gap balancing versus measured resection techniques in

total knee arthroplasty. *Bone Jt J.* 2017;99-B(2):151–158. https://doi.org/10.1302/0301-620X.99B2.BJJ-2016-0042. R2.

81. Dennis DA, Komistek RD, Kim RH, Sharma A. Gap balancing versus measured resection technique for total knee arthroplasty. *Clin Orthop Relat Res.* 2010;468(1):102–107. https://doi.org/10.1007/s11999-009-1112-3.

82. Daines BK, Dennis DA. Gap balancing vs. measured resection technique in total knee arthroplasty. *Clin Orthop Surg.* 2014;6:1–8.

83. Churchill JL, Mont MA, Khlopas A, Sultan AA, Harwin SF. Gap-balancing versus measured resection technique in total knee arthroplasty: A comparison study. *J Knee Surg.* 2017;31(1):13–16.

84. Cross MB, Nam D, Plaskos C, Sherman SL, Lyman S, Pearle AD, Mayman DJ. Recutting the distal femur to increase maximal knee extension during TKA causes coronal plane laxity in mid-flexion. *Knee.* 2012;19(6):875–879. https://doi.org/10.1016/j.knee.2012.05.007.

85. Nowakowski AM, Kamphausen M, Pagenstert G, Valderrabano V, Müller-Gerbl M. Influence of tibial slope on extension and flexion gaps in total knee arthroplasty: Increasing the tibial slope affects both gaps. *Int Orthop.* 2014;38(10):2071–2077. https://doi.org/10.1007/s00264-014-2373-3.

86. Walde TA, Bussert J, Sehmisch S, Balcarek P, Stürmer KM, Walde HJ, Frosch KH. Optimized functional femoral rotation in navigated total knee arthroplasty considering ligament tension. *Knee.* 2010;17(6):381–386. https://doi.org/10.1016/j.knee.2009.12.001.

87. Blakeney W, Beaulieu Y, Puliero B, Kiss M-O, Vendittoli P-A. Bone resection for mechanically aligned total knee arthroplasty creates frequent gap modifications and imbalances. *Knee Surg, Sports Traumatol, Arthrosc.* 2020;28(5):1532–1541. https://doi.org/10.1007/s00167-019-05562-8.

88. MacDessi SJ, Griffiths-Jones W, Chen DB, Griffiths-Jones S, Wood JA, Diwan AD, Harris IA. Restoring the constitutional alignment with a restrictive kinematic protocol improves quantitative soft-tissue balance in total knee arthroplasty: A randomized controlled trial. *Bone Jt J.* 2020;102(1):117–124. https://doi.org/10.1302/0301-620X.102B1.BJJ-2019-0674.R2.

89. Mihalko WM, Whiteside LA, Krackow KA. Comparison of ligament-balancing techniques during total knee arthroplasty. *J Bone Jt Surg Am.* 2003;85-A(Suppl 4):132–135.

90. Mullaji A, Sharma A, Marawar S, Kanna R. Quantification of effect of sequential posteromedial release on flexion and extension gaps. a computer-assisted study in cadaveric knees. *J Arthrop.* 2009;24(5):795–805. https://doi.org/10.1016/j.arth.2008.03.018.

91. Ferreira MC, Franciozi CES, Kubota MS, Priore RD, Ingham SJM, Abdalla RJ. Is the use of spreaders an accurate method for ligament balancing? *J Arthrop.* 2017;32(7):2262–2267. https://doi.org/10.1016/j.arth.2017.01.055.

92. Nagai K, Muratsu H, Matsumoto T, Miya H, Kuroda R, Kurosaka M. Soft tissue balance changes depending on joint distraction force in total knee arthroplasty. *J Arthrop.* 2014;29(3):520–524. https://doi.org/10.1016/j.arth.2013.07.025.

93. Basselot F, Gicquel T, Common H, Hervé A, Berton E, Ropars M, Huten D. Are ligament-tensioning devices interchangeable? A study of femoral rotation. *Orthop Traumatol: Surg Res.* 2016;102(4 Suppl):S213–S219. https://doi.org/10.1016/j.otsr.2016.02.001.

94. Mehliß V, Strauch Leira M, Serrano Olaizola A, Scior W, Graichen H. Proven accuracy for a new dynamic gap measurement in navigated TKA. *Knee Surg, Sports Traumatol, Arthrosc.* 2018;27(4):1189–1195. https://doi.org/10.1007/s00167-018-4989-0.

95. Kinsey TL, Mahoney OM. Balanced flexion and extension gaps are not always of equal size. *J Arthrop.* 2018;33(4):1062–1068. https://doi.org/10.1016/j.arth.2017.10.059.

96. Wada K, Hamada D, Takasago T, Nitta A, Goto T, Tonogai I, Tsuruo Y, Sairyo K. Joint distraction force changes the three-dimensional articulation of the femur and tibia in total knee arthroplasty: A cadaveric study. *Knee Surg, Sports Traumatol, Arthrosc.* 2019;28(5):1488–1496. https://doi.org/10.1007/s00167-019-05546-8.

97. Sugama R, Kadoya Y, Kobayashi A, Takaoka K. Preparation of the flexion gap affects the extension gap in total knee arthroplasty. *J Arthroplasty.* 2005;20(5):602–607. https://doi.org/10.1016/j.arth.2003.12.085.

98. Muratsu H, Matsumoto T, Kubo S, Maruo A, Miya H, Kurosaka M, Kuroda R. Femoral component placement changes soft tissue balance in posterior-stabilized total knee arthroplasty. *Clin Biomech.* 2010;25(9):926–930. https://doi.org/10.1016/j.clinbiomech.2010.06.020.

99. Mitsuyasu H, Matsuda S, Fukagawa S, Okazaki K, Tashiro Y, Kawahara S, Nakahara H, Iwamoto Y. Enlarged post-operative posterior condyle tightens extension gap in total knee arthroplasty. *J Bone Jt Surg [Br].* 2011;93B:1210–1216. https://doi.org/10.1302/0301-620X.93B9.25822.

100. Ahn JH, Woong BY. Comparative study of two techniques for ligament balancing in total knee arthroplasty for severe varus knee: Medial soft tissue release vs. bony resection of proximal medial tibia. *Knee Surg Relat Res.* 2013;25(1):13–18.

101. Song S, Gu KS, Je LY, Kim KII, Hee PC. An intraoperative load sensor did not improve the early postoperative results of posterior-stabilized TKA for osteoarthritis with varus deformities. *Knee Surg, Sports Traumatol, Arthrosc.* 2018;27(5):1671–1679. https://doi.org/10.1007/s00167-018-5314-7.

102. Aunan E, Kibsgård T, Röhrl SM. Minimal effect of patella eversion on ligament balancing in cruciate-retaining total knee arthroplasty. *Arch Orthop Trauma Surg.* 2017;137(3):387–392. https://doi.org/10.1007/s00402-017-2625-y.

103. Kamei G, Murakami Y, Kazusa H, Hachisuka S, Inoue H, Nobutou H, Nishida K, Mochizuki Y, Ochi M. Is patella eversion during total knee arthroplasty crucial for gap adjustment and soft-tissue balancing? *Orthop Traumatol: Surg Res.* 2011;97(3):287–291. https://doi.org/10.1016/j.otsr.2011.01.004.

104. Macdessi SJ, Gharaibeh MA, Harris IA. How accurately can soft tissue balance be determined in total knee arthroplasty? *J Arthrop.* 2019;34:290–294. https://doi.org/10.1016/j.arth.2018.10.003.

105. Manning WA, Blain A, Longstaff L, Deehan DJ. A load-measuring device can achieve fine-tuning of mediolateral load at knee arthroplasty but may lead to a more lax knee state. *Knee Surg, Sports Traumatol, Arthrosc.* 2018;27(7):2238–2250. https://doi.org/10.1007/s00167-018-5164-3.

106. Nielsen ES, Hsu A, Patil S, Colwell Jr CW, Lima DDD. Second-generation electronic ligament balancing for knee arthroplasty: A cadaver study. *J Arthrop.* 2018;33:2293–2300. https://doi.org/10.1016/j.arth.2018.02.057.

107. Wasielewski RC, Galat DD, Komistek RD. Correlation of compartment pressure data from an intraoperative sensing device with postoperative fluoroscopic kinematic results in TKA patients. *J Biomech.* 2005;38(2):333–339. https://doi.org/10.1016/j.jbiomech.2004.02.040.

108. Halder A, Kutzner I, Graichen F, Heinlein B, Beier A, Bergmann G. Influence of limb alignment on mediolateral loading in total knee replacement. *J Bone Jt Surg (Am).* 2012;94(11):1023–1029. https://doi.org/10.2106/JBJS.K.00927.

109. Hunt NC, Ghosh KM, Athwal KK, Longstaff LM, Amis AA, Deehan DJ. Lack of evidence to support present medial release methods in total knee arthroplasty. *Knee Surg, Sports Traumatol, Arthrosc.* 2014;22(12):3100–3112. https://doi.org/10.1007/s00167-014-3148-5.

110. Firer P, Gelbart B. Balancing of total knee arthroplasty by bone cuts achieves accurately balanced soft tissues without the need for soft tissue releases. *J ISAKOS.* 2018;3(5):263–268. https://doi.org/10.1136/jisakos-2018-000217.

111. Howell SM, Joshua DR, Maury LH. Kinematic Alignment in total knee arthroplasty definition, history, principle, surgical technique, and results of an alignment option for TKA what is kinematic alignment in TKA? *Arthropaedia.* 2014;1:44–53. http://33lfsllpawm41mkt63e2ts0a-wpengine.netdna-ssl.com/wp-content/uploads/2017/07/kinematic-alignment-in-total-knee-arthroplasty-definition-history-principle.pdf.

112. Morcos MW, Lanting BA, Webster J, Howard JL, Bryant D, Teeter MG. Effect of medial soft tissue releases during posterior-stabilized total knee arthroplasty on contact kinematics and patient-reported outcomes. *J Arthroplasty.* 2019;34(6):1110–1115. https://doi.org/10.1016/j.arth.2019.02.026.

113. Peters CL, Jimenez C, Erickson J, Anderson MB, Pelt CE. Lessons learned from selective soft-tissue release for gap balancing in primary total knee arthroplasty: An analysis of 1216 consecutive total knee arthroplasties. *J Bone Jt Surg - Ser A.* 2013;95(20):1–11. https://doi.org/10.2106/JBJS.L.01686.

114. Yagishita K, Muneta T, Ikeda H. Step-by-step measurements of soft tissue balancing during total knee arthroplasty for patients with varus knees. *J Arthrop.* 2003;18(3):313–320. https://doi.org/10.1054/arth.2003.50088.

115. Mullaji AB, Shetty GM. Correcting deformity in total knee arthroplasty. *Bone Jt J.* 2016;98-B(1_Supple_A):101–104. https://doi.org/10.1302/0301-620x.98b1.36207.

116. Masuda S, Miyazawa S, Yuya K, Kamatski Y, Tomohito H, Yoshiki O, Yuki O, Furumatsu T, Ozaki T. Posteromedial vertical capsulotomy selectively increases the extension gap in posterior stabilized total knee arthroplasty. *Knee Surg, Sports Traumatol, Arthrosc.* 2019;28(5):1419–1424. https://doi.org/10.1007/s00167-019-05511-5.

117. Zan P, Fan L, Liu K, Yang Y, Hu S, Li G. Reduction osteotomy versus extensive release on clinical outcome measures in simultaneous bilateral total knee arthroplasty. *Med Sci Monit.* 2017;23:3817–3823. https://doi.org/10.12659/MSM.905815.

118. Koh HS, In Y. Semimembranosus release as the second step of soft tissue balancing in varus total knee arthroplasty. *J Arthrop.* 2013;28(2):273–278. https://doi.org/10.1016/j.arth.2012.06.024.

119. Mullaji A, Shetty GM. Computer-assisted total knee arthroplasty for arthritis with extra-articular deformity. *J Arthrop.* 2009;24(8):1164–1169. https://doi.org/10.1016/j.arth.2009.05.005.

120. Mullaji A, Shetty G. Total knee arthroplasty for arthritic knees with tibiofibular stress fractures. classification and treatment guidelines. *J Arthrop*. 2010;25(2):295–301. https://doi.org/10.1016/j.arth.2008.11.012.

121. Mullaji AB, Singh A, Haidermota M. Arthritic knees with more than 10 valgus can have soft-tissue imbalance in flexion. *Knee Surgery, Sports Traumatology, Arthroscopy*. 2021. https://doi.org/10.1007/s00167-021-06798-z.

122. Watanabe M, Kuriyama S, Nakamura S, Nishitani K, Tanakaa Y, Sekiguchib K, Ito H, Matsuda S. Impact of intraoperative adjustment method for increased flexion gap on knee kinematics after posterior cruciate ligament-sacrificing total knee arthroplasty. *Clin Biomech*. 2019;63(April 2018):85–94. https://doi.org/10.1016/j.clinbiomech.2019.02.018.

123. Lustig S, Scholes CJ, Stegeman TJ, Oussedik S, Coolican MRJ, Parker DA. Sagittal placement of the femoral component in total knee arthroplasty predicts knee flexion contracture at one-year follow-up. *Int Orthop*. 2012;36(9):1835–1839. https://doi.org/10.1007/s00264-012-1580-z.

124. Okamoto Y, Otsuki S, Nakajima M, Jotoku T, Wakama H, Neo M. Sagittal Alignment of the femoral component and patient height are associated with persisting flexion contracture after primary total knee arthroplasty. *J Arthrop*. 2019;34(7):1476–1482. https://doi.org/10.1016/j.arth.2019.02.051.

125. Bellemans J, Vandenneucker H, Victor J, Vanlauwe J. Flexion contracture in total knee arthroplasty. *Clin Orthop Relat Res*. 2006;no. 452:78–82. https://doi.org/10.1097/01.blo.0000238791.36725.c5.

126. Koh IJ, Bum CC, Gwi KY, Cheol SS, Kyun KT. Incidence, predictors, and effects of residual flexion contracture on clinical outcomes of total knee arthroplasty. *J Arthrop*. 2013;28(4):585–590. https://doi.org/10.1016/j.arth.2012.07.014.

127. An VVG, Scholes CJ, Fritsch BA. Factors affecting the incidence and management of fixed flexion deformity in total knee arthroplasty: A systematic review. *Knee*. 2018;25(3):352–359. https://doi.org/10.1016/j.knee.2018.03.008.

128. Kim SH, Lim J-W, Jung H-J, Lee H-J. Influence of soft tissue balancing and distal femoral resection on flexion contracture in navigated total knee arthroplasty. *Knee Surg, Sports Traumatol, Arthrosc*. 2016;25(11):3501–3507. https://doi.org/10.1007/s00167-016-4269-9.

129. Athwal KK, Milner PE, Bellier G, Amis AA. Posterior capsular release is a biomechanically safe procedure to perform in total knee arthroplasty. *Knee Surg, Sports Traumatol, Arthrosc*. 2019;27(5):1587–1594. https://doi.org/10.1007/s00167-018-5094-0.

130. Baldini A, Scuderi G, Aglietti P, Chalnick D, Insall JN. Flexion—extension gap changes during total knee arthroplasty: Effect of posterior cruciate ligament and posterior osteophytes removal. *J Knee Surg*. 2004;17:69–72.

131. McEwen P, Balendra G, Doma K. Medial and lateral gap laxity differential in computer-assisted kinematic total knee arthroplasty. *Bone Jt J*. 2019;101-B(3):331–339. https://doi.org/10.1302/0301-620X.101B3.BJJ-2018-0544.R1.

132. Mihalko WM, Krackow KA. Anatomic and biomechanical aspects of pie crusting posterolateral structures for valgus deformity correction in total knee arthroplasty: A cadaveric study. *J Arthroplasty*. 2000;15(3):347–353. https://doi.org/10.1016/S0883-5403(00)90716-2.

133. Yang D, Shao H, Zhou Y, Tang H, Guo S. Location of the common peroneal nerve in valgus knees—is the reported safe zone for well-aligned knees applicable? *J Arthrop*. 2017;32(11):3539–3543. https://doi.org/10.1016/j.arth.2017.05.048.

134. Xu J, Liu H, Luo F, Lin Y. Common peroneal nerve "pre-release" in total knee arthroplasty for severe valgus deformities. *Knee*. 2020;27(3):980–986. https://doi.org/10.1016/j.knee.2020.02.012.

135. Buechel FF. A sequential three step lateral release for correcting fixed valgus knee deformities during total knee arthroplasty. *Clin Orthop Relat Res*. 1990;260:170–175.

136. Shetty GM, Mullaji A. Alignment in computer-navigated versus conventional total knee arthroplasty for valgus deformity. *SA Orthop J*. 2009;8(3):40–46.

137. Mullaji A, Lingaraju APP, Shetty GMM. Computer-assisted total knee replacement in patients with arthritis and a recurvatum deformity. *J Bone Jt Surg*. 2012;94 B(5):642–647. https://doi.org/10.1302/0301-620X.94B5.27211.

138. Mansour E, Whiteside LA. Ligament balancing in the valgus knee. *Semin Arthroplasty*. 2018;29(1):27–35. https://doi.org/10.1053/j.sart.2018.04.004.

139. Seo JG, Moon YW, Jo BC, Kim YT, Park SH. Soft tissue balancing of varus arthritic knee in minimally invasive surgery total knee arthroplasty: Comparison between posterior oblique ligament release and superficial MCL release. *Knee Surg Relat Res*. 2013;25(2):60–64. https://doi.org/10.5792/ksrr.2013.25.2.60.

140. Mehdikhani K, Moreno B, Reid JJ, Paz Nieves Ade, Yu Lee Y, Della Valle A. An algorithmic, pie-crusting medial soft tissue release reduces the need for constrained inserts patients with severe varus deformity undergoing total knee arthroplasty. *J Arthrop*.

2016;31(7):1465–1469. https://doi.org/10.1016/j.arth.2016.01.006.

141. Matsueda M, Gengerke TR, Murphy M, Lew WD, Gustilo RB. Soft tissue release in total knee arthroplasty: Cadaver study using knees without deformities. *Clin Orthop Relat Res.* 1999;no. 366:264–273. https://doi.org/10.1097/00003086-199909000-00034.

142. Nasab SHH, Smith CR, Schutz P, Damm P, Trepczynski A, List R, Taylor WR. Length-change Patterns of the collateral ligaments during functional activities after total knee arthroplasty. *Ann Biomed Eng.* 2020;48(4):1396–1406. https://doi.org/10.1007/s10439-020-02459-3.

143. Verdonk PCM, Pernin J, Pinaroli A, Ait SST, Neyret P. Soft tissue balancing in varus total knee arthroplasty: An algorithmic approach. *Knee Surg, Sports Traumatol, Arthrosc.* 2009;17(6):660–666. https://doi.org/10.1007/s00167-009-0755-7.

144. Boettner F, Renner L, Arana Narbarte D, Egidy C, Faschingbauer M. Total knee arthroplasty for valgus osteoarthritis: The results of a standardized soft-tissue release technique. *Knee Surg, Sports Traumatol, Arthrosc.* 2016;24(8):2525–2531. https://doi.org/10.1007/s00167-016-4054-9.

145. Xie K, Lyons ST. Soft tissue releases in total knee arthroplasty for valgus deformities. *J Arthrop.* 2017;32(6):1814–1818. https://doi.org/10.1016/j.arth.2017.01.024.

146. Miyasaka KC, Ranawat CS, Mullaji A. 10- to 20-Year followup of total knee arthroplasty for valgus deformities. *Clin Orthop Relat Res.* 1997;no. 345:29–37.

147. Apostolopoulos AP, Nikolopoulos DD, Polyzois I, Nakos A, Liarokapis S, Stefanakis G, Michos IV. Total knee arthroplasty in severe valgus deformity: Interest of combining a lateral approach with a tibial tubercle osteotomy. *Orthop Traumato: Surg Res.* 2010;96(7):777–784. https://doi.org/10.1016/j.otsr.2010.06.008.

148. Brilhault J, Lautman S, Favard L, Burdin P. Lateral femoral sliding osteotomy; lateral release in total knee arthroplasty for a fixed valgus deformity. *J Bone Jt Surg [Br].* 2002;84-B:1131–1137. https://doi.org/10.1007/s11610-007-0066-y.

149. Tucker A, O'Brien S, Doran E, Gallagher N, Beverland DE. Total knee arthroplasty in severe valgus deformity using a modified technique—A 10-year follow-up study. *J Arthrop.* 2019;34(1):40–46. https://doi.org/10.1016/j.arth.2018.09.002. e1.

150. Satish BRJ, Ganesan JC, Chandran P, Basanagoudar PL, Balachandar D. Efficacy and mid term results of lateral parapatellar approach without tibial tubercle osteotomy for primary total knee arthroplasty in fixed valgus knees. *J Arthrop.* 2013;28(10):1751–1756. https://doi.org/10.1016/j.arth.2013.04.037.

151. Nikolopoulos D, Michos I, Safos G, Safos P. Current surgical strategies for total arthroplasty in valgus knee. *World J Orthop.* 2015;6(6):469–482. https://doi.org/10.5312/wjo.v6.i6.469.

152. Wang B, Xing D, Jiao Li J, Zhu Y, Dong S, Zhao B. Lateral or medial approach for valgus knee in total knee arthroplasty—which one is better? A systematic review. *J Int Med Res.* 2019;47(11):5400–5413. https://doi.org/10.1177/0300060519882208.

153. Girard J, Amzallag M, Pasquier G, Mulliez A, Brosset T, Gougeon F, Duhamel A, Migaud H. Total knee arthroplasty in valgus knees: Predictive preoperative parameters influencing a constrained design selection. *Orthop Traumatol: Surg Res.* 2009;95(4):260–266. https://doi.org/10.1016/j.otsr.2009.04.005.

154. Mihalko WM, Woodard EL, Hebert CT, Crockarell JR, Williams JL. Biomechanical validation of medial pie-crusting for soft-tissue balancing in knee arthroplasty. *J Arthrop.* 2014;30:296–299. https://doi.org/10.1016/j.arth.2014.09.005.

155. Kwak D-S, In Y, Kyun Kim T, Suk Cho H, Jun Koh I. The pie-crusting technique using a blade knife for medial collateral ligament release is unreliable in varus total knee arthroplasty. *Knee Surg, Sports Traumatol, Arthrosc.* 2014;24(1):188–194. https://doi.org/10.1007/s00167-014-3362-1.

156. Amundsen SH, Meyers KN, Wright TM, Westrich GH. Variability in Elongation and failure of the medial collateral ligament after pie-crusting with 16- and 18-gauge needles. *J Arthrop.* 2018;33(8):2636–2639. https://doi.org/10.1016/j.arth.2018.03.021.

157. Meneghini RM, Daluga AT, Sturgis LA, Lieberman JR. Is the pie-crusting technique safe for MCL release in varus deformity correction in total knee arthroplasty? *J Arthrop.* 2013;28(8):1306–1309. https://doi.org/10.1016/j.arth.2013.04.002.

158. Bellemans J. Multiple Needle Puncturing: Balancing the Varus Knee. *Orthopaedics.* 2011;34(9):e510–e512. https://doi.org/10.3928/01477447-20110714-48.

159. Siong FT, Woo KT, Chan KS, Soo LE, Shahrul Azuan JM, Seuk LY. Efficacy and safety of functional medial ligament balancing with stepwise multiple needle puncturing in varus total knee arthroplasty. *J Arthrop.* 2019;35(2):380–387. https://doi.org/10.1016/j.arth.2019.09.005.

160. Ranawat AS, Chitranjan SR, Elkus M, Rasquinha VJ, Rossi R, Babhulkar S. Total knee arthroplasty for severe valgus deformity surgical technique. *J Bone Jt Surg.* 2004;86:2671–2676.

161. Clarke HD, Fuchs R, Scuderi GR, Norman Scott W, Insall JN. Clinical results in valgus total knee arthroplasty with the "pie crust" technique of lateral soft tissue releases. *J Arthrop.* 2005;20(8):1010–1014. https://doi.org/10.1016/j.arth.2005.03.036.

162. Kim MS, Koh IJ, Choi YJ, Kim YD, In Y. Correcting severe varus deformity using trial components during total knee arthroplasty. *J Arthrop.* 2017;32(5):1488–1495. https://doi.org/10.1016/j.arth.2016.11.043.

163. Kim MW, Koh IJ, Kim JH, Jong Jung J, In Y. Efficacy and safety of a novel three-step medial release technique in varus total knee arthroplasty. *J Arthrop.* 2015;30(9):1542–1547. https://doi.org/10.1016/j.arth.2015.03.037.

164. Orban H, Stan G, Dragusanu M, Adam R. Medial epicondyle osteotomy: A method of choice in severe varus knee arthroplasty. *Eur J Orthop Surg Traumatol.* 2012;22(7):579–583. https://doi.org/10.1007/s00590-011-0895-6.

165. Mullaji AB, Shetty GM. Surgical technique: Computer-assisted sliding medial condylar osteotomy to achieve gap balance in varus knees during TKA knee. *Clin Orthop Relat Res.* 2013;471(5):1484–1491. https://doi.org/10.1007/s11999-012-2773-x.

166. Mullaji AB, Shetty GM. Lateral epicondylar osteotomy using computer navigation in total knee arthroplasty for rigid valgus deformities. *J Arthrop.* 2010;25(1):166–169. https://doi.org/10.1016/j.arth.2009.06.013.

10

New Technology and Surgical Technique in TKA

Philip C. Noble, PhD, Shuyang Han, PhD, David Rodriguez-Quintana, MD, Adam M. Freehand, MD, Kenneth B. Mathis, MD, and Alexander V. Boiwka, MD

The critical determinants of successful, durable total knee arthroplasty (TKA) are correct positioning of the implanted components, acceptable alignment of the knee with weight-bearing, and restoration of normal stability during functional activities without the need for excessive muscular activation. Although the ideal values of component position, joint alignment, and knee stability remain topics of intense debate, there remains a general consensus that the success of surgeons in achieving the target values of each of these parameters is highly variable. Some authors[1] have speculated that this variability, and the disturbing incidence of outliers, contributes to the incidence of patient dissatisfaction with the outcome of TKA. This has led to the increasing adoption of computer-based technologies to augment or replace conventional manual instruments to provide confirmation of each patient's component placement and knee function within the operative setting. The case for computer assistance in TKA has been strengthened by the emergence of joint registries that highlight the true incidence of revision of joint arthroplasties and the striking effect of the age of the patient on the durability of the procedure. Joint registry data also show increased longevity of cases performed using computer navigation compared with conventional instrumentation. This supports the adoption of computer assistance in younger and more active patients in whom the need for correct positioning, alignment, and stability appears to be even more critical.

The emergence of computer-assisted technologies in TKA has also created opportunities for active instrumentation to provide feedback to the surgeon based on intraoperative measurements derived from each patient's knee. This information allows preoperative plans to be modified in response to the demands of each patient's soft tissue envelope and bony anatomy. This approach to personalization of each TKA is most evident in cases performed with sensor-based "smart" tibial trials and robotic surgical systems that allow the surgeon to measure compartmental loading, predict ligamentous laxity, and perform intraoperative correction if necessary.

This chapter reviews computer-based technologies that are commercially available to measure component position, joint alignment, knee stability, and compartment pressures. In addition, the chapter will review advances in robotically assisted TKA in which navigation and machining of the bony surfaces are integrated to further improve the accuracy and reliability of component placement and alignment.

SURGICAL NAVIGATION SYSTEMS IN TOTAL KNEE ARTHROPLASTY

Background

As the term "surgical navigation" suggests, the fundamental aim of computer-aided guidance technologies is to provide the operating surgeon with information defining the ideal or intended position and orientation of the prosthetic components with respect to the bony surfaces visible via the surgical incision. To make this possible, a predefined reference frame common to both the skeleton and implant is matched to the accessible features of the femur and tibia. This registration process can be performed using any anatomical or surface features digitized intraoperatively and any kinematic data inferred through the relative motion of the femur and the tibia. The simplest form of registration is performed using a calibrated probe to acquire the spatial coordinates of anatomical landmarks and bony surfaces required to define the reference frame within the surgical site. In theory this allows rapid registration with a minimum of data collection. However, most landmarks (e.g., the femoral epicondyles) are not singular points but are geometrical constructs (e.g., the center of a partial sphere), and so the accuracy and reproducibility of the registration process are dependent on the number of points collected and their relative spacing. For this reason, more sophisticated registration algorithms are "shaped-based," meaning that patches of data acquired intraoperatively from landmarks and bony surfaces are matched to the corresponding areas of bony models by statistical shape matching or through reference to large atlases of similar bones with precisely defined surfaces and anatomical axes. Even though both of these methods may be performed without preoperative imaging (image-free), the most accurate registration routines are based on patient-specific models derived from CT and/or MRI (image-based navigation). When these models have been created through segmentation and reconstruction of the imaging data, reference axes can be calculated and registration undertaken by performing standard shape-matching procedures.

Computer-Assisted Surgical Systems

It has been previously demonstrated that two of the most important factors associated with the longevity of TKA are accurate component placement and restoration of the mechanical alignment of the lower extremity.[2] Deviation of the mechanical axis by more than 3 degrees in the coronal plane has been correlated with accelerated component wear, loosening, instability, and poor implant survivorship.[2-8] Although traditional intramedullary and extramedullary cutting guides are readily available and easy to use, they have been associated with deviations greater than 3 degrees from planned mechanical alignment placement in up to 30% of procedures.[9] These errors are magnified in cases complicated by extraarticular deformity and unusual patient morphology. This experience has led to growing interest in computer-assisted surgery (CAS) over the past three decades to improve the accuracy and precision of bony resection, implant placement, and ligamentous

balancing. The first case of TKA in which computer navigation was used for the entire surgical procedure was performed by Krackow et al.[10] in August 1997. Currently, a wide variety of technologies exist to achieve these goals; these include patient-specific instrumentation, computer-assisted navigation systems, and, most currently, robotic systems.

CAS systems may be divided into three categories as defined by Picard et al.[11]: active robotic systems that are fully automated in the performance of surgical tasks (e.g., TSolution One, THINK Surgical), semiactive robotic systems that do not perform surgical tasks but may limit placement of tools or provide haptic feedback (e.g., Mako, Stryker), and passive systems that simply display alignment information (e.g., OrthAlign).

CAS navigation systems offer preoperative dynamic assessment of deformity, alignment, and kinematics and, as such, are classified as passive computer-assisted devices. Historically, navigation systems have been image-based (i.e., using imaging data derived from fluoroscopy, CT, or other modalities) and image-free (i.e., based on preconstructed computer models of knee anatomy).[12] Although image-based software remains prevalent in robotic-assisted systems, it quickly fell out of favor in CAS navigation because of its increased complexity and the associated financial burden of preoperative CT or MRI scans. Currently, imageless systems are the most widely studied and accepted for CAS navigation; they use kinematic or anatomical data that are collected intraoperatively to direct placement of cutting guides during implantation of off-the-shelf total knee implant designs (Table 10.1).

TABLE 10.1 List of Current Imageless Computer-Assisted Surgery (CAS) Navigation Total Knee Arthroscopy Systems	
CAS systems	Manufacturer
OrthoPilot/KneeSuite	Aesculap, Inc.
Knee3	Brainlab AG
ExactechGPS	Exactech
NaviPro Knee	Kinamed Incorporated
iMNS	Medacta International
KneeAlign	OrthAlign, Inc.
AchieveCAS	Smith & Nephew
NAV3i	Stryker
ORTHOsoft	Zimmer Biomet
iASSIST	Zimmer Biomet

Each navigation system has three basic components: a computer, a camera and trackers, and a direct line of sight between the arrays of trackers attached to the skeleton and a remotely positioned camera to measure the position and orientation of the femur and tibia to assess lower extremity movement, joint alignment, and instrument positioning in real time.[13] Trackers are fixed to the patient's femur and tibia often by pins, and a series of relevant anatomical landmarks are collected directly on the patient and processed through computer software to create a dynamic reference frame. The position of cutting guides and instruments are subsequently compared with this frame to enable the surgeon to customize the bone resection planes and final positioning of the implanted components.

Several tracking methods have been proposed based on electromagnetic, ultrasound, and stereoscopic technologies, but infrared optoelectronic tracking systems are the most common due to their reliability and ease of use. Validation studies of optoelectronic tracking systems have demonstrated high reliability and accuracy, with errors as low as 0.25 mm for translation and 1 degree for rotation, although measurement accuracy is correlated with the spatial location of the camera.[14] Active infrared light-emitting diode (LED) tracking uses an array of four to six diodes that are alternatively illuminated in a pattern detected by a charge-coupled device (CCD) camera (Fig. 10.1). Although accurate, active infrared technology relies on reusable electronic LED emitters within the surgical field that are reported to increase tracker weight, which leads to errors because of motion at

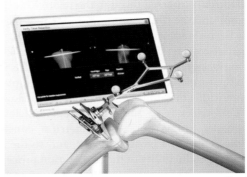

Fig. 10.2 Example of passive infrared tracker (Brainlab Knee3).

the bony fixation point.[15] Additional costs are also incurred due to battery requirements within each tracker. Alternatively, passive infrared tracking uses reflective spheres or discs that are affixed to a metal frame in a unique shape and registered by an infrared camera (Fig. 10.2). Although this method greatly lessens tracker weight, major costs are associated with the disposable reflective spheres/discs, and contamination of their reflective coating with tissue or bodily fluid markedly affects their accuracy.

Accuracy of CAS Systems in Terms of Limb and Component Alignment

Although there is continued debate regarding the optimal limb and component alignment in TKA, numerous studies have demonstrated that CAS navigation systems are more accurate, precise, and reproducible compared with conventional manual instrumentation using intramedullary or extramedullary guides.[14,16–33] Navigation systems have been shown to significantly improve postoperative mechanical limb alignment compared with traditional mechanical instrumentation.[17,20,21] In a metaanalysis performed by Mason et al.,[33] deviations in knee alignment greater than 3 degrees were reported in 9% of navigated TKAs versus 32% with conventional instrumentation. Similar improvements were also seen in the alignment of the femoral and tibial components themselves (Fig. 10.3). Coronal malalignment ≥3 degrees was seen in 5% of navigated femoral components and 4% of navigated tibial components versus 16% and 11%, respectively, in conventional TKA.[33] Sagittal femoral and tibial component alignment demonstrated greater discrepancies

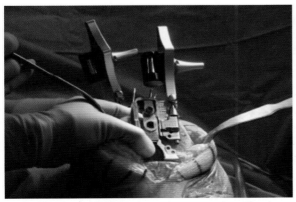

Fig. 10.1 Example of active infrared tracker (Stryker NAV3i).

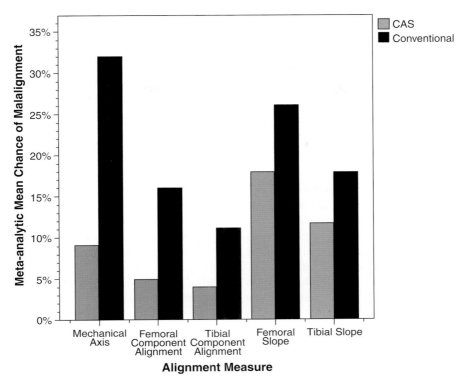

Fig. 10.3 Meta-analytic mean chance of malalignment at greater than 3 degrees. *CAS,* Computer-assisted surgery.

from target positioning, with both methods of component placement. In this case, malalignment ≥3 degrees occurred in 26% femoral and 18% of tibial components with conventional instrumentation compared with 8% and 12%, respectively, using CAS navigation.[33]

The effect of CAS navigation on rotational alignment has been less consistent. This is tied to the dependence of navigation systems on intraoperative identification of reference axes defining neutral rotation of the femur and the tibia. In separate studies analyzing postoperative CT images of TKA Chauhan et al.[20] and Stöckl et al.[26] demonstrated significant improvement in component rotation and decreased femoral/tibial rotational mismatch in cases performed with CAS navigation compared with conventional instrumentation. However, cadaveric studies reported by Siston et al. showed high variability in the rotational alignment of both the femoral[34] and tibial components,[35] regardless of whether navigation was used. Because the registration process is dependent on the precise location of bony landmarks, variations in spatial location arising from visual and

tactile cues, as commonly seen with the medial epicondylar sulcus, may have a profound effect on final surgical accuracy.[12,13,36]

Even though CAS navigation is commonly used in some countries such as Australia,[37] this technology has not received widespread global adoption in most of the world because of a variety of economic and ergonomic concerns. As with any new technology, the financial costs associated with CAS navigation were a primary deterrent to its initial adoption. Typically, these included the capital cost of the navigation system itself, the per-case cost of disposables (e.g., retroreflective arrarys), and the recurring cost of software and maintenance.[38] This does not take into account indirect costs attributable to the increased duration of operative procedures,[17] increased surgical instrument preparation and sterilization, and the need for additional intraoperative surgical assistance.[39] An analysis performed by Novak et al.[29] in 2007 estimated that CAS navigation led to an increase in upfront costs of approximately $1500 per case. However, they concluded that CAS navigation also had the potential to be a cost-effective or even cost-saving addition to TKA if improved component and limb alignment led to increased survivorship and reduced revision case load.

Regardless of financial barriers to adoption, ergonomic challenges have also been created by the bulk of the consoles, the line-of-sight limitation, and the addition of extra instruments. Furthermore, widespread acceptance was also deterred by concerns regarding the length of the CAS learning curve, coupled with the results of early studies reporting an increased incidence of complications such as fractures[40–42] and infection[10,12,25] associated with tracker pin sites. Even though later evidence did not confirm the initial concerns regarding increased complication rates,[43] skepticism was supported by other studies reporting limited advantages of CAS navigation compared with conventional instrumentation. Contrary to individual reports within the literature, a metaanalysis authored by Bauwens et al.[44] in 2007 demonstrated that CAS navigation did not significantly improve mechanical axis alignment, despite an average increase in operative time of 23%. This echoes the conclusions of numerous publications that have reported increases of 10 to 20 minutes in the duration of primary TKA procedures on average, furthering concerns for increased complication and infection risk and financial impact.[19–23,45–47]

To overcome some of the limitations associated with large-console CAS navigation systems, newer handheld accelerometer and gyroscope-based navigation systems have gained popularity. These imageless portable devices are supplied in a disposable, single-use format, and they use dynamic motion sensors to reference anatomical landmarks. Built-in displays provide digital feedback without the need for additional large, capital-intensive equipment within the operating room.[38,48–50] Furthermore, these systems avoid any line-of-sight issues and capital equipment and set-up costs, and they provide similar operative times and instrumentation to conventional methods.[51] However, these devices have a number of drawbacks, including significant cost and the inability to assess femoral and tibial component rotation.

Accelerometer-based Navigation Systems

Two accelerometer-based navigation (ABN) systems that are currently commercially available are the iASSIST (Zimmer Biomet, Warsaw, IN) and the OrthAlign (OrthAlign, Inc., Aliso Viejo, CA). Both systems

determine the center of rotation of the hip and the mechanical axis of the lower extremity to establish appropriate resection planes for the distal femur and proximal tibia. The iASSIST system uses small, disposable accelerometer-equipped "pods" and a local wireless network to assess limb alignment and direct cutting guides for optimal component positioning (Fig. 10.4).

In a prospective randomized controlled trial by Kinney et al.[52] iASSIST ABN demonstrated significant improvement over conventional instrumentation, with 4% of patients having a postoperative limb alignment of >3 degrees from the neutral mechanical axis compared with 36% with conventional instruments. Furthermore, studies have demonstrated no significant difference in the accuracy and precision of the iASSIST ABN compared with large-console CAS systems,[38,50] with no increase in operative time compared with conventional methods.[52] Although no initial capital equipment costs are incurred, a cost-based analysis for iASSIST ABN performed by Goh et al.[37] in 2016 found that an added cost of ABN was approximately $1000 per operation compared with the previously reported $1500 per case cost calculated by Novak et al.[29] for CAS navigation.

An alternative ABN system, the OrthAlign, provides dynamic measurement of the alignment of the distal femoral and tibial cutting blocks using a reference sensor and femoral and tibial jigs. The results are displayed on a display console within the single-use handheld device (Fig. 10.5).

This device has the added benefit of using open-platform software that allows it to be used with any design of knee prosthesis. A number of studies have demonstrated excellent accuracy and precision with the OrthAlign system[49,53,54] without the need for additional surgical time,[55] unlike large-console–based CAS navigation systems. In a retrospective analysis of cases performed with the OrthAlign ABN Nam et al.[51] reported 98% of tibial resections within 90 ± 2 degrees for coronal alignment and 96% within 3 ± 2 degrees for sagittal alignment. In addition, 96% of cases were within 90 ± 2 degrees for distal femoral alignment and 94% were within 0 ± 3 degrees for overall mechanical axis.[56] In a subsequent study comparing OrthAlign with a large-console imageless CAS system (AchieveCAS; Smith & Nephew, Memphis, TN), the OrthAlign ABN was found to be as accurate as, if not more so than, a large-console CAS system in regard to overall lower extremity, femoral,

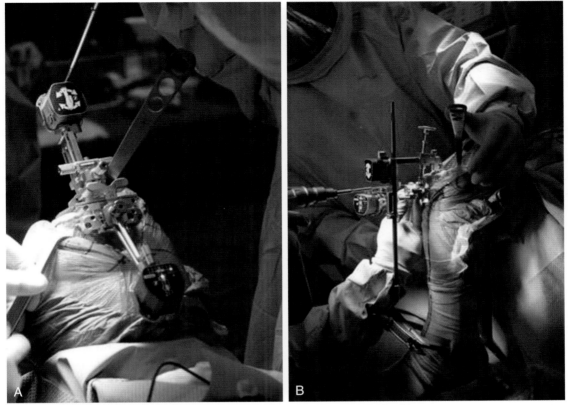

Fig. 10.4 Zimmer iASSIST handheld computer navigation system.

and tibial component alignment, particularly in valgus knees.[55]

Clinical Performance of Surgical Navigation Systems in TKA

Clinical Effectiveness (Complications and Survivorship)

The widespread use of navigation systems in knee arthroplasty has been slowed by the occurrence of specific complications associated with their use. These have been especially noted early in surgeons' learning curves even though inconsistent data are quite prevalent. Particular intraoperative complications associated with navigated arthroplasty include an increased incidence of femoral notching, periprosthetic fracture of the femur and tibia around pin insertion sites, increased surgical times, and procedure blood loss together with increased transfusion rates.

Anterior femoral notching in TKA is an avoidable complication in which the anterior femoral cut leads to violation of the anterior femoral cortex. Femoral notching in most studies has no major long-term effects on knee arthroplasty, but some studies have noted an increased risk of future periprosthetic fracture around a TKA femoral component.[57,58]

Factors that increase the risk of femoral notching include inappropriate femoral component sizing and rotation and inappropriate positioning on sagittal plane, leading to posterior displacement of the femoral component. In traditional navigation systems these variables are determined preoperatively and executed intraoperatively with expected reproducibility. Lee et al.[59] retrospectively reviewed 148 TKAs in 130 patients and compared conventional with navigated arthroplasty. They noted an increased rate of anterior femoral notching in the navigated cohort (5.7% vs. 16.7%, $P =$ .037). A similar difference in the incidence of anterior

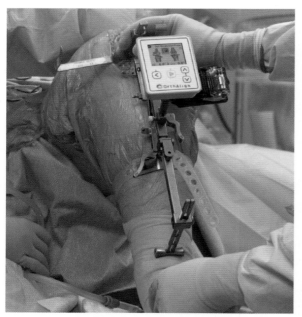

Fig. 10.5 OrthAlign handheld computer navigation system showing the display console, reference sensor, and tibial and femoral jigs.

notching was reported by Kim et al.[60] who, in a randomized control trial, observed notching in 11 TKAs (4%) performed with computer-assistance versus none in cases performed with conventional instrumentation (P = .046). The increased risk of femoral notching in navigated arthroplasties suggested less intraoperative awareness by the surgeon during anterior femoral cut and preparation or a combination of factors not noted by the authors of the available studies.

Acceptable durations of operative procedures and utilization of operating rooms (turnover) are of utmost importance to hospital efficiency and the productivity of busy surgical practices. Another significant barrier to widespread adoption of navigation or robotic technology is the perceived loss of operating room (OR) efficiency because of increased operative times. This is more acute during the early part of the surgeon's learning curve and tends to normalize with increased familiarity with the CAS system. Historically, increased surgical times have correlated with increased risk of infection, particularly when the length of the procedure exceeds 90 to 110 minutes.[61,62] The increased time required for placement of arrays, presurgical registration, and intraoperative planning can also extend the length of the procedure.

However, literature reports on the effect of CAS on operative duration and increased surgical times and complication rates are quite inconsistent. For example, Alcelik et al.[63] showed that surgical navigation improved component positioning and did increase operative duration (mean difference of 32 minutes; 95% confidence interval [CI], 20.97 to 43.15; P < .00001), but it had no effect on the rate of complications.

Most CAS navigation systems require attachment of tracker pins to the femur and tibia. At the case conclusion, tracking pin removal can introduce the possible risk of periprosthetic fracture because of the stress riser effect on the bone, though the reported incidence is very low.[40,64] A similar complication has been documented on medial unicompartmental arthroplasty, with extraarticular jig pins leading to stress fracture of the medial tibial plateau.[41,65] Management of these complications can be quite challenging, and in a patient expecting rapid recovery and with high activity expectations they can certainly prove devastating. Periprosthetic mid femur and tibia fractures have also been documented and can potentially occur around navigation tracker pin sites. By placing the trackers intraarticularly, a second incision is not needed, and muscle violation by the pin track and the stress riser can also be decreased. Smaller pins can potentially decrease the stress procedure on the bone, but they can lead to instability of the pins and compromise of the navigation workflow. Most reports of these tracker-induced fractures are in small case series and case reports in which the treatment consisted of protected weight-bearing and closed management.[40,64,66,67]

As CAS TKA does not require violation of the femoral canal, decreased surgical blood loss is an expected benefit, though the published evidence is mixed. Whereas some studies show a trend toward less intraoperative blood loss and less postoperative drainage in patients undergoing navigated TKA,[68,69] others show no change in the rate of transfusion.[70,71] In a registry study with 10,034 patients the group of 2008 patients treated with navigated TKA and the group of 8026 patients treated with conventional TKA showed no difference in surgical time but a statistically significant difference in perioperative transfusion rates (15.5% conventional vs. 9.7% navigated, P < .001).[72]

Long-term revision rates between conventional and navigated TKA are certainly inconsistent in the literature. One study based on data collected by the

Australian Orthopedic Association National Joint Replacement Registry examined the survivorship of navigated TKA in patients younger than 65 years of age and reported a cumulative revision rate of 7.8% (95% CI, 7.5 to 8.2) at 9 years postoperatively for conventional TKA compared with 6.3% (95% CI, 5.5 to 7.3) for navigated TKA.[73] In a retrospective study of 1121 consecutive primary TKA Schurr et al.[74] noted that all case revision rates averaged 4.7% for conventional TKA and 2.3% for navigated procedures ($P = .012$), with a dramatic reduction in the rate of aseptic revision (1.9% vs. 0.1%, $P = .024$). However, other studies report very minimal or no difference in the durability of conventional and navigated TKA.[75, 76]

Patient Outcomes (Pain, Function, and Satisfaction)

Long-term functional success after TKA has been defined in terms of correction of preoperative deformity, optimal radiographic implant positioning, and return to pain-free, age-related function. The widespread adoption of patient-reported outcome measures (PROMs) in total joint arthroplasty now enables surgeons to measure the pain, function, and quality of life experienced by their patients in an efficient manner. Moreover, PROMs data provide a basis for the implementation of patient-centered care and evidence-based decision making. PROMs also have the potential to serve as a measure of surgeon quality and could dictate future reimbursement algorithms (quality of service).

A patient's perception of the success of the procedure and their satisfaction with the outcome is tied to pain perception and return to function in the immediate postoperative period and afterward. This section will evaluate whether computer-assisted navigation has shown progress in positively or negatively affecting immediate postoperative pain and implant- or surgery-related complications and long-term patient-reported outcomes after TKA.

Despite the great promise of CAS systems in improving the accuracy and reproducibility of TKA, showing any difference in functional outcome, PROMs, or pain between conventional and navigated TKA. At 15-year follow-up, in a randomized trial of patients with same-day bilateral knee arthroplasties, Kim et al.[60] reported on 296 patients and showed no difference in functional scores, postoperative arc of motion, and revision rate between conventional and navigated knees. No changes in radiographic alignment parameters were shown between the groups.[60] Similar conclusions were reported in two studies with functional outcome measures as their endpoint; Harvie et al.[77] and Spencer et al.[78] were unable to show differences in functional outcomes even though statistically significant differences in overall alignment were noted at 5 years. This lack of clinical outcome difference in most likely secondary to the long-standing success rate of TKA.

ROBOTIC SYSTEMS IN TKA

Background

Robotic surgical systems can be divided into three categories based on the degree of control provided to the operating surgeon: active and autonomous, semiactive, and passive.[79,80] In active systems the robot autonomously executes the preplanned surgical procedure without physical guidance from the surgeon, who assumes the role of an observer monitoring the progress of the robotic device. Semiactive systems provide intraoperative feedback to the surgeon during the operation, usually in the form of auditory (beeping), tactile (vibration), and visual information, as a means of assisting the surgeon in positioning the components more accurately while avoiding overresection of bone stock. In passive systems the robotic system provides guidance and positions instruments (e.g., cutting blocks) while all or part of the procedure is carried out under the surgeon's direct control.

Robotic systems are also differentiated by the source of data used to create the individualized surgical plan. These are classified as either image-based or imageless. In image-based systems a patient-specific three-dimensional (3D) computer model of the patient's bony anatomy is created preoperatively through reconstruction of data derived from CT or MRI (Fig. 10.6). During preoperative planning the surgeon uses these models to determine bone resection depth, component size, implant alignment, and so on (see Fig. 10.6). To enable replication of these resections during surgery, the computer models and the patient's joint surfaces must be spatially matched (i.e., registered) before the robot can execute the preoperative plan. In imageless systems these steps are performed intraoperatively by predicting the surface coordinates of the femur and tibia using accessible areas of the bony surfaces and various anatomical landmarks. This information is used as a basis for predicting

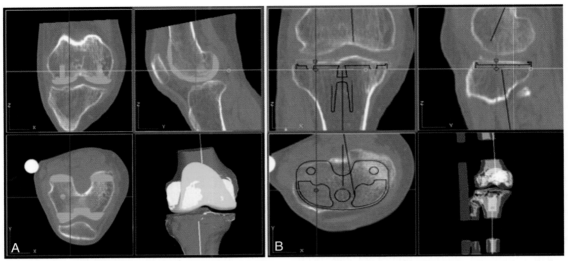

Fig. 10.6 Image-based preoperative planning is performed in a virtual environment to determine the size and alignment of the (A) femoral and (B) tibial components using the ROBODOC knee system.

the patient's bony morphology by scaling preexisting detailed anatomical models that have been collected preoperatively.

Systems Approved for TKA

Many robotic TKA platforms have been developed and used in clinical settings worldwide (Table 10.2). This has occurred in conjunction with a dramatic increase in peer-reviewed publications related to robotic technology in TKA.[79,81–84] In the United States the Food and Drug Administration (FDA) has given approval for the use of a number of new robotic systems for TKA with varying features and functions. Some of the common contemporary robotic systems used for TKA include (1) Mako (Stryker, Mahwah, NJ), (2) OMNIBotics (Corin Group, Cirencester, UK), (3) NAVIO (Smith & Nephew, London, UK), (4) ROSA (Zimmer Biomet, Warsaw, IN), (5) VELYS (Johnson & Johnson/DePuy Synthes, Warsaw, IN), and (6) TSolution One (ROBODOC) (THINK Surgical, Inc., Fremont, CA).

TABLE 10.2	Historic and Contemporary Robotic Systems Used for Total Knee Arthroscopy			
Robotic System	**Resection Type**	**Preop Imaging**	**Control**	**FDA Approval**
Mako	Semiactive	Pre-op CT	Haptic feedback	Aug. 2015
OMNIBotics	Passive	Imageless	Manual (robotically positioned cutting guide)	Sept. 2017
NAVIO	Semiactive	Imageless	Robotic-assisted nonhaptic	Jun. 2017
ROSA	Semiactive	Pre-op X-ray or imageless	Manual (robotically positioned cutting guide)	Jan. 2019
ROBODOC/TSolution One	Active	Pre-op CT	Autonomous control	Oct. 2019
Velys	Semiactive	Imageless	Robotic-assisted nonhaptic	Jan. 2021
CORI	Semiactive	Imageless	Robotic-assisted nonhaptic	Nov. 2021
MBARS	Active	Imageless	Autonomous control	NA
CASPAR	Active	Pre-op CT	Autonomous control	NA
Acrobot/Sculptor	Semiactive	Pre-op CT	Active-constraint	NA
PiGalileo	Passive	Imageless	Manual	NA

FDA, US Food and Drug Administration; *NA,* not applicable; *Pre-op,* preoperative.

The next section will review the individual features of the robotic platforms approved for clinical use in TKA.

Mako Robotic Arm System

The Mako robotic arm system (originally named Rio) is an image-based semiactive system widely used in clinical practice for robotic-assisted unicompartmental knee arthroplasty (UKA) and total hip arthroplasty (Fig. 10.7). Mako TKA system was granted 510(k) market clearance by the FDA in 2015. As an image-based robotic system, a preoperative patient-specific model derived from a CT scan is used to plan component sizing and implant positioning. Intraoperatively, the patient's limb is secured within a mobile leg holder boot, and the preoperative models and the planned implant components are registered to the patient's anatomy. The patient's knee is then moved through the arc of flexion from 0 to 90 degrees. During this maneuver, shims are placed within the medial and lateral compartments to determine the correct adjustment of the native joint space required for correct alignment and joint balancing. Once the desired 3D plan has been created, the surgeon can make the corresponding cuts with a conventional surgical saw that is mounted on the robotic arm. Haptic feedback generated by the system helps the surgeon to control the force and direction of saw blade within the confines of the predefined resection zone.[79,82,83] An additional safety feature automatically stops the device when there is rapid or jerking movement to prevent bone and soft tissue injury. The system allows the surgeon to execute the preoperative plan with precision, but if this plan is flawed, the system cannot compensate for it.[85]

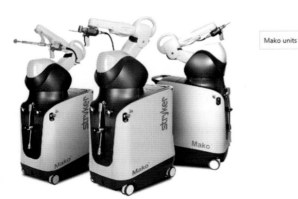

Fig. 10.7 Mako robotic arm system.

Many studies have been published examining different aspects of the Mako robotic system, ranging from its accuracy and cost effectiveness to its effect on clinical outcomes and patient satisfaction. In UKA applications a series of clinical and cadaveric studies have demonstrated that the robotic system provides greater accuracy than conventional manual instruments in terms of posterior slope of the tibial cut and alignment of the implanted components.[86–89] In a cohort of 120 UKA patients 62 prepared with robotic-assistance and 58 with conventional instrumentation, large differences were observed in the percentage of cases placed within 2 degrees of the target alignment of the femoral components (sagittal angle: 57% vs. 26%, $P = .0008$; coronal angle: 70% vs. 28%, $P = .0001$; axial angle: 53% vs. 31%, $P = .0163$).[86] Even larger differences were reported for placement of the tibial component (sagittal angle: 80% vs. 22%, $P = .0001$; axial angle: 48% vs. 19%, $P = .0009$). Moreover, the group reported that the use of the robotic system resulted in significantly lower pain and greater Knee Society Score (KSS) points at 3-month follow-up and higher rate of patient satisfaction at 2-year follow-up.[90]

In TKA applications similar findings regarding clinical outcome and accuracy were observed in several studies. At 6-month follow-up, Marchand et al.[91] compared the outcomes of 20 Mako-assisted and 20 manual TKAs in terms of pain score, functional score, and patient satisfaction. The robotic cohort showed significantly higher pain score (3 ± 3 vs. 5 ± 3, $P < .05$) and higher patient satisfaction (14 ± 8 vs. 7 ± 8 points, $P < .05$). In a prospective multicenter comparative study of 150 Mako-assisted TKAs and 102 manual TKAs[92] early results showed that the robotic cohort had equal or greater improvements in 9 out of 10 components of the KSS at 3 months postoperatively. Specifically, improvements were seen in the walking and standing (6.0 vs. 4.8 points), standard activities (11.4 vs. 10.1 points), advanced activities (6.2 vs. 4.6 points), functional activities total score (22.8 vs. 21.2 points), pain with walking (4.3 vs. 4.1 points), total symptom score (10.5 vs. 10.3 points), satisfaction score (17.0 vs. 15.5 points), and the expectation score (4.8 vs. 4.0 points).

In terms of coronal alignment, the Mako system has demonstrated accuracy in correcting knees with deformities of 9 to 15 degrees varus or valgus before TKA.[93] Sultan et al.[94] compared the posterior condylar offset ratio (PCOR) and the Insall-Salvati ratio in 43 Mako TKAs (mean age, 67 years; range, 46 to 79 years) and

39 manual TKAs (mean age, 66 years; range, 48 to 78 years) at 4 to 6 weeks postoperatively. The patients in the robotic group had smaller mean differences in PCOR (0.49 vs. 0.53, $P = .024$) than the manual group, which has been shown to correlate with better range of motion at 1 year after TKA. The number of patients with an Insall-Salvati index outside of the normal range was also lower in the robotic cohort (4 vs. 12), that is, patients in the robotic group were less likely to develop restricted flexion and overall range of motion. There are also data showing smaller errors in bone cuts and component positioning relative to preoperative plans after the use of the Mako robotic arm system.[95]

As with most new surgical technologies, there is a learning curve associated with the Mako TKA system before surgeons are able to reach the same level of efficiency as with conventional TKAs. An analysis of 240 Mako-assisted TKAs performed by two surgeons indicated that the operative procedure was significantly longer during the first 20 cases. Thereafter, operative times were comparable between robotic TKA and conventional manual TKA for both surgeons.[96] In another study Kayani et al.[97] assessed the learning curve by using a set of surrogate operative and radiographic markers in 60 consecutive conventional TKAs and 60 Mako-assisted TKAs. The results showed that the Mako system was associated with a learning curve of seven cases for operative time and surgical team anxiety level. Moreover, the authors reported that there was no penalty in changing from conventional to robotic instrumentation in terms of femoral and tibial implant positioning, limb alignment, posterior condylar offset ratio, posterior tibial slope, or restoration of the joint line.

Robotic technology is associated with substantial installation and maintenance costs and costs related to preoperative imaging, increased operative times, training of the surgical team, updating of computer software and servicing contracts, and purchase of consumables. A Markov decision analysis published in 2016 estimated that the direct cost of the Mako UKA platform with the service contract exceeded $1.362 million.[98] Conversely, a comparison of the 90-day episode-of-care cost of 519 Mako-assisted TKA and 2595 conventional TKA estimated that robotic assistance led to an average saving of US $2391 per case ($18,568 vs. $20,960, $P < .0001$) when index costs, length-of-stay, discharge disposition, and readmissions were included in the analysis.[99]

A substantial component of the cost of the episode of care in both cohorts was postacute services, with robotic TKA accruing fewer costs than manual TKA ($5234 vs. $6978, $P < .0001$). Although the authors did not take into account other clinical factors, such as the type and duration of anesthesia, the anticoagulation prescribed, and other risk factors, the study is large and properly powered, with strict inclusion criteria. It compares 90-day costs and potentially contributing cost-related factors between robotic-assisted TKA and conventional TKA patients.

OMNIBotics

OMNIBotics is an imageless platform that consists of a bone-modeling module (Bone Morphing), a ligament-balancing robot (BalanceBot), and a resection robot (OMNIBot) to perform TKA (Fig. 10.8). A patient-specific 3D model of the joint is created intraoperatively using bone-morphing technology, which registers sparse point data with a 3D statistical deformable model.[100]

The BalanceBot ligament-balancing device is then used to measure ligament tension and the resultant gaps throughout the midflexion range. Taking into account the mechanical axis, the 3D bone morphology, and the tibiofemoral gaps, the position of the implant is planned on the navigation system, and the device is mounted to the femur fixation base and locked into varus/valgus and internal/external rotation. A single cutting guide is then aligned in the sagittal plane for each of the five femoral cuts to allow the surgeon make resections[101,102] (Fig. 10.9). OMNIlife Science, Inc. was acquired by the international Corin Group in 2019.

Several studies have shown increased efficiency and accuracy of bone resection in cases performed with the iBlock robotic cutting guide compared with conventional cutting guides during TKA.[103–106] Suero et al.[103] compared the results of 30 TKA patients in whom the iBlock was used for femoral resection versus 64 cases performed with manual cutting blocks.

The results showed reduced variability in limb alignment (standard deviation: 1.7 vs. 2.7 degrees, $P = .0091$) and tourniquet time (76 vs. 91 minutes, $P = .008$) in cases performed with robotic assistance. In another study the same authors evaluated the accuracy and postoperative limb alignment in 100 knees using iBlock for femoral resection. The authors reported that the femoral and tibial component alignment was within 3 degrees of neutral alignment in 98% of cases, and final limb

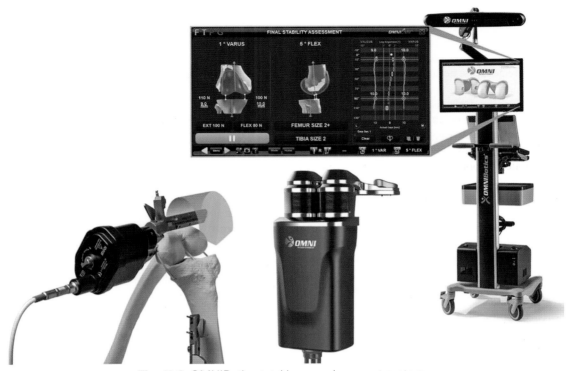

Fig. 10.8 OMNIBotics total knee replacement system.

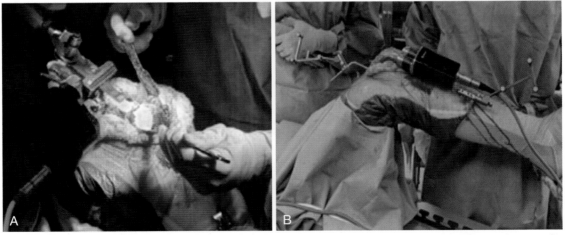

Fig. 10.9 (A) Resection of the femur using the OMNIBot and (B) acquiring the final tibiofemoral gap using the BalanceBot.

alignment was restored to within 3 degrees in 87% of cases.[105] In a cadaveric study the use of iBlock reduced the time required for femoral preparation from an average of 13.8 minutes to 5.5 minutes ($P < .001$) while achieving more accurate bone resections in all anatomical planes.[104] Similar findings regarding bone resection were reported by Ponder et al.[106]

Regarding soft tissue balancing, Koenig et al.[107] compared the final intraoperative coronal balance obtained throughout the knee range of motion (0 to 90 degrees) in 27 OMNIBotics-assisted TKAs and 25 TKAs performed with standard trials and manual instrumentation. The robotic-assisted cases showed a statistically significant difference in the gaps between the two groups at higher flexion angles (60 to 90 degrees of flexion). Overall, 78% to 86% of robotic cases were balanced to within 2 mm compared with 65% to 76% without robotic assistance.

Regarding patient-reported outcomes and patient satisfaction, Revenga et al.[108,109] and Hernández-Vaquero et al.[110] collected the Europe KSS, Western Ontario and McMaster Universities Osteoarthritis Index (WOMAC), and the 12-item Short Form Health Survey (SF-12) scores of 892 patients (343 OMNIBotics vs. 549 conventional) at 2-year follow-up. The OMNIBotics group showed greater improvement in the KSS score; the WOMAC pain, stiffness, and function subscores; and the SF-12 physical function score. In another series of studies Keggi et al.[111,112] reported early patient satisfaction with OMNIBotics-assisted TKA in 29 knees. All patients were either "fully satisfied" (86%) or "partly satisfied" (14%) with their surgery. In an ongoing prospective study comparing patient satisfaction and outcomes in OMNIBotics-assisted TKA and conventional TKA,[102] the KSS satisfaction score 6 months postoperatively improved by 19 points in the robotic group, which was twice the improvement of those receiving conventional TKA. At 1 year after OMNIBotics-assisted TKA, the authors reported greater improvement in knee function, pain reduction, satisfaction, and quality of life

There is a learning curve associated with the use of iBlock. It took an average of 15 extra minutes during the first 10 cases and 5 extra minutes during the second 10 cases without compromising accuracy.[105] Keggi et al.[111,112] demonstrated a reduction of 27 minutes in skin-to-skin time after the first seven cases, from 84 to 57 minutes. Moreover, compared with conventional TKA, robotic assistance extended the duration of TKA

by an average of only 3.3 minutes.[108-110] In a subsequent study Koenig et al.[113] reported that severe varus and valgus deformity >10 degrees was corrected in all 128 cases within 2 to 3.5 degrees of neutral position, with an additional 2.9 to 4.8 minutes of operative time. Licini and Meneghini[114] investigated the effect of robot use on blood loss. The robotic TKAs demonstrated less hourly drain output ($P = .02$), hemoglobin change ($P = .001$), and estimated blood loss ($P = .001$) compared with conventional instrumentation.

NAVIO Surgical System

NAVIO is a handheld, imageless, semiactive robotic system that combines surgical planning, navigation, and intraoperative visualization (Fig. 10.10). The system has been approved by the FDA for TKA and for unicondylar and patellofemoral knee arthroplasty.[82-84] This system is composed of a mobile computer cart that includes a surgeon-controlled graphical user interface, a passive infrared camera tracking system, a handheld burring device with robotic control of the cutting function, and a point probe that functions to calibrate the handpiece and to characterize patient anatomy[115] (Fig. 10.11). NAVIO relies on intraoperative 3D images to create a virtual model of the osseous knee and to guide bone resection. Unlike the Mako system, the NAVIO system does not rely on haptic feedback. Rather, it has a handheld end-cutting burr that can extend and retract during the procedure so that only the planned bone is removed. Specifically, the system monitors the position of the burring tool with respect to the patient's lower extremity; when the edge of the desired bone resection volume is approached, the system retracts the burr tip to avoid overresection of bone, thereby ensuring accuracy and safety.[79] The NAVIO TKA system is compatible

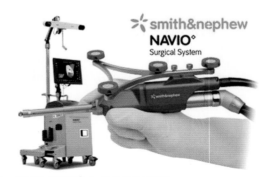

Fig. 10.10 NAVIO surgical system.

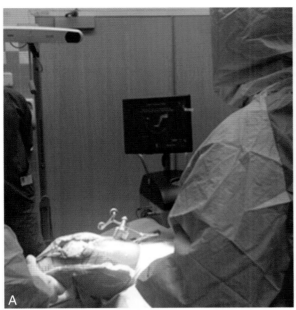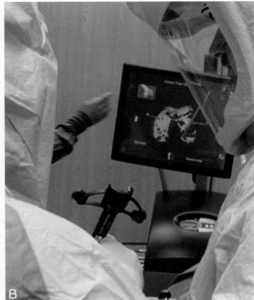

Fig. 10.11 (A) Soft tissue and ligament laxity characterization through full range of motion. (B) Use of the point probe to map out the articular surface of the femur.

with a wide portfolio of implants for TKA, including the JOURNEY II, LEGION, and GENESIS total knee implants.

The NAVIO surgical system has demonstrated high accuracy for bone preparation and gap balancing in TKA. In the first attempt to evaluate its accuracy in TKA, Casper et al.[115] carried out a cadaveric study in 18 knees using the robotic system. The results showed that the overall femur varus/valgus mean orientation error was −0.1 ± 0.9 degrees, the tibial varus/valgus error was −0.2 ± 0.9 degrees, and the posterior slope error for the tibial component was −0.2 ±1.3 degrees. However, the femoral implant flexion/extension error was −2.0 ± 2.2 degrees. Jaramaz et al.[116] measured the translational, angular, and rotational differences between the planned and achieved positions of components implanted in cadaveric and synthetic bones with the NAVIO TKA system. The root mean square errors of femoral varus/valgus, rotation, and distal resection were 0.7 degrees, 0.7 degrees, and 0.86 mm, respectively. The root mean square errors of tibial posterior slope, varus/valgus, and resection depth were 0.88 degrees, 0.69 degrees, and 0.68 mm, respectively, suggesting accurate implementation of the surgical plan using the NAVIO system.

Currently, there are limited complication, outcome, and learning curve data available.

ROSA Knee System

The ROSA knee system, as shown in Fig. 10.12, gained FDA approval in January 2019. This robotic system offers a computer software program to convert two-dimensional (2D) radiographic images into a 3D patient-specific bone model, allowing virtual planning on implant positioning and ligament balancing before execution. Then, the cutting jig is placed in the desired location as determined by the surgical plan, and the surgeon performs the cuts using manual instruments.[82,117] The ROSA knee system supports the Persona, Vanguard, and NexGen implant families.

The system accuracy in term of the depth and angle of bony resection has been validated in a cadaveric study of 30 knees.[117] The authors found that, compared with the planned cut, the depth, frontal, and sagittal angles of bone cut performed using the robotic system were on average within 1 ± 1 degree. Except for the femoral sagittal angle (−0.95 ± 0.88 degrees), there was no difference between the planned angles and the measured values; these were close to 0 degrees and were not significantly different from

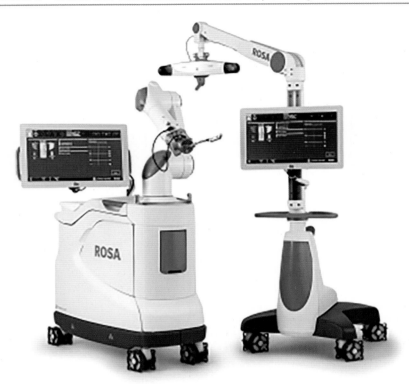

Fig. 10.12 The ROSA knee system.

0 degrees. In terms of the resection thickness, the mean difference between the planned and measured values was not significantly different from 0 mm in all but two measurements, namely distal femoral condyle (0.3 mm) and medial tibial plateau (0.66 mm). In addition, Seidenstein et al.[118] carried out a cadaveric study to compare the accuracy and reproducibility of ROSA to conventional instrumentation. The results showed that final limb alignment (hip-knee-ankle angle) had an accuracy of 0.8° ± 0.6°, with 100% of cases within 3° of the targeted neutral alignment. In addition, the accuracy of bone resection was below 0.6°, except for the femur flexion (1.3° ± 1.0°) and there were fewer outliers for ROSA Knee cases for all bone resection angles.

ROBODOC and THINK TSolution One Surgical System

The ROBODOC system (CUREXO Technology, Fremont, CA) is an autonomous milling system based on preoperative CT scans (Fig. 10.13). It consists of three components: a 3D preoperative planning workstation, a surgical robot, and a computer control unit used for precise cavity and surface preparation.

The initial ROBODOC system was designed for femur preparation in cementless total hip replacement. In both hip and knee applications the robotic system executes the preoperative cut plan without active feedback from the operating surgeon. The first TKA system was installed in Germany after being approved for sale in the European Union.[119] In 2014 the original company (CUREXO Technology) changed its name to THINK Surgical, Inc. A newer version of the ROBODOC system named TSolution One surgical system was approved by the FDA on October 8, 2019, for the use in TKA.

The results of the first 100 TKA cases showed that bone resection was good enough to allow cementless implantation in 76% of cases with no cases of varus malpositioning.[120] The accuracy of the system was also demonstrated in a 25-patient study with a mean coronal mechanical alignment of −0.4 ± 1.7 degrees and 100% accuracy in matching the size of the implant selected during preoperative planning.[121] In a 4-year follow-up of 72 knees

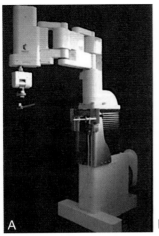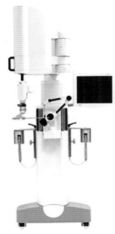

Fig. 10.13 (*Left*) ROBODOC. (*Right*) TSolution One surgical system.

Park and Lee[122] reported differences in the coronal femoral angle (97.7 vs. 95.6 degrees, $P < .01$), sagittal femoral angle (0.2 vs. 4.2 degrees, $P < .01$), and sagittal tibial angles (85.5 vs. 89.7 degrees, $P < .01$) of robotic versus conventional TKA. In a 10-year follow-up study of cruciate-retaining TKA, Yang et al.[123] assessed the clinical and radiological results of the ROBODOC system in comparison with a group prepared with conventional instrumentation TKA. The robotic cohort had significantly fewer outliers in terms of excessive deviation from the mechanical axis (8.5% vs. 31%) and fewer radiolucent lines (0% vs. 14%) than the conventional TKA group.

In terms of clinical outcome measures, Yang et al.[123] reported no significant intergroup differences in Hospital for Special Surgery (HSS) knee score (88.7 vs. 87.2, $P = .79$), WOMAC score (7.6 vs. 11.5, $P = .12$), Visual Analog Scale (VAS) pain score (1.1 vs. 1.2, $P = 0.51$), and range of motion (132.6 vs. 131.0 degrees, $P = .92$) at 10-year follow-up. Similar conclusions were reached by Cho et al.[124] who reported outcomes in 155 robotic TKAs versus 196 conventional jig-based NexGen TKAs, at a minimum 10-year follow-up. They reported no difference in WOMAC, Oxford Knee Score (OKS), KSS, or SF-12 scores. However, Liow et al.[125] reported higher 36-item Short Form Health Survey (SF-36) quality-of-life measures in 31 robotic TKAs than in 29 conventional jig-based TKAs at 2-year follow-up. At a longer term,[123] the survival rate in robotic TKA group and conventional group was not significantly different at 5 years (98.5% vs. 97.6%, $P > .05$) and 10 years (97.1% vs. 92.3%, $P > .05$).

In addition, there was an obvious learning curve associated with the ROBODOC TKA system; operating time decreased from 130 minutes for the first case to an average of 90 to 100 minutes after 27 cases.[120,121,126] Overall, robot-assisted implantation increased operative times by approximately 25 minutes (95 vs. 70 minutes).[126] Jacofsky et al.[79] noted that the time needed for planning, registration, and milling is greater than many other robotic systems.

VELYS Robotic-Assisted Solution

The VELYS TKA system is released by Johnson & Johnson/DePuy-Synthes in January 2021. To the best of our knowledge, the system has been referred to as Orthotaxy in the previous development stage. Unlike other surgical robotic systems, VELYS is compact and is attached to the operating table.[125] The system does not require preoperative CT imaging. Like other semi-active systems, the cutting guide is locked into position according to preoperative planning, allowing the surgeon to perform all bony cuts using an oscillating saw. Because the robot will not require surgeons to use disposable instruments, savings compared to other robotic systems are projected to range from $1500 to $2500 per procedure. Moreover, the system is designed to be used without the assistance of an additional technician, potentially saving additional cost and possibly shortening the learning curve associated with introduction of the system into clinical use.[127] The reduced footprint of the VELYS system minimizes space requirements in the operating room. In an internal report of Johnson & Johnson[128] the dimensions of the VELYS were compared to the Mako system, which included carts, robotic arms, arrays, cameras, and other components. This comparison showed that the OR footprint of the VELYS system (robot plus satellite station) is 32% smaller than the Mako system (1165 in^2 vs. 1715 in^2), while the reduction due to the device itself was 80% (336 in^2 vs. 1715 in^2 for Mako).

TECHNOLOGIES ADDRESSING LIGAMENT BALANCING

Numerous studies and reports from joint registries have shown that symptoms arising from knee instability are a major source of failure of TKAs, making up 18% to 22% of revisions, after aseptic loosening and infection.[129,130] From a biomechanical perspective, this means that when the patient performs some activity, the knee is placed in a position where there is insufficient resistance to the forces acting on the articulating surfaces to prevent them from slipping until the stretched soft tissues and/or the articulation itself create sufficient resistance to stop motion. In practice, this generally means that too much load is passing through one compartment compared with the other, possibly to the extent that contact is lost between the prosthetic components in the unloaded compartment. Although clinical instability is multifactorial, the causes are primarily surgical and relate to the positioning of the components and the retention of soft tissues.

One of the fundamental beliefs of arthroplasty surgeons is that the most successful knee arthroplasty is one that restores the normal loading and motion of the native joint. This includes loading of both compartments during physiological activity without excessive demand on the muscles and ligaments stabilizing the joint. To achieve this goal, surgeons classically assess the laxity of the joint through its response to manual varus and valgus loading throughout the range of motion with the trial implants in place.[131] As this method is not standardized, relies upon the tactile feel of the surgeon, and requires visibility of the joint line, its reproducibility is expected to be highly dependent on the skill and experience of the surgeon. In practice, this makes the technique of joint balance challenging to teach and achieve on a consistent basis without some form of objective measurement. As a result, training of surgeons may suffer in terms of consistency and efficiency, and the outcome of knee arthroplasty is expected to be variable, especially early in each surgeon's career.[132,133]

As these decisions are made intraoperatively, it is generally believed that the presence of instability could be detected, and potentially corrected, by measuring the relative values of the reaction forces passing through the medial and lateral compartments during a maneuver generating load across the joint. This assumption is supported by the work of Wasielewski et al.[134] who recorded tibiofemoral contact pressures intraoperatively in 38 TKA patients during flexion-extension of the knee and then correlated their findings with outcome scores and fluoroscopy examinations performed at 6 and 10 months postoperatively. The authors found a correlation between inappropriate or paradoxical postoperative kinematics recorded at follow-up and the presence of abnormal compartment pressures and distributions recorded intraoperatively. In addition, patients with

similar pressures in both the medial and lateral compartments of their TKA throughout a range of motion did not exhibit condylar liftoff values greater than 1.0 mm during a deep knee bend at postoperative follow-up.

Knee balance during TKA is often assessed by measuring the displacement of the medial and lateral joint lines under standardized conditions of distraction.[133] This may be obtained using lamina spreaders to independently distract the medial and lateral compartments with the knee positioned in both extension and 90 degrees of flexion. Using this method, the surgeon attempts to apply equal amounts of tension, as judged manually by the resistance of the spreader. Once this is achieved, the degree of balance of the joint may be assessed by measuring the medial and lateral opening of the joint and the alignment of the extremity. This method has a number of shortcomings, including the fact that measurements are not performed over the motion arc of the joint and the degree of joint opening is affected by the point of application of the distraction force to the surfaces of the femur and tibia. In addition, devices of this design limit the freedom of translation and rotation of the femur on the tibia during distraction. This can lead to erroneous measurements and an unbalanced joint when the prosthetic components have been implanted.

Implant manufacturers have addressed some of these concerns through the introduction of spring-loaded and pneumatic actuators that can be used directly with the native femur or trial components throughout the range of motion of the knee during application of a fixed value of distraction force.[135,136] These modifications have been shown to increase the accuracy and reproducibility of conventional mechanical distraction instruments. Commercial systems using these principles include the BalanceBot ligament-balancing device[137,138] and the XpandOrtho electronic balancing device (Exactech, Gainesville, FL).[139,140] The BalanceBot has been described in the earlier section of this chapter dealing with robotic surgical systems. The XpandOrtho electronic balancing device generates distraction of the joint by means of an inflatable chamber that is expanded through the introduction of air under pressure. As the femoral and tibial surfaces are uniformly loaded, the joint space assumes an equilibrium position that is measured with electromagnetic sensors. As the knee is flexed, the system monitors the medial and lateral opening of the joint and the angle of knee flexion. The accuracy and utility of this device has been verified in cadaveric specimens[141]; however, it is not yet commercially available.

An alternative approach is to measure the location and magnitude of contact pressures within the medial and lateral compartments after placement of the trial components. This principle is applied by the VERASENSE Knee System (OrthoSensor, Inc., Dania Beach, FL), which deploys an instrumented polymeric replica of the tibial insert with force sensors embedded within its medial and lateral articulating surfaces.[142] After the trial components and the patella have been reduced, the knee can be moved through its range of motion with additional application of varus/valgus loading to gauge laxity. During these maneuvers, the location and magnitude of the loads within each tibiofemoral compartment are recorded and wirelessly transmitted to a computer display that graphically depicts the points of contact between the femoral condyles and the load-sensing insert. This enables the surgeon to set the rotation of the tibial baseplate by placing the knee in extension and then rotating the baseplate until the medial and lateral contact points are parallel to the mediolateral axis of the knee. The compartmental load data recorded by the VERASENSE device during ranging of the knee allow the surgeon to assess the degree to which normal knee kinematics are restored by the proposed position and alignment of the tibial and femoral components. To assess the soft tissue balance, varus/valgus moments are applied to the knee in extension and 10 and 45 degrees of flexion to check for the presence of laxity of the collateral ligaments. In the balanced TKA medial and lateral contact pressures are similar in magnitude, are centrally located, and display appropriate rollback with knee flexion, remaining approximately parallel to the transverse axis of the knee from 0 to 90 degrees.

Additional testing can be performed to evaluate loading of the posterior cruciate ligament (PCL) by applying a posteriorly directed force to the knee when placed in 90 degrees of flexion with the hip in neutral rotation. Under these conditions, contact points in balanced knees fall within the middle of the posterior third of the tibial insert and display less than 10 mm of posterior excursion during application of the posterior drawer test. Conversely, in the case of an unbalanced knee, medial and lateral compartment pressures differ by more than 15 pounds and are often displaced from the central third of the bearing surface. For example, in the case of a knee that is tight in flexion the peak contact pressures will be

elevated and located more posteriorly on the surface of the tibial inserts, prompting the surgeon to loosen the PCL through "pie crusting" techniques or to open up the back of the knee by recutting the tibial osteotomy to increase its posterior slope.[143–145] In the converse situation excessive laxity of the PCL may be detected by monitoring the anteroposterior translation of the tibial contact points during a posterior drawer test. This may be corrected by inserting a thicker or more constrained tibial insert, or by converting from a cruciate-retaining to a posterior-stabilizing implant.

The accuracy of sensor measurements in determining the degree of balance of the knee is difficult to establish. However, the studies of Chu et al.[146] performed in total knee replacement cases have shown that an array of outcome variables, including the pain, function, and satisfaction subscores of the KSS, were not affected by changes in loading of the medial and lateral compartments ranging from approximately 30% to 70% of the total joint load (i.e., the sum of the medial and lateral loads). A true randomized clinical trial has not been reported comparing the results of treatment and control groups of patients whose knees were balanced using a sensor device versus those whose knees were balanced manually. Possibly the closest approximation of this research design is a single group multicenter study of 135 patients who underwent primary total knee replacement using sensor-guided balancing of the knee. This study has been reported in various publications after different periods of follow-up,[144,147–149] including 6 and 12 months postoperatively. In retrospect 17 knees (13%) were classified as unbalanced, based on the observation that the difference between medial and lateral compartmental loads exceeded 15 lbs in extension (10 degrees), midflexion (45 degrees), or at 90 degrees of flexion. This load value subsequently emerged as the threshold for differentiating between a balanced and unbalanced TKA in clinical application of the sensor device.

A notable difference in patient outcomes was observed between the balanced and unbalanced groups at 1-year follow-up, as reflected in a difference of 23.3 points in the average values of the KSS (179 ± 17.2 points and 156 ± 23.4 points, respectively, $P < .001$). In terms of KSS subscales, the difference between the balanced and unbalanced groups was 96.4 versus 87.8 points for pain ($P < .001$) and 82.4 versus 68.3 points for function ($P = .022$). The major weakness of this study is that it is not known what the outcome of the unbalanced group would have been if measures were taken to ensure that each knee was left in a balanced condition.

In one interesting study by Cho et al.[150] 84 patients underwent TKA using the same implant design with either a measured resection technique (ROBODOC, $n = 34$) or a modified gap balancing technique ($n = 50$). After placement of the trial femoral and tibial components, compartment pressures were measured with a VERASENSE sensor during mobilization of the limb from full extension to full flexion. If compartment loads differed by more than 15 pounds, the knee was considered imbalanced, and soft tissue releases and/or additional bone resection was performed and the compartment loads were remeasured. In 30 patients (36%) the knee was found to be balanced after initial preparation, whereas the remaining 54 cases required additional releases and/or bone resection, which achieved a balanced condition in all but five cases (6%). Much higher percentages of knees have been reported to meet this definition of balanced when the transepicondylar axis is used to set the rotation of the femoral component.[151]

The learning curve associated with sensor balancing has been studied in two ways. Gharaibeh et al.[152] examined a consecutive series of 90 TKA cases performed after the introduction of sensor balancing and recorded compartmental pressures achieved at flexion angles of 10, 45, and 90 degrees. The authors found that the incidence of unbalanced knees, defined by a difference of more than 15 pounds between the medial and lateral compartmental loads, was 8% to 11% of the first 45 cases versus 0% of the second group of 45 cases. The duration of the learning curve, defined by the elimination of unbalanced knees, was approximately 30 cases. Lakra et al.[153] reported an analysis of the duration of primary TKA cases performed before and after introduction of the sensor balancing technology. Initial use of the technology increased the duration of the procedure by an average of 10.5 minutes (11%) over the course of the first 41 cases, at which point the use of sensors had no effect on the length of the procedure. Additional concerns have been raised regarding the reproducibility of compartmental pressure measurements performed with this device, especially near extension (10 degrees of flexion).[154] In a study of 33 TKA procedures compartmental pressures were performed three times on each TKA. For the first two measurements, the examiner was blinded to the pressure recordings, whereas for the third measurement the compartmental pressures were visible. The investigators reported that the intraclass correlation coefficient between the blind measurements was poor in 2 of the 12 (17%), moderate in 4 of 12 (33%), and good in 6 of 12 (50%) measurements. Similar results were reported for comparison of the blinded and visible pressures. This observation may be the result of inadvertent varus or valgus loading of the knee or creep of the articular surfaces during measurement of compartmental pressures.[154]

REFERENCES

1. Kahlenberg CA, Nwachukwu BU, McLawhorn AS, Cross MB, Cornell CN, Padgett DE. Patient satisfaction after total knee replacement: A systematic review. *HSS J.* 2018;14(2):192–201. doi:10.1007/s11420-018-9614-8.
2. Attar FG, Khaw FM, Kirk LM, et al. Survivorship analysis at 15 years of cemented press-fit condylar total knee arthroplasty. *J Arthroplasty.* 2008;23:344–349.
3. Fang DM, Ritter MA, Davis KE. Coronal alignment in total knee arthroplasty: Just how important is it? *J Arthroplasty.* 2009;24:39–43.
4. Bachmann M, Bolliger L, Ilchmann T, et al. Long-term survival and radiological results of the Duracon total knee arthroplasty. *Int Orthop.* 2014;38:747–752.
5. Berend ME, Ritter MA, Meding JB, et al. Tibial component failure mechanisms in total knee arthroplasty. *Clin Orthop Relat Res.* 2004;428:26–34.
6. Perillo-Marcone A, Taylor M. Effect of varus/valgus malalignment on bone strains in the proximal tibia after TKR: An explicit finite element study. *J Biomech Eng.* 2007;129:1–11.
7. Ritter MA, Davis KE, Meding JB, et al. The effect of alignment and BMI on failure of total knee replacement. *J Bone Jt Surg Am.* 2011;93:1588–1596.
8. Rossi R, Rosso F, Cottino U, et al. Total knee arthroplasty in the valgus knee. *Int Orthop.* 2014;38:273–283.
9. Blakeney WG, Khan RJ, Wall SJ. Computer-assisted techniques versus conventional guides for component alignment in total knee arthroplasty: a randomized controlled trial. *J Bone Jt Surg Am.* 2011;93:1377–1384.
10. Krackow KA, Bayers-Thering M, Phillips MJ, et al. A new technique for determining proper mechanical axis alignment during total knee arthroplasty: progress toward computer-assisted TKA. *Orthopedics.* 1999;22:698–702.
11. Picard F, Deakin A, Balasubramanian N, et al. Minimally invasive total knee replacement: techniques and results. *Eur J Orthop Surg Traumatol.* 2018;28:781–791.
12. Krackow KA, Phillips MJ, Bayers-Thering M, et al. Computer-assisted total knee arthroplasty: navigation in TKA. *Orthopedics.* 2003;26:1017–1023.

13. Krackow KA. Fine tuning your next total knee: computer assisted surgery. *Orthopedics*. 2003;26: 971–972.

14. Pitto RP, Graydon AJ, Bradley L, et al. Accuracy of a computer-assisted navigation system for total knee replacement. *J bone Jt Surg Br volume*. 2006;88:601–605.

15. Picard F, Gregori A, Deakin A. Total knee replacement navigation: The different techniques. In: *The Knee Joint*. Springer, Paris; 2012:867–878.

16. Barrett WP, Mason JB, Moskal JT, et al. Comparison of radiographic alignment of imageless computer-assisted surgery vs conventional instrumentation in primary total knee arthroplasty. *J Arthroplasty*. 2011;26: 1273–1284.e1271.

17. Bathis H, Perlick L, Tingart M, et al. Alignment in total knee arthroplasty. A comparison of computer-assisted surgery with the conventional technique. *J bone Jt Surg Br*. 2004;86:682–687.

18. MacDessi SJ, Jang B, Harris IA, et al. A comparison of alignment using patient specific guides, computer navigation and conventional instrumentation in total knee arthroplasty. *Knee*. 2014;21:406–409.

19. Bolognesi M, Hofmann A. Computer navigation versus standard instrumentation for TKA: A single-surgeon experience. *Clin Orthop Relat Res*. 2005;440:162–169.

20. Chauhan SK, Scott RG, Breidahl W, et al. Computer-assisted knee arthroplasty versus a conventional jig-based technique. A randomised, prospective trial. *J bone Jt Surg Br*. 2004;86:372–377.

21. Haaker RG, Stockheim M, Kamp M, et al. Computer-assisted navigation increases precision of component placement in total knee arthroplasty. *Clin Orthop Relat Res*. 2005;433:152–159.

22. Hart R, Janecek M, Chaker A, et al. Total knee arthroplasty implanted with and without kinematic navigation. *Int Orthop*. 2003;27:366–369.

23. Jenny JY, Boeri C. Computer-assisted implantation of total knee prostheses: A case-control comparative study with classical instrumentation. *Comput Aided Surg*. 2001;6:217–220.

24. Saragaglia D, Picard F, Chaussard C, et al. Computer-assisted knee arthroplasty: comparison with a conventional procedure. Results 50 cases a prospective randomized study. *Rev Chir Orthop Reparatrice Appar Mot*. 2001;87:18–28.

25. Sparmann M, Wolke B, Czupalla H, et al. Positioning of total knee arthroplasty with and without navigation support. A prospective, randomised study. *J bone Jt Surg Br*. 2003;85:830–835.

26. Stöckl B, Nogler M, Rosiek R, et al. Navigation improves accuracy of rotational alignment in total knee arthroplasty. *Clin Orthop Relat Res*. 2004;426:180–186.

27. Anderson KC, Buehler KC, Markel DC. Computer assisted navigation in total knee arthroplasty: comparison with conventional methods. *J Arthroplasty*. 2005;20:132–138.

28. Keyes BJ, Markel DC, Meneghini RM. Evaluation of limb alignment, component positioning, and function in primary total knee arthroplasty using a pinless navigation technique compared with conventional methods. *J Knee Surg*. 2013;26:127–132.

29. Novak EJ, Silverstein MD, Bozic KJ. The cost-effectiveness of computer-assisted navigation in total knee arthroplasty. *J Bone Jt Surg Am*. 2007;89:2389–2397.

30. Bae DK, Yoon KH, Song SJ, et al. Comparative analysis of radiologic measurement according to TKR using computer assisted surgery and conventional TKR. *J Korean Orthop Assoc*. 2005;40:398–402.

31. Bae DK, Yoon KH, Song SJ, et al. Intraoperative versus postoperative measurement in total knee arthroplasty using computer-assisted orthopaedic surgery (CAOS): Accuracy of CAOS. *J Korean Orthop Assoc*. 2005;40:168–173.

32. Decking R, Markmann Y, Fuchs J, et al. Leg axis after computer-navigated total knee arthroplasty: a prospective randomized trial comparing computer-navigated and manual implantation. *J Arthroplasty*. 2005;20:282–288.

33. Mason JB, Fehring TK, Estok R, et al. Meta-analysis of alignment outcomes in computer-assisted total knee arthroplasty surgery. *J Arthroplasty*. 2007;22:1097–1106.

34. Siston RA, Patel JJ, Goodman SB, et al. The variability of femoral rotational alignment in total knee arthroplasty. *J Bone Jt Surg Am*. 2005;87:2276–2280.

35. Siston RA, Goodman SB, Patel JJ, et al. The high variability of tibial rotational alignment in total knee arthroplasty. *Clin Orthop Relat Res*. 2006;452:65–69.

36. Yau WP, Leung A, Chiu KY, et al. Intraobserver errors in obtaining visually selected anatomic landmarks during registration process in nonimage-based navigation-assisted total knee arthroplasty: A cadaveric experiment. *J Arthroplasty*. 2005;20:591–601.

37. AOANJRR. *Hip, Knee & Shoulder Arthroplasty: 2017 Annual Report*. Adelaide: Australian Orthopaedic Association National Joint Replacement Registry; 2017:188.

38. Goh GS, Liow MH, Lim WS, et al. Accelerometer-based navigation Is as accurate as optical computer navigation in restoring the joint line and mechanical axis after total knee arthroplasty: A prospective matched study. *J Arthroplasty*. 2016;31:92–97.

39. Picard F, Clarke J, Deep K, Gregori A. Computer assisted knee replacement surgery: is the movement mainstream? *Orthop Musc Syst*. 2014 June;15:3(2).

40. Ossendorf C, Fuchs B, Koch P. Femoral stress fracture after computer navigated total knee arthroplasty. *Knee.* 2006;13:397–399.

41. Seon JK, Song EK, Yoon TR, et al. Tibial plateau stress fracture after unicondylar knee arthroplasty using a navigation system: two case reports. *Knee Surg Sports Traumatol Arthrosc.* 2007;15:67–70.

42. Wysocki RW, Sheinkop MB, Virkus WW, et al. Femoral fracture through a previous pin site after computer-assisted total knee arthroplasty. *J Arthroplasty.* 2008;23:462–465.

43. Brown MJ, Matthews JR, Bayers-Thering MT, et al. Low incidence of postoperative complications with navigated total knee arthroplasty. *J Arthroplasty.* 2017;32:2120–2126.

44. Bauwens K, Matthes G, Wich M, et al. Navigated total knee replacement. A meta-analysis. *J Bone Jt Surg Am.* 2007;89:261–269.

45. Friederich N, Verdonk R. The use of computer-assisted orthopedic surgery for total knee replacement in daily practice: A survey among ESSKA/SGO-SSO members. *Knee Surg Sport Traumatol Arthrosc.* 2008;16:536–543.

46. Stulberg SD, Loan P, Sarin V. Computer-assisted navigation in total knee replacement: results of an initial experience in thirty-five patients. *J Bone Jt Surg Am.* 2002;84-A(Suppl 2):90–98.

47. Stulberg SD. How accurate is current TKR instrumentation? *Clin Orthop Relat Res.* 2003;416: 177–184.

48. Scuderi GR, Fallaha M, Masse V, et al. Total knee arthroplasty with a novel navigation system within the surgical field. *Orthop Clin North Am.* 2014;45:167–173.

49. Nam D, Cody EA, Nguyen JT, et al. Extramedullary guides versus portable, accelerometer-based navigation for tibial alignment in total knee arthroplasty: A randomized, controlled trial: Winner of the 2013 HAP PAUL Award. *J Arthroplasty.* 2014;29:288–294.

50. Desseaux A, Graf P, Dubrana F, et al. Radiographic outcomes in the coronal plane with iASSIST versus optical navigation for total knee arthroplasty: A preliminary case-control study. *OTSR.* 2016;102:363–368.

51. Nam D, Jerabek SA, Haughom B, et al. Radiographic analysis of a hand-held surgical navigation system for tibial resection in total knee arthroplasty. *J Arthroplasty.* 2011;26:1527–1533.

52. Kinney MC, Cidambi KR, Severns DL, et al. Comparison of the iAssist handheld guidance system to conventional instruments for mechanical axis restoration in total knee arthroplasty. *J Arthroplasty.* 2018;33:61–66.

53. Nam D, Jerabek SA, Cross MB, et al. Comparison of the iAssist handheld guidance system to conventional instruments for mechanical axis restoration in total knee arthroplasty. *Comput Aided Surg.* 2012;17:205–210.

54. Bugbee WD, Kermanshahi AY, Munro MM, et al. Accuracy of a hand-held surgical navigation system for tibial resection in total knee arthroplasty. *Knee.* 2014;21:1225–1228.

55. Nam D, Weeks KD, Reinhardt KR, et al. Accelerometer-based, portable navigation vs imageless, large-console computer-assisted navigation in total knee arthroplasty: a comparison of radiographic results. *J Arthroplasty.* 2013;28:255–261.

56. Nam D, Nawabi DH, Cross MB, et al. Accelerometer-based computer navigation for performing the distal femoral resection in total knee arthroplasty. *J Arthroplasty.* 2012;27:1717–1722.

57. Puranik HG, Mukartihal R, Patil SS, et al. Does femoral notching during total knee arthroplasty influence periprosthetic fracture. A prospective study. *J Arthroplasty.* 2019;34:1244–1249.

58. Zalzal P, Backstein D, Gross AE, et al. Notching of the anterior femoral cortex during total knee arthroplasty characteristics that increase local stresses. *J Arthroplasty.* 2006;21:737–743.

59. Lee JH, Wang SI. Risk of anterior femoral notching in navigated total knee arthroplasty. *Clin Orthop Surg.* 2015;7:217–224.

60. Kim YH, Park JW, Kim JS. 2017 Chitranjan S. Ranawat Award: Does computer navigation in knee arthroplasty improve functional outcomes in young patients? A randomized study. *Clin Orthop Relat Res.* 2018;476: 6–15.

61. Bovonratwet P, Shen TS, Ast MP, et al. Reasons and risk factors for 30-day readmission after outpatient total knee arthroplasty: A review of 3015 cases. *J Arthroplasty.* 2020;35:2451–2457.

62. Ravi B, Jenkinson R, O'Heireamhoin S, et al. Surgical duration is associated with an increased risk of periprosthetic infection following total knee arthroplasty: A population-based retrospective cohort study. *EClinicalMedicine.* 2019;16:74–80.

63. Alcelik IA, Blomfield MI, Diana G, et al. A comparison of short-term outcomes of minimally invasive computer-assisted vs minimally invasive conventional instrumentation for primary total knee arthroplasty: A systematic review and meta-analysis. *J Arthroplasty.* 2016;31:410–418.

64. Hoke D, Jafari SM, Orozco F, et al. Tibial shaft stress fractures resulting from placement of navigation tracker pins. *J Arthroplasty.* 2011;26(504):e505–e508.

65. Ji JH, Park SE, Song IS, et al. Complications of medial unicompartmental knee arthroplasty. *Clin Orthop Surg.* 2014;6:365–372.

66. Jung HJ, Jung YB, Song KS, et al. Fractures associated with computer-navigated total knee arthroplasty. A report of two cases. *J Bone Jt Surg Am.* 2007;89:2280–2284.

67. Massai F, Conteduca F, Vadala A, et al. Tibial stress fracture after computer-navigated total knee arthroplasty. *J Orthop Traumatol.* 2010;11:123–127.

68. Hinarejos P, Corrales M, Matamalas A, et al. Computer-assisted surgery can reduce blood loss after total knee arthroplasty. *Knee Surg Sports Traumatol Arthrosc.* 2009;17:356–360.

69. Kalairajah Y, Simpson D, Cossey AJ, et al. Blood loss after total knee replacement: effects of computer-assisted surgery. *J bone Jt Surg Br.* 2005;87:1480–1482.

70. Gholson JJ, Duchman KR, Otero JE, et al. Computer navigated total knee arthroplasty: Rates of adoption and early complications. *J Arthroplasty.* 2017;32:2113–2119.

71. Jhurani A, Agarwal P, Aswal M, et al. Computer navigation has no beneficial effect on blood loss and transfusion in sequential bilateral total knee arthroplasty. *J Orthop Surg (Hong Kong).* 2019;27 2309499019832440.

72. Liodakis E, Antoniou J, Zukor DJ, et al. Navigated vs conventional total knee arthroplasty: Is there a difference in the rate of respiratory complications and transfusions? *J Arthroplasty.* 2016;31:2273–2277.

73. de Steiger RN, Liu YL, Graves SE. Computer navigation for total knee arthroplasty reduces revision rate for patients less than sixty-five years of age. *J Bone Jt Surg Am.* 2015;97:635–642.

74. Schnurr C, Gudden I, Eysel P, et al. Influence of computer navigation on TKA revision rates. *Int Orthop.* 2012;36:2255–2260.

75. Roberts TD, Clatworthy MG, Frampton CM, et al. Does computer assisted navigation improve functional outcomes and implant survivability after total knee arthroplasty? *J Arthroplasty.* 2015;30:59–63.

76. Antonios JK, Kang HP, Robertson D, et al. Population-based survivorship of computer-navigated versus conventional total knee arthroplasty. *J Am Acad Orthop Surg.* 2020;28:857–864.

77. Harvie P, Sloan K, Beaver RJ. Computer navigation vs conventional total knee arthroplasty: five-year functional results of a prospective randomized trial. *J Arthroplasty.* 2012;27:667–672.e661.

78. Spencer JM, Chauhan SK, Sloan K, et al. Computer navigation versus conventional total knee replacement: no difference in functional results at two years. *J bone Jt Surg Br.* 2007;89:477–480.

79. Jacofsky DJ, Allen M. Robotics in arthroplasty: A comprehensive review. *J Arthroplasty.* 2016;31:2353–2363.

80. Netravali NA, Shen F, Park Y, et al. A perspective on robotic assistance for knee arthroplasty. *Adv Orthop.* 2013;2013:970703.

81. Agarwal N, To K, McDonnell S, et al. Clinical and radiological outcomes in robotic-assisted total knee arthroplasty: A systematic review and meta-analysis. *J Arthroplasty.* 2020;35 3393–3409.e2.

82. Kayani B, Haddad FS. Robotic total knee arthroplasty: Clinical outcomes and directions for future research. *Bone Jt Res.* 2019;8:438–442.

83. Kayani B, Konan S, Ayuob A, et al. Robotic technology in total knee arthroplasty: A systematic review. *EFORT Open Rev.* 2019;4:611–617.

84. Mont MA, Khlopas A, Chughtai M, et al. Value proposition of robotic total knee arthroplasty: What can robotic technology deliver in 2018 and beyond? *Expert Rev Med Devices.* 2018;15:619–630.

85. Lang JE, Mannava S, Floyd AJ, et al. Robotic systems in orthopaedic surgery. *J bone Jt Surg Br.* 2011;volume 93:1296–1299.

86. Bell SW, Anthony I, Jones B, et al. Improved accuracy of component positioning with robotic-assisted unicompartmental knee arthroplasty: Data from a prospective, randomized controlled study. *J Bone Jt Surg Am.* 2016;98:627–635.

87. Citak M, Suero EM, Citak M, et al. Unicompartmental knee arthroplasty: Is robotic technology more accurate than conventional technique? *Knee.* 2013;20:268–271.

88. Iñiguez M, Negrin R, Duboy J, et al. Robot-assisted unicompartmental knee arthroplasty: Increasing surgical accuracy? A cadaveric study. *J Knee Surg.* 2019;34:628–634.

89. Lonner JH, John TK, Conditt MA. Robotic arm-assisted UKA improves tibial component alignment: A pilot study. *Clin Orthop Relat Res.* 2010;468:141–146.

90. Conditt M. *Short to Mid-Term Survivorship of Robotically Guided Unicompartmental Knee Arthroplasty.* Kona, HI: 2nd Annual Pan Pacific Orthopaedic Congress; 2015.

91. Marchand RC, Sodhi N, Khlopas A, et al. Patient satisfaction outcomes after robotic arm-assisted total knee arthroplasty: A short-term evaluation. *J Knee Surg.* 2017;30:849–853.

92. Khlopas A, Sodhi N, Hozack WJ, et al. Patient-reported functional and satisfaction outcomes after robotic-arm-assisted total knee arthroplasty: Early results of a prospective multicenter investigation. *J Knee Surg.* 2020;33(7):685–690.

93. Marchand RC, Khlopas A, Sodhi N, et al. Difficult cases in robotic arm-assisted total knee arthroplasty: A case series. *J Knee Surg.* 2018;31:27–37.

94. Sultan AA, Samuel LT, Khlopas A, et al. Robotic-arm assisted total knee arthroplasty more accurately restored the Posterior Condylar Offset Ratio and the Insall-Salvati Index compared to the manual technique; a cohort-matched study. *Surg Technol Int.* 2019;34:409–413.

95. Hampp EL, Chughtai M, Scholl LY, et al. Robotic-arm assisted total knee arthroplasty demonstrated greater accuracy and precision to plan compared with manual techniques. *J Knee Surg*. 2019;32:239–250.

96. Sodhi N, Khlopas A, Piuzzi NS, et al. The learning curve associated with robotic total knee arthroplasty. *J Knee Surg*. 2018;31:17–21.

97. Kayani B, Konan S, Huq SS, et al. Robotic-arm assisted total knee arthroplasty has a learning curve of seven cases for integration into the surgical workflow but no learning curve effect for accuracy of implant positioning. *Knee Surg Sports Traumatol Arthrosc*. 2019;27:1132–1141.

98. Moschetti WE, Konopka JF, Rubash HE, et al. Can robot-assisted unicompartmental knee arthroplasty be cost-effective? A Markov decision analysis. *J Arthroplasty*. 2016;31:759–765.

99. Cool CL, Jacofsky DJ, Seeger KA, et al. A 90-day episode-of-care cost analysis of robotic-arm assisted total knee arthroplasty. *J Comp Eff Res*. 2019;8:327–336.

100. Stindel E, Briard JL, Merloz P, et al. Bone morphing: 3D morphological data for total knee arthroplasty. *Comput Aided Surg*. 2002;7:156–168.

101. Lu TW, Chen HL, Chen SC. Comparisons of the lower limb kinematics between young and older adults when crossing obstacles of different heights. *Gait Posture*. 2006;23:471–479.

102. Koenig JA, Plaskos C. Total knee arthroplasty technique: OMNIbotics. In *Robotics in Knee and Hip Arthroplasty* 2019 (pp. 167–183). Springer, Cham.

103. Suero EM, Plaskos C, Dixon PL, et al. Adjustable cutting blocks improve alignment and surgical time in computer-assisted total knee replacement. *Knee Surg Sports Traumatol Arthrosc*. 2012;20:1736–1741.

104. Koulalis D, O'Loughlin PF, Plaskos C, et al. Sequential versus automated cutting guides in computer-assisted total knee arthroplasty. *Knee*. 2011;18:436–442.

105. Koenig JA, Suero EM, Plaskos C. Surgical accuracy and efficiency of computer-navigated TKA with a robotic cutting guide–report on the first 100 cases. In *Orthopaedic Proceedings* 2012 Oct (Vol. 94, No. SUPP_XLIV, pp. 103–103). The British Editorial Society of Bone & Joint Surgery.

106. Ponder CE, Plaskos C, Cheal EJ. Press-fit total knee arthroplasty with a robotic-cutting guide: proof of concept and initial clinical experience. In *Orthopaedic Proceedings* 2013 Aug (Vol. 95, No. SUPP_28, pp. 61–61). The British Editorial Society of Bone & Joint Surgery.

107. Koenig JA, Shalhoub S, Chen EA, Plaskos C. Accuracy of soft tissue balancing in robotic-assisted measured-resection TKA using a robotic distraction tool. *CAOS*. 2019 Oct 26;3:210–214.

108. Revenga C. *Robotics and Navigation. 2-Year Follow-up in Navigated TKR. Results of a Multi-Centre Study. Prague, Czech Republic*: 16th EFORT Annual Congress; 2015.

109. Revenga C. *2-Year Follow-up of iBlock: Robotic Assisted Surgery Versus Navigation in Total Knee Arthroplasty. Results of a Multicenter Study. Geneva*: 17th EFORT Annual Congress; 2016.

110. Hernández-Vaquero D, Fernández-Carreira J, Revenga-Giertych C, et al. The use of PS or CR models is not sufficient to explain the differences in the results of total knee arthroplasty. Study of interactions. *J Adv Med Med Res*. 2015;12:1–9.

111. Keggi JM, Plaskos C. *Learning curve and early patient satisfaction of robotic assisted total knee arthroplasty*. Boston, MA: International Society for Technology in Arthroplasty; 2016.

112. Keggi JM, Plaskos C. *Surgical efficiency and early patient satisfaction in imageless robotic-assisted total knee arthroplasty*. New York City, NY: International Congress for Joint Reconstruction Transatlantic Orthopaedic Conference; 2016.

113. Koenig JA, Plaskos C. Influence of pre-operative deformity on surgical accuracy and time in robotic-assisted TKA. In *Orthopaedic Proceedings* 2013 Aug (Vol. 95, No. SUPP_28, pp. 62–62). The British Editorial Society of Bone & Joint Surgery.

114. Licini DJ, Meneghini RM. Modern abbreviated computer navigation of the femur reduces blood loss in total knee arthroplasty. *J Arthroplasty*. 2015;30:1729–1732.

115. Casper M, Mitra R, Khare R, et al. Accuracy assessment of a novel image-free handheld robot for total knee arthroplasty in a cadaveric study. *Comput Assist Surg (Abingdon)*. 2018;23:14–20.

116. Jaramaz B, Mitra R, Nikou C, et al. Technique and accuracy assessment of a novel image-free handheld robot for knee arthroplasty in bi-cruciate retaining total knee replacement. *EPiC Ser Health Sci*. 2018;2:98–101.

117. Parratte S, Price AJ, Jeys LM, et al. Accuracy of a new robotically assisted technique for total knee arthroplasty: A cadaveric study. *J Arthroplasty*. 2019;34:2799–2803.

118. Seidenstein A, Birmingham M, Foran J, Ogden S. Better accuracy and reproducibility of a new robotically-assisted system for total knee arthroplasty compared to conventional instrumentation: a cadaveric study. *Knee Surg Sports Traumatol Arthrosc*. 2021 Mar;29(3):859–866.

119. Bargar WL. Robots in orthopaedic surgery: Past, present, and future. *Clin Orthop Relat Res*. 2007;463:31–36.

120. Börner M, Wiesel U, Ditzen W. Clinical Experiences with ROBODOC and the Duracon Total Knee.

Navigation and Robotics in Total Joint and Spine Surgery. Berlin, Heidelberg: Springer Berlin Heidelberg; 2004:362–366.

121. Liow MH, Chin PL, Tay KJ, et al. Early experiences with robot-assisted total knee arthroplasty using the DigiMatch ROBODOC(R) surgical system. *Singap Med J*. 2014;55:529–534.

122. Park SE, Lee CT. Comparison of robotic-assisted and conventional manual implantation of a primary total knee arthroplasty. *J Arthroplasty*. 2007;22:1054–1059.

123. Yang HY, Seon JK, Shin YJ, et al. Robotic total knee arthroplasty with a cruciate-retaining implant: A 10-year follow-up study. *Clin Orthop Surg*. 2017;9:169–176.

124. Cho KJ, Seon JK, Jang WY, et al. Robotic versus conventional primary total knee arthroplasty: Clinical and radiological long-term results with a minimum follow-up of ten years. *Int Orthop*. 2019;43:1345–1354.

125. Liow MHL, Goh GS, Wong MK, et al. Robotic-assisted total knee arthroplasty may lead to improvement in quality-of-life measures: A 2-year follow-up of a prospective randomized trial. *Knee Surg Sports Traumatol Arthrosc*. 2017;25:2942–2951.

126. Song EK, Seon JK, Park SJ, et al. Simultaneous bilateral total knee arthroplasty with robotic and conventional techniques: A prospective, randomized study. *Knee Surg Sports Traumatol Arthrosc*. 2011;19:1069–1076.

127. Schache AG, Blanch P, Rath D, et al. Differences between the sexes in the three-dimensional angular rotations of the lumbo-pelvic-hip complex during treadmill running. *J Sport Sci*. 2003;21:105–118.

128. https://www.jnjmedicaldevices.com/sites/default/files/2021-11/167459-210217%20DSUS_VRAS_MAKO%20Footprint%20Study.pdf.

129. Sharkey PF, Hozack WJ, Rothman RH, et al. Insall Award paper. Why are total knee arthroplasties failing today? *Clin Orthop Relat Res*. 2002;404:7–13.

130. Lombardi Jr. AV, Berend KR, Adams JB. Why knee replacements Fail 2013: Patient, surgeon, implant? *Bone Jt J*. 2014;96-B:101–104.

131. Kuster MS, Bitschnau B, Votruba T. Influence of collateral ligament laxity on patient satisfaction after total knee arthroplasty: A comparative bilateral study. *Arch Orthop Trauma Surg*. 2004;124:415–417.

132. Elmallah RK, Mistry JB, Cherian JJ, et al. Can we really "feel" a balanced total knee arthroplasty? *J Arthroplasty*. 2016;31:102–105.

133. Griffin FM, Insall JN, Scuderi GR. Accuracy of soft tissue balancing in total knee arthroplasty. *J Arthroplasty*. 2000;15:970–973.

134. Wasielewski RC, Galat DD, Komistek RD. An intraoperative pressure-measuring device used in total knee arthroplasties and its kinematics correlations. *Clin Orthop Relat Res*. 2004;427:171–178.

135. D'Lima DD, Colwell CW. Intraoperative measurements and tools to assess stability. *J Am Acad Orthop Surg*. 2017;25(Suppl 1):S29–S32.

136. Plaskos C, Levalee S, Champleboux G. Guiding Device for Bone Cutting. *US Pat*. US 2006/0200161 A1. September 7, 2006.

137. Plaskos C., Levalee S., Rit J. 2016. Robotic Guide Assembly for use in Computer-Aided Surgery. *US Pat*. 9421019B2. August 23, 2016.

138. Shalhoub S, Moschetti WE, Dabuzhsky L, et al. Laxity profiles in the native and replaced knee-application to robotic-assisted gap-balancing total knee arthroplasty. *J Arthroplasty*. 2018;33:3043–3048.

139. D'Lima DD, Patil S, Steklov N, et al. An ABJS Best Paper: Dynamic intraoperative ligament balancing for total knee arthroplasty. *Clin Orthop Relat Res*. 2007;463:208–212.

140. Nielsen ES, Hsu A, Patil S, et al. Second-generation electronic ligament balancing for knee arthroplasty: A cadaver study. *J Arthroplasty*. 2018;33:2293–2300.

141. Nielsen ES, Hsu A, Patil S, Colwell CW, D'Lima DD. Second-generation electronic ligament balancing for knee arthroplasty: A cadaver study. *J Arthroplasty*. 2018;33(7):2293–2300.

142. Gustke K. Use of smart trials for soft-tissue balancing in total knee replacement surgery. *J bone Jt Surg Br*. 2012;94:147–150.

143. Bellemans J. Multiple needle puncturing: Balancing the varus knee. *Orthopedics*. 2011;34:e510–e512.

144. Gustke KA, Golladay GJ, Roche MW, et al. A new method for defining balance: Promising short-term clinical outcomes of sensor-guided TKA. *J Arthroplasty*. 2014;29:955–960.

145. Siong FT, Kim TW, Kim SC, et al. Efficacy and safety of functional medial ligament balancing with stepwise multiple needle puncturing in varus total knee arthroplasty. *J Arthroplasty*. 2020;35:380–387.

146. Chu LM, Meere PA, Oh C, et al. Relationship between surgical balancing and outcome measures in total knees. *Arthroplasty Today*. 2019;5:197–201.

147. Gustke KA. Soft-tissue and alignment correction: the use of smart trials in total knee replacement. *Bone Jt J*. 2014;96-B:78–83.

148. Gustke KA, Golladay GJ, Roche MW, et al. Primary TKA patients with quantifiably balanced soft-tissue achieve significant clinical gains sooner than unbalanced patients. *Adv Orthop*. 2014;2014:628695.

149. Gustke KA, Golladay GJ, Roche MW, et al. Increased satisfaction after total knee replacement using sensor-guided technology. *Bone Jt J*. 2014;96-B:1333–1338.

150. Cho KJ, Seon JK, Jang WY, et al. Objective quantification of ligament balancing using VERASENSE in measured resection and modified gap balance total knee arthroplasty. *BMC Musculoskelet Disord.* 2018;19:266.

151. Nodzo SR, Franceschini V, Gonzalez Della Valle A. Intraoperative load-sensing variability during cemented, posterior-stabilized total knee arthroplasty. *J Arthroplasty.* 2017;32:66–70.

152. Gharaibeh MA, Chen DB, MacDessi SJ. Soft tissue balancing in total knee arthroplasty using sensor-guided assessment: is there a learning curve? *ANZ J Surg.* 2018;88:497–501.

153. Lakra A, Sarpong NO, Jennings EL, et al. The learning curve by operative time for soft tissue balancing in total knee arthroplasty using electronic sensor technology. *J Arthroplasty.* 2019;34:483–487.

154. van der Linde JA, Beath KJ, Leong AKL. The reliability of sensor-assisted soft tissue measurements in primary total knee arthroplasty. *J Arthroplasty.* 2018;33:2502–2505.e2512.

11

Cement Technique

William M. Mihalko, MD, PhD and Joseph Cline, MD

"There is no excuse for poor cement technique!" This quote was heard quite often from Dr. Krackow, and in every case he paid close attention to detail during this step of the total knee arthroscopy (TKA) procedure. Much has changed since the first edition of this textbook, but the polymethylmethacrylate (PMMA) that is used today is the essentially the same as that used in the early 1990s. Many more surgeons are now using a higher viscosity cement, but the one addition that has changed is the more frequent use of antibiotics in the cement. The advantages of adding antibiotics are not a topic for this chapter, and most agree that its use in higher-risk individuals is most likely beneficial. There has also been a surge in the use of cementless fixation in primary TKA, but to date registry information continues to show good long-term survivorship for cemented primary TKA.

Cement can be classified according to viscosity. Low-, medium-, and high-viscosity cements are available from a number of manufacturers. The type of cement surgeons use is greatly influenced by their training and what they have been used to over their residency and fellowship. Dr. Krackow's preference was always a low-viscosity cement. For operating room (OR) efficiency, many surgeons have switched to higher viscosity options because of a shorter time to a "working phase." No matter the choice, surgeons must be familiar with the manufacturer's recommendations for mixing, the working window recommendations, and the need to have a team approach in which everyone in the OR understands the importance of each step of the cementation procedure. An adequate number of assistants to ensure retractors are held in place and an OR technician who has been adequately trained in the manufacturer's procedures to optimally mix and prepare the cement are essential.

STEP 1: EXPOSURE

Proper exposure and retractor placement are essential so that all surfaces to be cemented can be properly prepared. We prefer to have the knee hyperflexed with medial and lateral soft-tissue sleeve retractors and the patella everted. The addition of a posterior cruciate ligament (PCL) type retractor to sublux the tibia forward also is recommended. Adequate exposure of the tibia to allow seating of the baseplate without interference from the femoral surfaces should be ensured (Fig. 11.1).

STEP 2: BONE SURFACE PREPARATION

Any areas on the tibia or distal femur (especially the lateral condyle of a valgus deformed knee) that are sclerotic should be drilled to ensure mechanical penetration into the area for fixation. We find a 2-mm drill bit to be sufficient for this step. Pulse lavage of the tibia/femur and patellar surfaces is then carried out to the point that no "blush" of blood or remnant of fatty fluid from the intramedullary contents is evident. A thorough drying of the surfaces and the keel preparation of the tibia are then carried out, and dry sponges are placed to keep these surfaces dry until ready for cementation (see Fig. 11.1). Adding a small-tip suction to a tibial bone block pin site can aid in keeping any marrow contents from rising to the surface during this drying time. If an intramedullary rod was used for femoral

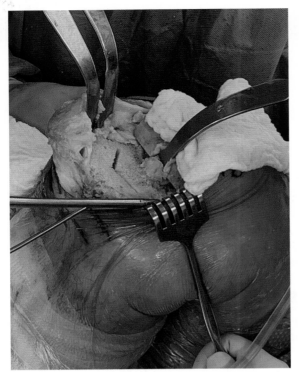

Fig. 11.1 Exposure of entire cancellous bone bed of the tibia should be obtained and the bone cleaned by pulse lavage until no blush from residual blood is evident.

instrumentation, a bone block of the canal also can help keep surfaces dry. Dr. Krackow routinely used thrombin- or epinephrine-soaked sponges on the cancellous bone to enhance drying of the marrow contents.

STEP 3: CEMENT MIXING

Although many surgeons likely take this step for granted, it is extremely important to understand the steps that the manufacturer recommends for the brand of PMMA being used. Some recommend that the liquid monomer go first into the vacuum mixer, whereas others recommend that the powder polymer go in first. Some brands of cement do not recommend mixing lot numbers into the same mixer (most surgeons use two large batches of cement for a primary TKA). Attention to detail matters in this step. Regardless of cement type, we always recommend vacuum mixing and the use of a gun to pressurize the cement into the cancellous bone bed.

STEP 4: CEMENT APPLICATION ONTO IMPLANT SURFACES

It is optimal to make sure application to the metallic implant surfaces is carried out first and that this is done in the first or middle-third time window for the manufacturer's recommended length of working time after mixing is complete. Biomechanical studies have shown that if cement is applied onto the implant surfaces in the latter third of the recommended working window, bond strength to the implant is significantly decreased.[1,2] In this earlier working window the cement may have a sheen to it, and it will better bond to the implant surface. It also will stick to gloves at this point. This is one reason we recommend the use of the gun to apply the cement to the implant surface without touching it at this phase (Fig. 11.2A–B).

STEP 5: BONE SURFACE PRESSURIZATION

There should be a final inspection of the bony surfaces to ensure that there are no marrow contents or irrigation fluid present. While the cement is being prepared, a small metal tip suction placed into the proximal tibial cancellous bone can aid in keeping the cut surface dry and free of marrow contents that can weaken the cement-implant interface (see Fig. 11.1). When dry surfaces are confirmed, the keel and then the tibial cut surface are pressurized (Fig. 11.3). We use the spatula included in most mixing sets to push the cement into the cancellous trabeculae as well. The tibial baseplate is then impacted with care to seat the implant in a symmetrical fashion (Fig. 11.4). This is important to keep the bony envelope of the keel preparation intact and also to ensure equal pressurization of the bony surfaces as the implant is completely impacted. The extruded cement is "cut" (not pulled away) circumferentially from the edges of the baseplate with an elevator.

The femoral surface is then pressurized. Some surgeons like to place a horseshoe of cement on the femoral prepared bony surfaces and then press the cement into the cancellous bone. Dr. Krackow always made certain that he pressurized the cement into the posterior condylar bone cut surfaces as well. We use the spatula to push cement into the cancellous bone in the posterior condylar bone surface (Fig. 11.5). If the cement is not pressurized into the anterior cut under the flange of the implant, there is a tendency for the cement to not penetrate at all

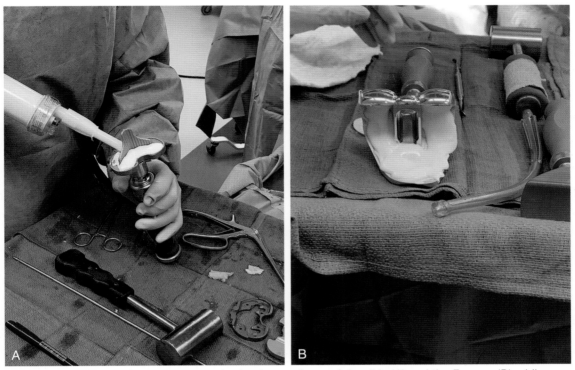

Fig. 11.2 Getting the cement onto the implant surfaces of the tibia (A) and the Femure (B) while the cement is in the initial working window ("sticky" phase) will ensure optimal bonding to the implant.

and just extrude from under the implant, resulting in suboptimal fixation. Again, the femoral component is seated in a symmetrical fashion to ensure equal pressurization of the bony surfaces during insertion. All of the extruded cement is then cut away from the edges of the implant, with specific care to ensure that the remnants of cement around the posterior condyles are cleared. A trial insert that is 2-mm thicker than what was trialed is placed to keep a compression force across the implant, cement, and bone interfaces, and the knee is held in extension while the cement completely sets. We do not recommend flexing the knee while the cement is setting. This can put asymmetrical forces on the tibial baseplate interface and affect the long-term strength of the cement interface.

The patellar button is then cemented and inserted, and it is held with a compression clamp. Again, the extruded cement is cut away from the edges of the implant, and the clamp is kept in place until the cement is completely set.

STEP 6: LET THE CEMENT COMPLETELY SET

It is important to keep the knee in extension during the setting phase of the PMMA. If the knee is taken through a range of motion or if soft-tissue balancing is tested before complete setting of the cement, movement in the cement mantle can produce stress risers and a propensity for early loosening. The surgeon should resist the urge to irrigate too early or to insert the final polyethylene before complete setting, because both of these maneuvers can affect the strength of the cement-implant interface. Many polyethylene locking mechanisms can impart a shear force to the baseplate in the anterior-posterior direction, and insertion should not be performed until the cement has completely finished its setting phase.

When done properly, the cemented interfaces will be seen as penetrating all bony cut surfaces along the implant interface. When this is verified on postoperative radiographs, the cemented interface should have

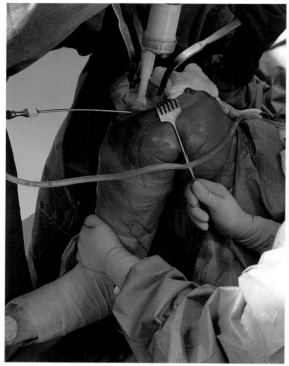

Fig. 11.3 Using the gun allows for pressurization of the cancellous bone bed.

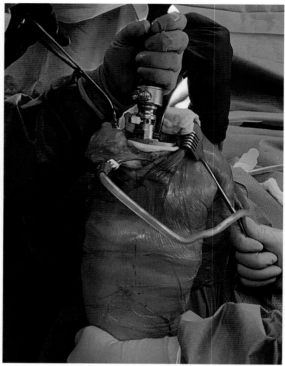

Fig. 11.4 Impacting the implant until fully seated and then cutting the excess cement from the periphery is performed to assure no cement is pulled away from the implant bone interface.

a good chance for survivorship over the long term (15+ years).[3–5]

BIOMECHANICAL STUDIES

Multiple biomechanical studies have supported the discussed techniques because of their ability to provide improved implant stability at both the bone-cement and cement-implant interfaces.[6–9] In their cadaver study of tibial baseplate failures Nagel et al.[6] demonstrated that a threshold cement penetration of 1.1 mm was required for failure of the proximal tibial bone compared with failure at the cement-bone interface in a test of pullout strength. The techniques described have been demonstrated to provide improved cement penetration into trabecular bone. Schlegel et al.[7] showed that high-pressure pulsatile lavage resulted in better cement penetration compared with low-pressure irrigation in cadaver tibiae, with mean 1.32-mm penetration in the

lavage group compared with 0.79 mm in the bulb irrigation group. This depth resulted in improved median pullout strength of 1275 N compared with 568 N in the bulb-irrigated tibiae. Of note, all the failures in the pulse lavage group occurred at the cement-implant interface, whereas failure of five of the six tibiae in the bulb irrigation group occurred at the bone-cement interface. An in vivo study of TKAs cemented using syringe irrigation compared with high-pressure lavage by Ritter et al.[8] showed a statistically significant higher incidence of radiolucency around the tibial stem in the group treated with syringe irrigation at 5-year follow-up ($P < .001$).

Use of a pressurizing cement gun rather than finger-packing cement on the tibia was also shown to lead to a statistically significant increase in cement penetration of cancellous bone by Vanlommel et al.[10] in a Sawbones model, lending further stability to the implant. In their study use of the cement gun led to

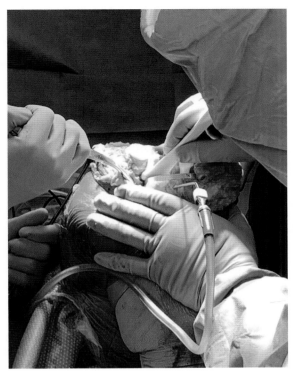

Fig. 11.5 Applying cement on the femur in a horseshoe fashion and using the spatula to pressurize the posterior condylar cancellous bone bed and all surfaces is carried out last. Once impacted the cement is cut from the interface in the same manner as for the tibia but care needs to be taken that all cement is removed from the top of the posterior condyles as well.

an average penetration of 5.6 mm of the proximal tibia compared with the finger-packing technique, which on average only reached 3.8 mm. Billi et al.[1] showed that adding cement to the keel of the tibial component rather than just the tray also increased strength to failure, with mean increases of 153% and 147% in their acyclic knee model with two studied cements.

The importance of clean cement and implant surfaces also has been proven biomechanically. In a study examining the effect of marrow fat contamination of the cement-implant interface in an acrylic model Billi et al.[1] demonstrated a decrease in failure strength of 99% and 97% in the two cements tested compared with samples with no contamination. Adding cement to the tibial tray immediately while still having fat contamination on the tibial cement resulted in fat at the cement-cement

interface and a mean decrease in strength of 65% and 43% in their two samples.

Timing of cement application also has been studied extensively in regard to strength of fixation. Billi et al[1]. examined the effect of early and late cement application to tibial components compared with the normal, manufacturer-recommended time. Whereas early cementation resulted in an increased load to failure of 48% and 72% in the two cements studied, late cementation caused a similar decrease in strength of 47% and 73% compared with the samples cemented in the standard, recommended time frame. Grupp et al.[2] similarly showed a trend of decreasing strength of the implant interface with increasing cement times in an acrylic knee model, although the trend reached statistical significance when the later third of the recommended working time was used to apply high-viscosity cement to the implant (Cobalt, DJO Surgical, Vista, CA; Palacos, Zimmer-Biomet Inc, Warsaw IN; DePuy HVC, Depuy Inc., Warsaw, IN).

LONG-TERM RESULTS

The long history of cemented TKA has allowed study of its survivorship and mechanisms of failure. In a postmortem study of 12 implanted TKAs that examined the cement-trabecular bone interdigitation Miller et al.[11] found that increased time since implantation was correlated with higher trabecular bone resorption and decreased cement interdigitation depth. A contact fraction was generated as a marker of retained fixation by randomly generating points at the interface and determining whether there was cement-bone contact at these points. They found a contact fraction of less than 10% in knees that had been in place more than 10 years compared with a contact fraction of 40.9% in cadaver knees at initial evaluation. Similarly, the five knees that had been in place for more than 10 years had on average an interdigitation depth of 0.4 mm compared with 1.13 mm in the seven knees that had been in place for less than 10 years. Despite this evidence of loss of cement-bone fixation with time, cemented TKA has an excellent track record for survivorship. In a review by Montonen et al.[12] of several cemented cruciate-retaining TKA designs in the Finnish Arthroplasty Register and NZOA Joint Registry 10-year survival rates ranged between 94% and 96% for the cruciate-retaining designs with all-cause revision as the endpoint.

A review of the New Zealand joint registry by Nugent et al.[4] demonstrated similarly high rates of survivorship at 10 years, with cemented total knees at 97%. They also compared cemented TKA to uncemented and hybrid TKA designs and found cemented implants to have equivalent Oxford Knee Scores at 10-year follow-up, with higher survival rates (97% vs. 94.5%) compared with uncemented designs. They found a revision rate of 0.47 per 100 component years for cemented TKA compared with 0.74 per 100 component years for uncemented implants. Overall, cemented TKA has demonstrated excellent long-term results and retention. With the increased study of various cement techniques, these outcomes should continue to improve.[3–5]

Some who advocate cementless fixation point to the evidence on decreasing trabecular contact and cement penetration depth after 10 years as a reason to use a biological interface. Some reports note that pain scores tend to rise between 10 and 15 years after cemented primary TKA.[5]

In summary, a cement-implant interface seems to remain a durable option for primary TKA. Proper technique must be adhered to during the procedure to ensure longevity of the fixation. This can be the weak link of the procedure because, if not done properly, it can doom the total joint arthroplasty to early aseptic loosening and untimely revision surgery.

REFERENCES

1. Billi F, Kavanaugh A, Schmalzried H, Schmalzried TP. Techniques for improving the initial strength of the tibial tray-cement interface bond. *Bone Joint J.* 2019; 101-B(1_Supple_A):53–58. https://doi.org/10.1302/0301-620X.101B1.BJJ-2018-0500.R1.

2. Grupp TM, Schilling C, Schwiesau J, Pfaff A, Altermann B, Mihalko WM. Tibial implant fixation behavior in total knee arthroplasty: a study with five different bone cements. *J Arthroplasty.* 2020;35(2):579–587. https://doi.org/10.1016/j.arth.2019.09.019.

3. Sartawi M, Zurakowski D, Rosenberg A. Implant survivorship and complication rates after total knee arthroplasty with a third-generation cemented system: 15-year follow-up. *Am J Orthop (Belle Mead NJ).* 2018;47(3). https://doi.org/10.12788/ajo.2018.0018. 10.12788/ajo.2018.0018.

4. Nugent M, Wyatt MC, Frampton CM, Hooper GJ. Despite improved survivorship of uncemented fixation in total knee arthroplasty for osteoarthritis, cemented fixation remains the gold standard: an analysis of a national joint registry. *J Arthroplasty.* 2019;34(8): 1626–1633. https://doi.org/10.1016/j.arth.2019.03.047.

5. Rodriguez JA, Bhende H, Ranawat CS. Total condylar knee replacement: a 20-year followup study. *Clin Orthop Relat Res.* 2001;388:10–17.

6. Nagel K, Bishop NE, Schlegel UJ, Püschel K, Morlock MM. The influence of cement morphology parameters on the strength of the cement-bone interface in tibial tray fixation. *J Arthroplasty.* 2017;32(2):563–569. https://doi.org/10.1016/j.arth.2016.08.013.

7. Schlegel UJ, Siewe J, Delank KS, et al. Pulsed lavage improves fixation strength of cemented tibial components. *Int Orthop.* 2011;35(8):1165–1169. https://doi.org/10.1007/s00264-010-1137-y.

8. Ritter MA, Herbst SA, Keating EM, Faris PM. Radiolucency at the bone-cement interface in total knee replacement. The effects of bone-surface preparation and cement technique. *J Bone Joint Surg Am.* 1994;76(1):60–65. https://doi.org/10.2106/00004623-199401000-00008.

9. Grupp TM, Saleh KJ, Holderied M, et al. Primary stability of tibial plateaus under dynamic compression-shear loading in human tibiae—Influence of keel length, cementation area and tibial stem. *J Biomech.* 2017; 59:9–22.

10. Vanlommel J, Luyckx JP, Labey L, Innocenti B, De Corte R, Bellemans J. Cementing the tibial component in total knee arthroplasty: which technique is the best? *J Arthroplasty.* 2011;26(3):492–496. https://doi.org/10.1016/j.arth.2010.01.107.

11. Miller MA, Goodheart JR, Izant TH, Rimnac CM, Cleary RJ, Mann KA. Loss of cement-bone interlock in retrieved tibial components from total knee arthroplasties. *Clin Orthop Relat Res.* 2014;472(1):304–313. https://doi.org/10.1007/s11999-013-3248-4.

12. Montonen E, Laaksonen I, Matilainen M, et al. What is the long-term survivorship of cruciate-retaining TKA in the Finnish registry? *Clin Orthop Relat Res.* 2018 Jun; 476(6):1205–1211. https://doi.org/10.1007/s11999.0000000000000202.

Postoperative TKA Considerations

12

Avoiding Peri- and Postoperative Management After Total Knee Arthroplasty

Evgeny Dyskin, MD, PhD

Surgical complication is defined as "any undesirable, unintended and direct result of an operation affecting the patient, which would not have occurred had the operation gone as well as could reasonably be hoped." (p. 942)[1]

The rate of complications or adverse events after primary total knee arthroplasty (TKA) ranges from 6.1% to 37.1% depending on geography, economic status, and inclusion criteria. The cost of readmissions and rehospitalizations resulting from complications has reached $7.1 billion.[2,3]

Initially, classifications of surgical adverse events were developed by general surgeons and later applied to the field of orthopedics.[4] A descriptive list of the 22 most pertinent complications after TKA was created by the consensus of experts.[5]

There are numerous postoperative complications. However, deep periprosthetic joint infection, stiffness, instability, and mechanical failure of an endoprosthesis top the list and remain the leading causes of failure after TKA.[6]

The etiology of deep joint sepsis is multifactorial and includes numerous nonmodifiable and modifiable conditions. Acute postoperative wound complications, hematoma formation, postoperative blood transfusions, prolonged hospital stays, and hematogenous disseminations from endogenous and exogenous (e.g., indwelling urinary catheters) sources have been related to the development of deep periprosthetic infections.

WOUND ISSUES

Severity of wound problems can range from quickly resolved sanguinous drainage and superficial skin eschars to full-thickness capsular necrosis with exposed endoprosthesis and generalized sepsis.

Postoperative wound drainage is a common problem after TKA because of the close proximity of a bulky implant and naturally tenuous soft tissue coverage. Drainage affects 0.33% to 10% of patients undergoing TKA. The drainage is considered substantial when it soaks more than 2×2 cm area of gauze, and lasts more than 72 hours after surgery.[7] Tense subcutaneous hematomas and intra-articular fluid escape through capsular defects that can manifest as relatively benign "rose wine" appearing leakage through slightly dehisced edges of the inferior portion of the surgical wound. In many cases the drainage resolves after spontaneous evacuation of a superficial hematoma; however, it can also lead to backflow implant seeding through direct communication with deep joint space.

Onset of drainage varies from immediate soaking through the dressings in a postoperative area to several hours or days after an increase in physical activity. The classic rule of "no patient who has a draining wound should be discharged from the hospital" has become less relevant as contemporary TKA has moved to outpatient settings. In an outpatient setting the surgeon should provide the patient and visiting nursing personnel with explicit wound care instructions. Substantial wound drainage (as described previously) prompts immediate evaluation in the surgeon's office, where the wound and the joint are inspected for signs of dehiscence, subcutaneous fluctuating hematoma, and tense hemarthrosis. Moderate amounts of serosanguinous drainage, good approximation of skin edges with minimal necrosis, and presumable good integrity of the capsule indicate nonoperative management with sterile, compressive, absorbent dressings; immobilization in extension; rest; and discontinuation of physical therapy. The efficacy of a novel treatment modality, negative pressure wound therapy, remains unproven; furthermore, it can potentially delay time of surgical débridement.[8]

Manual or ultrasound-guided aspiration of substantial intraarticular and subcutaneous fluid collections is possible under strict aseptic conditions in the medical office or in a radiology suite settings.

Considerations are also given for adjustment or even discontinuation of chemical anticoagulation therapy, but mechanical prophylaxis needs to be continued. Reflexive preventive administration of antibiotics is strongly discouraged because of minimal efficacy and potential association with serious complications such as adverse systemic effects, emerging bacterial antibiotic resistance, and beclouding of deep joint infection.[7,9]

Drainage related to excessive local bleeding and chemical anticoagulation usually stops within 5 to 7 days. Drainage, lasting more than a week is unlikely to stop and requires surgical intervention to prevent backflow contamination. If left untreated, drainage can be associated with as much as a 50% increase in deep periprosthetic infection rates. Surgical The procedure starts with careful wound exploration, débridement and evacuation of subcutaneous fluid collections. Static and dynamic examination of capsular repair is performed to detect fluid egress through the defects. If the capsule is intact and tense hemarthrosis is present, the knee can be aspirated from outside of the wound to decompress the joint and obtain material for microbiological analysis. In that case the skin is closed over a drain without opening the deep space. If the joint capsule is compromised, the surgeon proceeds further with arthrotomy, synovectomy, tibial insert exchange, implant-bone interface débridement, irrigation, and watertight monofilament capsular closure over a closed-suction drain. Multiple cultures must be collected to detect deep joint infection and guide antibiotic therapy.

Periarticular skin and deep soft tissue necrosis represents another complication after TKA. Etiology includes preexisting skin compromises caused by steroid intake, poor surgical technique, forceful wound retraction, tourniquet usage, and excessive anticoagulation, particularly with vitamin K antagonists. Prognosis and management depend on the depth of necrosis. When skin breakdown is superficial and does not involve the capsule, local wound care with delayed staged excisional débridement remains the standard of care. Deep soft tissue necrosis with capsular involvement requires aggressive surgical débridement and advanced soft tissue coverage procedures, such as local and free musculocutaneous flaps with early plastic surgery involvement.

Patients after TKA retain a 1% to 10% life-long risk of deep periprosthetic joint infection. The majority of complications (60% to 70%) happens within the first 2 years after surgery. The mechanism of late infection remains unclear; however, hematogenous seeding from remote sources has been noted in 6% of patients who have documented bacteremia. Microbiological suspects range from a variety of gram-negative and gram-positive species, but *Staphylococcus aureus* represents 30% to 40% of remote seeding cases. Traditionally, orthopedic surgery and dental governing bodies advocated for a 2-year-long prophylactic administration of antibiotics before invasive dental and surgical procedures. Recommendations were based on anecdotal data, underpowered cohort studies, and clinical analogy with endocarditis.[10] Broad-spectrum antibiotics from the cephalosporin, aminoglycoside, macrolide, and fluoroquinolone families have been used to cover gram-positive and gram-negative species. For example, oral intake of 600 mg of clindamycin, 2 g of amoxicillin, 2 g of cephalexin, or 800 mg of erythromycin was recommended 1 hour before a dental procedure. Genitourinary and gastrointestinal interventions required intravenous administration of 80 mg of gentamycin or 2 g of ampicillin.[11] Recent evidence from rigorous studies was unable to identify increased risk of deep joint infection after oral procedures; furthermore, preprocedural antibiotic prophylaxis failed to prevent the development of subsequent periprosthetic infection. Currently, the American Academy of Orthopedic Surgeons is unable to recommend for or against the use of oral antibiotics and even encourages providers to discontinue routine prophylaxis before dental procedures. Patients are encouraged to maintain good oral hygiene.[8,12] Routine antimicrobial prophylaxis is also not recommended before genitourinary or lower gastrointestinal endoscopy. The topic of postoperative prophylaxis with antibacterial agents remains highly controversial, suggesting that management needs to be individualized based on each patient's needs.

POSTOPERATIVE RADIOGRAPHIC ANALYSES

Radiography is an essential part of a follow-up process after TKA. It helps to monitor mechanical well-being of the endoprosthesis and to ensure early detection of complications that are still clinically asymptomatic, such as structural wear and breakdown, loosening with progressive malalignment, instability, and disruption of the extensor apparatus. Radiographic findings are used to modify a follow-up schedule and contemplate preemptive treatment to prevent further mechanical damage and preserve long-term knee function.

A systematic approach is required to detect subtle changes. Ideal postoperative radiographs include three standard views of the knee obtained under weight-bearing conditions: anteroposterior, lateral, and skyline views of the patellofemoral joint. It is also advisable to acquire weight-bearing anteroposterior images of the entire lower extremity (bone-length, hip-to-ankle radiographs) once a year. Weight load unmasks the joint's alignment, ligamentous laxity, and tibial plastic wear.[13]

Each radiograph is analyzed for implant positioning, structural competence, relationships among different components of the endoprosthesis, maintenance of bone-prosthesis interface, and integrity of the adjacent osseous and soft tissue envelope.

The term "implant positioning" assumes relationships between the mechanical axis of the extremity (alignment) and its corresponding bony structures (bone coverage). The mechanical axis of the extremity is drawn on anteroposterior standing radiographs and ideally should be perpendicular to the joint line and pass through the center of the knee. The relationship to the anatomical axis can also be used if only short anteroposterior radiographs are available. Medial distal femoral anatomical and medial proximal tibial angles should be approximately 95 degrees and 90 degrees, respectively. It is important to remember that these measures can be skewed by the presence of abnormal tibial and femoral curves. Coronal malalignment may result in asymmetrical stress redistribution along mechanical interfaces, increased polyethylene wear, and early component loosening.[14–16]

Sagittal plane alignment assessment includes analysis of posterior tibia slope and the flexion-extension relationship of the femoral component to the distal aspect of the femur on a lateral radiograph. The femoral component should be in a neutral position, demonstrating appropriate posterior offset to ensure proper balance of collateral ligaments. Hyperextension of a femoral component increases the chances of notching the anterior femoral cortex and may result in a periprosthetic fracture and decreased knee flexion. Hyperflexion can lead to internal impingement between the patella and proud anterior flange of the femur, manifesting as stiffness, knee pain, and locking of the patellofemoral articulation.

The amount of anteroposterior slope of a tibial component depends on the design. Most cruciate-retaining baseplates require 3 to 7 degrees of posterior slope to ensure appropriate femoral roll back, whereas posterior-stabilized tibial trays are implanted with a 0 degree slope to prevent instability of the peg in the femoral box during flexion. Excessive anterior or posterior inclination of a baseplate can lead to instability in extension or flexion.

The prosthesis should follow natural anatomy and sit snugly on cortical surfaces. Undersized components tend to subside, whereas oversized components incline to impinge against soft tissues, leading to pain and stiffness. A small lateral projection of a femoral component is acceptable; however, anterior and medial overhang of a femoral component and posterior overhang of a tibial tray should be avoided.

Patellar alignment directly and indirectly reflects the state of an extensor apparatus of the knee, and it is best evaluated on lateral and skyline views. On a good lateral radiograph, the patella aligns against the middle portion of the femoral component with its inferior pole corresponding to the tibiofemoral joint line. Sagittal stance of the patella in relation to the tibiofemoral joint can be described via various formulae, based on ratios between the length of the infrapatellar tendon and the vertical size of the patella (e.g., Insall-Salvati and Caton-Deschamps ratio). An excessively raised tibiofemoral joint line, scarring of an infrapatellar tendon, or a tear of the quadriceps tendon lead to a low-lying patella (patella baja). Patella baja can affect knee kinematics and result in pain and stiffness, whereas high-standing patella (patella alta) can represent acute or chronic tears of the infrapatellar tendon.

Femoral and tibial components should maintain anatomical relationships with congruent matching through the radiolucent shadow of the polyethylene insert. The patellar component should occupy the medial two-thirds of the patellar bone stump and perfectly match the groove of the anterior femoral flange on a skyline view. Lateral position of the patella predisposes it to maltracking and subluxation and can reflect axial malrotation of femoral and tibial pieces.

Parameters, such as bone-component apposition, presence of radiolucent lines, and condition of a cement mantle, are used to describe the quality of prosthetic fixation and assess stability of a prosthesis.

Ideally, press-fit components should maintain intimate contact with corresponding osseous surfaces without interposed radiolucent lines. In cases of cemented fixation uniform 2 to 3 mm cement penetration into distal femoral and proximal tibial metaphyseal cancellous bone is desired.

Radiographic follow-up after TKA requires weight-bearing anteroposterior, lateral, and skyline views. Radiographs are often obtained at 6 weeks, 3 months, 6 months, 1 year, and then every 2 years after surgery. Radiographic goniometry is performed on standing bone-length radiographs as a reference for future follow-up measurements.[17] Particular attention is paid to maintenance of the alignment, condition of the bone-prosthesis interface and cement mantle, and congruence of tibiofemoral and patellofemoral articulations.

Changes in the alignment can be due to subsidence, mechanical wear of the components, alterations in bony anatomy, or changes in limb rotation compared with previous radiographs. Because of force distribution and asymmetrical density of proximal tibial and distal femoral metaphyseal bones, the tibial component typically subsides into varus and extension whereas the femoral component drifts into more flexed position. Instability of the patellar button manifests as lateral subluxation and asymmetrical rotation of the component along the longitudinal axis, observed on a skyline view, or complete dislodgement of the component.

Ideally, the bone-prosthesis interface is characterized by a fluent transition between opposing surfaces; however, the picture is often complicated by the presence of radiolucent lines beneath components of the endoprosthesis. Their importance depends on size, thickness, and progression. Lines can be complete (surrounding the entire component), partial, stable or progressive. Thin (less than 1 mm) stable lucencies, adjacent to the tibial tray and the stem, are acceptable as long as they appear and remain stable within the first 6 months for cemented implants and the first 2 years for cementless implants. Increase in size and development of focal lucencies thicker than 2 mm may signify aseptic or septic loosening of the component. Assessment of the radiolucent lines remains mostly subjective because current scoring systems are unreliable and overly sophisticated for practical usage.[17–19]

Tibial insert wear can lead to instability, osteolysis, and mechanical damage caused by direct contact between metallic parts of the prosthesis. The plastic piece maintains a uniform, at least 8-mm thick, radiolucent space between femoral and tibial components. Progressive uniform or asymmetrical narrowing of the joint space represents polyethylene wear. In cases of plastic insert dissociation and fragmentation direct contact between femoral and tibial components occurs, and a shadow of the liner can be seen outside of its normal position.

Tibial, femoral, and patellar bone stocks can be affected by fractures and osteolysis. Osteolysis usually manifests as a radiolucent lesion adjacent to the prosthetic components. Typical locations include the posterior femoral condyles, the edge of a tibial tray or stem, areas around the patellar button, or fixation pegs or screws. Osteolysis is typically associated with polyethylene wear.

Any change in the alignment of the extremity and prosthetic components, progression of radiolucent lines, changes in size and shape of a joint space, or focal lesions in supporting osseous structures should raise concern and warrant correlation with clinical symptoms and further investigation into potential underlying conditions, such as infection or aseptic loosening. The patient requires more frequent follow-up visits or even early revision surgery to avoid irreparable damage to the prosthesis and anatomical structures of the knee.

Patients after TKA carry a small, but nonnegligible, risk of adverse events; therefore they need lifelong follow-up to ensure appropriate function of the endoprosthesis and to prevent complications.

POSTOPERATIVE FOLLOW-UP VISITS

Each follow-up visit requires clinical and radiographic assessment of the soft tissue envelope, knee function, and mechanical integrity of the endoprosthesis. A typical follow-up schedule includes appointments at 2 and 6 weeks, 3 and 6 months, 1 and 2 years, and every 2 years thereafter.

The goal of the first visit is to ensure appropriate progress of wound healing, adequacy of pain control, and compliance with physical therapy. Radiographs are usually not required during the first appointment. Pain usually subsides to a moderate level at this point; however, the patient may still require additional support with oral opioid medications in tapering dosages for another 2 to 4 weeks. The patient usually ambulates with an appreciable antalgic limp using assistive walking devices. The wound must be completely clean and dry with well-approximated and viable skin edges. If any drainage is noticed at the 2-week visit, irrigation and débridement to prevent deep infection should be considered. The knee at this point may be moderately swollen and tender to palpation. Range of motion varies at this first visit, but there should be a minimal flexion contracture (5 to 10 degrees) and flexion to 90 degrees. If flexion is <90 degrees, an earlier second visit at 4 or 5 weeks can be scheduled. Then if there is no further improvement, manipulation under anesthesia should be considered.

The main milestone of a 6-week appointment is to demonstrate at least 90 degrees of flexion and full extension; otherwise, manipulation under anesthesia is recommended during the next 2 weeks.[20] The first set of standard radiographs is obtained during this visit. Long-leg standing imaging is also possible during this visit if the patient is comfortable enough to stand with a fully extended knee.

By 3 months, patients approach maximum active range of motion of the knee and transition to independent ambulation.[21] If the knee remains unacceptably stiff, a surgical intervention can be discussed because improvements are typically minimal past the 3-month mark. The topic of functional range of motion remains debatable; however, in Western culture the achievement of full extension and 110 degrees of flexion is considered as a success after TKA.[20]

Pain and swelling usually completely resolve and the patient's level of physical activity gradually increases 6 to 12 months after surgery. It is important to notice any negative change in objective or subjective symptoms. Spontaneously increased pain, swelling, a feeling of instability, and change in alignment should raise a red flag and trigger further investigations into the cause of the symptoms.

RETURN TO PREVIOUS ACTIVITIES

The majority of previously employed patients return to work after TKA.[22] The length of disability depends on individual progress of recovery and physical requirements of the job. Patients working sedentary jobs are allowed to return whenever they can safely get to work, usually within 6 weeks after surgery. It is important for patients to be able to periodically elevate the operated extremity and walk around during business hours.

Patients can return to light-duty jobs that require more standing and walking whenever they can ambulate without a limp, which is generally around 12 weeks after surgery.

Patients performing heavy-duty work require longer rehabilitation, up to 6 months after surgery. Obviously, individual exceptions are possible.

Return to driving entails discontinuation of opioid pain medications and ability to safely accelerate and decelerate the vehicle. Subjective safe brake response is required after right-sided surgery; as for left TKA, the decision is deferred to the patient.[22]

POSTOPERATIVE PAIN CONTROL

TKA is associated with intense postoperative pain. For the majority of patients, the worst pain period occurs during the first 2 weeks after surgery while the patients are at home. Almost half of the patients describe pain as severe and extreme during that time.[23] Postoperative pain control is affected by economic pressure for early hospital discharge and public scrutiny perceiving opioids as a frequent path to addiction.

Pain management after TKA actually starts before surgery by setting appropriate expectations, educating, and reducing consumption of long-acting opioids in patients who have a history of chronic pain. It is important to establish risk factors for chronic pain after TKA such as poor mental health, presence of multiple medical comorbidities, high-intensity knee pain, pain elsewhere, history of chronic pain, or pain catastrophizing.[24]

Postoperative pain is controlled via pharmacological and nonpharmacological techniques. Pharmacological interventions remain the first line of treatment and include consumption of weak short-acting oral opioids, acetaminophen, nonsteroidal antiinflammatory drugs, COX-2 inhibitors, and gabapentinoids. Opioid medications are reserved for moderate to severe pain; their usage should be gradually tapered off by the 6-week mark after surgery.

Nonpharmacological modalities are heavily supported; they include cryotherapy, compressive dressings, elevation of the extremity, physical therapy with possible inclusion of electrotherapy, and acupuncture.

Pain after TKA usually plateaus 3 to 6 months after surgery; however, 16% to 33% of patients report chronic pain and discomfort lasting past their anticipated recovery time.[24] From a surgeon's perspective, chronic pain can be classified as surgery-related and surgery-unrelated types. Surgery-related pain originates from complications after TKA and malfunction of the endoprosthesis. Infection, prosthesis loosening, instability, internal impingement because of oversizing and malpositioning of the components, and localized nerve injuries frequently manifest with pain. Surgery-unrelated issues include pain originating from the ipsilateral hip or lumbar spine, vascular obstruction, and other generalized or poorly understood problems such as complex regional pain syndrome, fibromyalgia, and metabolic neuropathy. Management of those conditions is usually deferred to specialists in appropriate fields of medicine. Pain management consultation is occasionally required.

CONCLUSION

Patients require lifelong follow-up with regular radiographic examination after TKA in order to detect subtle changes and prevent avoidable complications. Standard postoperative antibiotic prophylaxis remains highly controversial, and routine prophylaxis before dental procedures is not currently recommended. Postoperative pain management includes pharmacological and nonpharmacological approaches with judicious use of oral opioid medications.

REFERENCES

1. Sokol DK, Wilson J. What is a surgical complication? *World J Surg.* 2008;32(6):942–944.
2. Huddleston J, et al. Adverse events in total knee arthroplasty: A national Medicare study. *J Arthroplasty.* 2009;24(2):e6.
3. Raddaoui K, et al. Perioperative morbidity in total knee arthroplasty. *Pan Afr Med J.* 2019;33:233.
4. Iorio R, et al. Stratification of standardized TKA complications and adverse events: A brief communication. *Clin Orthop Relat Res.* 2014;472(1):194–205.
5. Healy WL, et al. Complications of total knee arthroplasty: Standardized list and definitions of the Knee Society. *Clin Orthop Relat Res.* 2013;471(1):215–220.
6. Le DH, et al. Current modes of failure in TKA: Infection, instability, and stiffness predominate. *Clin Orthop Relat Res.* 2014;472(7):2197–2200.
7. Simons MJ, Amin NH, Scuderi GR. Acute wound complications after total knee arthroplasty: Prevention and management. *J Am Acad Orthop Surg.* 2017;25(8):547–555.
8. Siqueira MB, et al. Role of negative pressure wound therapy in total hip and knee arthroplasty. *World J Orthop.* 2016;7(1):30–37.
9. Daines BK, Dennis DA, Amann S. Infection prevention in total knee arthroplasty. *J Am Acad Orthop Surg.* 2015;23(6):356–364.
10. Tande AJ, Patel R. Prosthetic joint infection. *Clin Microbiol Rev.* 2014;27(2):302–345.
11. Illingworth KD, et al. How to minimize infection and thereby maximize patient outcomes in total joint arthroplasty: A multicenter approach: AAOS exhibit selection. *J Bone Joint Surg Am.* 2013;95(8):e50.
12. Slullitel PA, et al. Is there a role for antibiotic prophylaxis prior to dental procedures in patients with total joint arthroplasty? A systematic review of the literature. *J Bone Jt Infect.* 2020;5(1):7–15.
13. Kumar N, et al. How to interpret postoperative X-rays after total knee arthroplasty. *Orthop Surg.* 2014;6(3):179–186.
14. Li Z, et al. Polyethylene damage increases with varus implant alignment in posterior-stabilized and constrained condylar knee arthroplasty. *Clin Orthop Relat Res.* 2017;475(12):2981–2991.
15. Ritter MA, et al. The effect of alignment and BMI on failure of total knee replacement. *J Bone Joint Surg.* 2011;93(17):1588–1596.
16. Lee BS, et al. Femoral component varus malposition is associated with tibial aseptic loosening after TKA. *Clin Orthop Relat Res.* 2018;476(2):400–407.
17. Cyteval C. Imaging of knee implants and related complications. *Diagn Interv Imaging.* 2016;97(7-8):809–821.
18. Meneghini RM, et al. Development of a modern knee society radiographic evaluation system and methodology for total knee arthroplasty. *J Arthroplasty.* 2015;30(12):2311–2314.
19. Bach CM, et al. Radiographic assessment in total knee arthroplasty. *Clin Orthop Relat Res.* 2001;385:144–150.
20. Manrique J, Gomez MM, Parvizi J. Stiffness after total knee arthroplasty. *J Knee Surg.* 2015;28(02):119–126.
21. Bade MJ, Kohrt WM, Stevens-Lapsley JE. Outcomes before and after total knee arthroplasty compared to healthy adults. *J Orthop Sports Phys Ther.* 2010;40(9):559–567.
22. Lombardi AV, et al. Do patients return to work after total knee arthroplasty? *Clin Orthop Relat Res.* 2014;472(1):138–146.
23. Chan E, et al. Acute postoperative pain following hospital discharge after total knee arthroplasty. *Osteoarthr Cartil.* 2013;21(9):1257–1263.
24. Wylde V, et al. Chronic pain after total knee arthroplasty. *EFORT Open Rev.* 2018;3(8):461–470.

13

Complications of Total Knee Arthroplasty and Evidence Basis for Outcomes of Knee Arthroplasty

Mohan K. Puttaswamy, MD and John M. Tarazi, MD

The scientific basis for total knee arthroscopy (TKA) has had an interesting and exciting journey over the last five decades. A few pragmatic and visionary surgeons laid foundational principles, moderated the designs, and founded this specialty. I have no doubt that Dr. Krackow was among those select few. Dr. Krackow believed in an equitable distribution of opportunity and propagation of knowledge across borders for the benefit of humanity. The eclectic bunch of fellows from various backgrounds whom he encouraged and recruited stands testimony to that philosophy. His prescience in recording audio during patient counseling and providing one tape to the patient and retaining one for internal documentation is a genius technique to avoid long-term dissonance if there are adverse outcomes and to encourage family members to partake in decision making in absentia. He encouraged intellectual debate and insisted on hands-on training of fellows and residents with paternal firmness and rigorous academic pursuit. His patient-counseling strategy always began with no assumption of patient knowledge of disease pathology and progressed on to the usage of metal and plastic to accomplish pain relief described in simple language. He combined science, humor, and grace to convey information, and his sartorial taste communicated class and confidence in his surgical skills. This compendium is a tribute to a great human being, excellent teacher, and a master artisan.

Patients who have knee arthritis present mostly with a painful, stiff knee with or without deformity with significant limitations in the quality of life (QOL). The expectation after a knee arthroplasty is a long-lasting, pain-free functional range to full range of motion (ROM) with no deformity. The surgeon's role is to educate the patient about the possibility of success and help define a successful outcome from the patient's perspective. *The desirable outcomes after knee arthroplasty are symptomatic relief, recovery of function and restoration of desirable alignment.* One of the important aspects of the surgical discussions with patients involves reviewing the risk of surgical complications. *Knee arthroplasty surgery does provoke anxiety in some patients and a candid discussion helps to clear doubts about the surgery.* Evidence-based discussion on complications eases anxiety and helps with objective decision making.

Each surgeon's philosophy of patient counseling evolves over time, with contributions from mentors, patient behavior, societal expectation, and cultural imperatives. The fundamental question is how much information is too much for the patient in decision-making. The surgical discussion has ethical, moral, and legal dimensions. The information provided should be factually accurate and balanced about the advantages, limitations, and success rates.

OUTCOMES

Patient satisfaction is an important factor in the outcomes assessment of TKA in end-stage arthritis. There are many tools that assess total knee outcomes, but recently the patient-reported outcome measures (PROMs), where there is direct patient reporting rather than an indirect assessment, have increased in importance. The orthopedic registries are an important source of decision-making. At present, there is a heterogeneity between the registry and PROMs used in a particular country. European quality five-dimension health survey–three level (EQ-5D-3L), European quality five-dimensional health survey–five level (EQ-5D-5L), 36-item Short Form Health Survey (SF-36), 12-item Short Form Health Survey (SF-12), and Patient-Reported Outcomes Measurement Information System (PROMIS) have all been used in general functional improvement assessment. The Oxford Knee Score (OKS), Knee Injury and Osteoarthritis Outcome Score (KOOS), Western Ontario and McMaster Universities Arthritis Index (WOMAC), University of California Los Angeles (UCLA) activity score, and Visual Analog Scale (VAS) for pain are used in the focused assessment of knee functional outcome. The 2011 Knee Society Score (KSS) included patient expectation and functional activity in addition to information that has to be assessed by the clinician, which was an improvement from its previous version. Although useful for patient counseling, synthesizing information from registry data represents a challenge as a different indexes are used by different registries. The New Zealand (NZOA) Joint Registry has 20-year patient satisfaction data measured by Oxford-12 Knee Score scale from 0 to 48, and the data are categorized as excellent outcomes (>41), good outcomes (34–41), fair outcomes (27–33), and poor outcome (<27).[1] Table 13.1 summarizes the serial outcomes using the OKS.

The American Joint Replacement Registry has shown that 88.5% of patients at 1-year postoperative follow-up had meaningful improvement in KOOS score.[2] During 2017, the Swedish Knee Arthroplasty Registry demonstrated that 87% of patients at 1-year follow-up were very satisfied or satisfied with TKA as assessed by the VAS.[3] In a study of satisfaction using OKS at 1 year postsurgery in 10,000 patients who underwent surgery in England and Wales the National Joint Registry noted that 81.8% (6625 of 8095) were satisfied, 11.2% (904 of 8095) were unsure, and 7.0% (566 of 8095) were not satisfied.[4]

In a systematic review of 208 studies and 95,560 patients Kahlenberg et al.[5] determined that the median reported percentage of satisfied patients was 88.9%. The same study also showed that the most commonly reported predictor of satisfaction was a higher absolute postoperative patient-reported functional score. Preoperative anxiety and/or depression was the most common preoperative predictor of dissatisfaction, and persistent pain was the most common postoperative predictor of dissatisfaction. Certain activities are easier than others in the postoperative period. In a study by Bourne et al.[6] using WOMAC scoring for pain relief in 1703 patients 72% were satisfied with their ability to go up or down stairs compared with 85% with walking on a flat surface and 84% with sitting or lying. For restored function, patients were least satisfied with getting in or out of a bus or car (70%) and ascending stairs (73%) compared with rising from a bed (82%), lying in a bed (84%), and performing light domestic duties (83%). For overall satisfaction, which was used as the proxy for the satisfaction outcome, 81% (1375) of patients claimed that they were satisfied or very satisfied and 19% (328) were very dissatisfied, dissatisfied, or neutral. The same study also showed that the strongest contributing variables to patient dissatisfaction after primary TKA using odds ratios (ORs) were expectations not met (10.79), a low 1-year WOMAC (2.59), a low preoperative WOMAC pain score while sitting or lying (2.49), and a complication requiring hospital admission (1.99).

With the available data, it is safe to say that 75% to 89% of patients are satisfied after TKA. It has also been shown that expectations not being met is a critical factor in the lack of postoperative satisfaction, and presurgical discussion should include clear goal setting of achievable objectives.

COST-EFFECTIVENESS

Many patients are worried about the cost-effectiveness and QOL improvement in financial terms concerning TKA. Many studies are looking into the cost-effectiveness of TKA and have concluded that TKA is a cost-effective surgery in improving QOL. A study by Losina et al.[7] showed an incremental cost of $18,300 per quality-adjusted life year gained, and they concluded that TKA

TABLE 13.1	Twenty-Year Satisfaction Outcome Using the Oxford Knee Score				
Time	6 months	5 years	10 years	15 years	20 years
Number of patients	29,816	11,768	6572	2364	128
Excellent or good outcomes	75%	84%	82%	79%	75%
Average score	37.65	40.5	39.96	39.39	39.04

is a highly cost-effective procedure for the management of end-stage knee osteoarthritis (OA) among Medicare-aged persons compared with nonoperative management. In a systematic review of 23 studies Kamaruzaman et al.[8] concluded that TKA and total hip arthroplasty are cost-effective and should be recommended for the management of patients with end-stage knee and hip OA. Surgeons can convey to their patients that TKA is a cost-effective surgical procedure to improve QOL.

COMPLICATIONS

In 2013 the Knee Society TKA Complications Workgroup published a list of 22 important complications that have a bearing on the outcome of TKA.[9] They can be classified as relating to the surgical procedure, to certain processes, and to the property of the materials used (Table 13.2). This classification helps not only with patient communication regarding the rationale for complications but also with the possible strategies to minimize them. Certain complications such as neurovascular injury, ligament injury, and extensor mechanism disruption are operator-dependent and can be reduced by strict attention to detail.

Nerve and Vessel Injury

Nerve and vessel injury can be caused by direct injury, pressure effect, or secondary damage. Patients who have preexisting flexion or valgus deformity, prolonged tourniquet usage, or rheumatoid arthritis are at increased risk for nerve palsy, primarily of the peroneal nerve.[14] Jacob et al.[10] found that the majority (62%) of

neurological deficits completely resolved during the median follow-up of 5.1 years, with an additional 36% of patients reporting partial recovery.

Vascular injuries are a rare but devastating complication of TKA. The popliteal vessels are vulnerable to excessive manipulation, direct injury during bony cuts and during posterior midline soft tissue dissection, and cement polymerization. In a large population database study by Lin et al.[15] there were 15 direct vascular injuries in 111,497 patients, and the primary risk factor was surgeon volume; there was a higher risk of injury in procedures performed by surgeons with lower volume.

Extensor Mechanism Complications

The extensor mechanism complications can include quadriceps tendon and patellar tendon rupture, patellar or tibial tuberosity fracture, or subluxation of the patellofemoral joint. Extensor mechanism rupture can occur in 0.17% to 2.5% of cases as seen in a study by Schoderbek et al.[13] Extensor mechanism disruption is a difficult problem with complicated surgical solutions. The risk factors that predispose to the extensor mechanism dysfunction are inflammatory joint disease, diabetes mellitus, hyperthyroidism, and repeated corticosteroid injections into the knee joint.[13,16,17]

Bleeding

Bleeding is a well-known side effect of TKA. With transfusion rates varying from 2.5% to 35.3%, significant postoperative anemia can warrant a blood transfusion.[18-21] Postoperative allogeneic blood transfusion (ALBT) has been shown to be associated with an increased incidence

TABLE 13.2 **Common Complications After Total Knee Arthroscopy**		
Procedure (Intraoperative)	**Process (Medium to Long Term)**	**Property (Mechanical Factors)**
Bleeding	Instability and dislocations	Osteolysis
Wound complications	Malalignment	Loosening
Nerve (0.79%)[10] and vessel injury (0.08%)[11]	Stiffness	Wear
Medial collateral ligament injury (MCL) (2.6%)[12]	Periprosthetic fracture	
	Deep venous thrombosis	
	Extensor mechanism disruption (0.17%–2.5%)[13]	
	Reoperation, revision, readmission	
	Infection	
	Death	

of early postoperative confusion (OR = 3.44), cardiac arrhythmia (OR = 5.90), urinary catheterization (OR = 1.60), incidence of deep infection (OR = 4.03), and mortality (OR = 2.35).[22] Anemia in the postoperative period is not a benign condition and has the potential to be preventable and correctable. Strategies available are listed in Table 13.3. Of all the surgical strategies, intraarticular and intravenous (IV) tranexamic acid (TXA) has been known to significantly reduce blood loss. In a systematic review it was found that TXA reduced total blood loss by a mean of 591 mL.[23]

Wound Complications

The knee is a superficially located joint with minimal soft tissue covering. In a study by Galat et al.[26] 59 out of 17,784 patients required surgical intervention within 30 days of TKA. More importantly, the need for immediate surgical intervention increased the subsequent need for surgeries by 8 to 10 times. Diabetes, obesity, presurgical albumin <3.5 g/dL, and anemia all increase the risk of superficial surgical site infection (SSI).[27]

Ligament Injury

The medial collateral ligament (MCL) medially stabilizes the knee joint. Disruption of this ligament can affect the functional and long-term outcomes of TKA. Although studies have shown that it is uncommon, adverse outcomes can occur if not recognized and managed appropriately. In a study by Leopold et al.[12] 2.6%

of patients were reported to have a midsubstance damage or avulsion of the MCL from the femoral and tibial attachment. The management of an MCL injury consists of end-to-end repair with nonabsorbable material, varus/valgus constrained insert, reconstruction of the MCL using semitendinosus graft, or suture anchor repair of avulsions.[28]

Instability

Instability after TKA is one of the most common causes for revision TKA.[29] Effective gap balancing is imperative for successful TKA outcomes. The Australian Orthopedic Association National Joint Replacement Registy (AOANJRR) has shown that 0.4% of primary TKA warrant a revision surgery at 5 years because of instability.[30] The sagittal balance of the flexion and extension spaces is not as important as the coronal varus/valgus gap balancing. Patients must recognize that certain factors are determined by the surgeon, such as symmetrical gaps after bony cuts and appropriate ligament releases. However, patients who have advanced deformity with bony defects, rheumatoid arthritis, uncemented TKA, and neuromuscular arthritis are at a higher risk for instability.

Suboptimal Alignment

The issue of alignment and the outcome of TKA is a topic of intense discussion. Some studies point to the direct relationship between suboptimal alignment and poor outcomes with a higher risk of revision, whereas other studies do not show any significant differences. A systematic review of studies published from 2000 to 2014 found that suboptimal alignment may be correlated with outcomes.[31] Currently, there are no clear guidelines regarding the ideal alignment in the sagittal and coronal planes. The rotational alignment of the implants and its effect on outcomes is better defined. In a systematic review by Valkering et al.[32] it was found that a positive correlation of 0.44 (95% confidence interval [CI], 0.27 to 0.59) for tibial rotation and of 0.68 (95% CI, 0.64 to 0.73) for femoral rotation would indicate that a higher degree of external rotation coincides with a higher total KSS. The same review also determined that TKA revision for an internal malrotation of the tibial component of 4.3 degrees and for an internal malrotation of the femoral component of 7.1 degrees resulted in marked improvement, but because of certain limitations, it is difficult to give a cutoff value for revision TKA. However, standard

TABLE 13.3	**Anemia Prevention Strategies in Total Knee Arthroscopy**
Iron deficiency anemia	Iron deficiency calculated by standard formula Single dose of intravenous (IV) iron ± erythropoietin and multivitamin; 4 weeks before surgery based on dosage calculation
Intraoperative blood loss	1. IV/Intraarticular tranexamic acid administration to prevent blood loss[23] 2. Surgical technique with fibrin tissue adhesive[24] 3. Hypotensive anesthesia[25]
Postoperative blood loss	1. Compression dressing 2. Clamping of drain 3. Cryotherapy[24]

principles of external rotation of both femoral and tibial components are crucial to achieve satisfaction and avoid complications.

The coronal plane alignment of TKA is 90 degrees to mechanical axis alignment, with ±3 degrees as tolerance for a predictable outcome in TKA. Two articles published simultaneously in *Clinical Orthopaedics and Related Research* in 1985 discussed differing philosophies of coronal plane alignment. Insall et al.[33] was an advocate for cemented fixation and mechanical alignment. Alternatively, Hungerford and Krackow[34] advocated for uncemented fixation and anatomical alignment, where the knee is aligned in 2 to 3 degrees of varus similar to the natural knee alignment and primarily relied on uncemented fixation.

Major amounts of resources are expended on achieving target alignment with technology, which includes computer-assisted orthopedic surgery in TKA (CAOS), patient-specific instrumentation (PSI), and robotic-assisted TKA. In a 10-year follow-up study the robotic TKA reduced the outliers and improved accuracy; however, there was no difference in the functional outcome of either conventional jig-based or robotic TKA.[35] Similarly, in a systematic review of robotic TKA, Kayani et al.[36] concluded that there are no differences in medium- to long-term functional outcomes between conventional jig-based TKA and robotic TKA. In a meta-analysis of 23 studies, it was found that CAOS reduced femoral component outlier's rate by 87% and for the tibial implant a reduction in outlier's rate of approximately 80% but concluded that clinical significance of these findings though has to be proven in the future.[37] In a metaanalysis by Kizaki et al.[38] PSI in TKA did not improve PROMs, surgery time, or complication rates compared with standard TKA. Although the current consensus is that technology has allowed for innovative changes to performing a TKA, clinical or functional outcomes may not improve.

Stiffness

Stiffness is a painful limitation in functional ROM after a TKA. The exact definition of stiffness varies according to studies, but most commonly it can be defined as the presence of flexion contracture with available ROM of the knee being <70 degrees that leads to functional limitations. Stiffness has been reported as a complication 1.3% to 5.3% of the time.[39,40] Risk factors associated with stiffness are preoperative ROM (the most important risk factor), diabetes, lung disease, smoking, and previous

surgery on the knee joint.[41] Surgeon-determined factors can contribute to stiffness in TKA and can include component size mismatch, mal-alignment, or improper ligament balancing.[42] The treatment for stiffness consists of identifying the primary cause and intervening appropriately. In the early postoperative period and up to 3 months after surgery stiffness is managed by manipulation under anesthesia (MUA); long-standing stiffness is managed by arthroscopic arthrolysis or revision surgery if there is an identifiable cause of implant mal-alignment.[41]

Periprosthetic Fracture

Periprosthetic fractures are fractures of the femur or tibia within 15 cm of the knee joint or 5 cm from the end of the prosthesis and any patellar fractures post- TKA.[43] According to multiple studies, fractures are seen primarily in the femur, with an incidence of 0.1% to 2.5% compared with an incidence of 0.4% and 0.68% in the tibia and patella, respectively.[44–46] The risk factors are mentioned in Box 13.1. The treatment of periprosthetic fractures is predicated on bone integrity and stability of the implant fixation.

Deep Venous Thrombosis

Deep venous thrombosis (DVT) can be a predictable complication after TKA. Given the importance of DVT, there are various regimens available to prevent this complication. The incidence without prophylaxis is 40% to 84%.[48,49] In a large database survey of more than 600,000 patients the incidence of in-hospital pulmonary embolism was 0.36% even with prophylaxis.[50] All patients are offered prophylaxis in order to reduce the incidence of DVT. Before 2012, there was a divergence in the guidelines between the American Academy of

---

BOX 13.1   Risk Factors for Periprosthetic Fractures[47]

Osteopenia
Old age
Rheumatoid arthritis
Corticosteroid usage
Epilepsy
Parkinsonism
Surgical technique with femoral notching in posterior referencing
Patellar resurfacing
Posterior stabilized femoral implant design

TABLE 13.4 **Major Guidelines for Perioperative Prevention of Deep Venous Thrombosis**	
National Institute of Health and Care Excellence (UK) NICE[51]	Aspirin (75–150 mg) for 14 days Low molecular weight heparin (LMWH) for 14 days Rivaroxaban 10 mg Apixaban and dabigatran as second-line treatment if the above are not effective
American College of Chest Physicians (ACCP)[52]	1B recommendation for usage of aspirin, LMWH, rivaroxaban, apixaban, dabigatran, warfarin, low-dose unfractionated heparin at least for 10–14 days can be extended to 35 days Preference for LMWH over other agents
American Association of Orthopaedic Surgeons (AAOS)[53]	"We suggest the use of pharmacologic agents and/or mechanical compressive devices for the prevention of venous thromboembolism in patients undergoing elective hip or knee arthroplasty, and who are not at elevated risk beyond that of the surgery itself for venous thromboembolism or bleeding." "Current evidence is unclear about which prophylactic strategy (or strategies) is/are optimal or suboptimal. Therefore, we are unable to recommend for or against specific prophylactics in these patients." Recommends physician and patient consensus on individual basis

Orthopaedic Surgeons (AAOS) and American College of Chest Physicians (ACCP), leading to controversy regarding the most effective methods and goals of prophylaxis. There is a convergence of thought with present guidelines and certain drugs such as aspirin that are acceptable chemoprophylaxis agents. In addition, the guidelines recommend the postoperative usage of mechanical measures such as stockings and intermittent pneumatic compression devices for at least 18 hours a day. The current recommendations for DVT chemoprophylaxis are mentioned in Table 13.4.

Mortality

TKA does improve QOL, but there is a minimal risk of perioperative mortality after TKA. In a systematic review of over 1.75 million TKA cases it was found that 30- and 90-day mortality was 0.20% and 0.39%, respectively.[54] In this same review the leading cause of death was cardiovascular disease. Other risk factors for mortality include age >70 years, use of cemented TKA, and simultaneous bilateral TKA.[55]

Wear and Osteolysis

Wear occurs when a soft bearing surface such as polyethylene (PE) is susceptible to repetitive motion causing mechanical damage to the structural integrity. The inflammatory response to the loss of PE particles is largely responsible for periimplant osteolysis. Wear in total knee implant is due to a combination of rolling,

sliding, and rotational motion leading to delamination and fatigue failure of the PE.[56] Implant- and manufacturing-related risk factors for wear are mentioned in Box 13.2. The activity level of the patient determines the amount of wear, however, good surgical practice with proper gap balancing and restoration of the mechanical axis can lead to symmetrical loading of the liner surface, resulting in less wear. Highly cross-linked polyethylene (HXLPE) versus conventional polyethylene (CPE) is a topic of controversy with conflicting data regarding outcomes. HXLPE considerably increases the cost of TKA. Some outcome studies support its usage, whereas other studies have shown no improvement. A 10-year

---

BOX 13.2 Implant And Mechanical Factors[59]

Compression-moulded polyethylene is better than extruded manufacturing.[60]

Method of sterilization: Currently all sterilization is done in oxygen-free environment to avoid free radicals.

Highly cross-linked polyethylene (HXLPE): Role is controversial in total knee arthroscopy.

Thickness of polyethylene should be at least 8 mm (lesser thickness leads to greater wear).

Conformity of the liner and the femoral component: Greater conformity leads to lesser articular side wear.

All polyethylene tibia have lesser wear than modular.

Highly polished cobalt-chrome tray has lesser wear than titanium base plate.

follow-up data Australian joint registry demonstrated that the cumulative revision rate was 5.8% (95% CI, 5.7 to 6.0) for non–cross-linked PE and 3.5% (95% CI, 3.2 to 3.8) for cross-linked polyethylene, therefore showing a significant reduction in revision rate for HXLPE liners.[57] In a study of 550,658 TKA in the National Joint Registry of England, Wales, and Northern Ireland the unadjusted aseptic revision rates were significantly lower after procedures performed with CPE (n = 513, 744) compared with those performed with HXLPE.[58] The revision rate for CPE was 0.29 (95% CI, 0.28 to 0.30) compared with 0.38 (95% CI, 0.35 to 0.42; P < .01) for HXPLE. The authors concluded that HXPLE might have a role in a specific patient population, such as in patients with an age <60 years old and body mass index >35 kg/m².

Aseptic Loosening

Aseptic loosening is the process of a gradual loosening of the implant-bone interface in the absence of infection; it accounts for 29.8% of revisions of TKA and is the most common cause of revision knee arthroplasty.[61] In the AOANJRR, there was a progressive reduction in the rate of revisions for aseptic loosening during 2013 to 2018, with a 1.3% for 1999 to 2005, a 0.9% for the years 2006 to 2012, and an overall, 5-year cumulative revision of 0.6%.[62]

Aseptic loosening can be the result of inadequate initial fixation, mechanical loss of fixation over time, or biological loss of fixation caused by particle-induced osteolysis around the implant.[63] The wear particles of either polymethylmethacrylate or PE lead to inflammatory cytokine response and progressive loosening of the biological interface between the bone and implant. Other causes of aseptic loosening can include stress shielding by metal, micromotion at the bone-implant interface, high fluid pressure, and genetic variation.[64]

Prosthetic Joint Infection

Infection is a devastating complication after TKA. It reduces the QOL of the patient and significantly increases the cost of care to society. In the Australian registry report of 2019 the 1-year, 3-year, and 5-year cumulative risk percentage for infection was 0.5%, 0.8%, and 0.9%, respectively.[62] Given the increase in the expected number of projected TKA, emerging antibiotic resistance is a major concern with infection. In a review of 679,010 primary knee replacements performed between 2003 and 2013 in England and Wales

TABLE 13.5 Patient Characteristics Associated With Higher Risk of Revision

Patient Characteristics	Risk Ratio
Male	1.8
Chronic pulmonary disease	1.2
Diabetes	1.4
Liver disease	2.2
Rheumatic and connective tissue disease	1.5
Total knee arthroscopy for trauma	1.9
Previous septic arthritis	4.9
Posteriorly stabilized fixed bearing knee	1.4
General anesthesia	1.1

with a median follow-up of 4.6 years the risk ratio for revision was higher in patients with certain characteristics, which are mentioned in Table 13.5.[65] Eighty percent of patients who are candidates for an arthroplasty procedure have modifiable risk factors. The most common are obesity (46%), anemia (29%), malnutrition (26%), and diabetes (20%).[66] Fig. 13.1 shows the modifiable and nonmodifiable risk factors associated with prosthetic joint infection (PJI). As mentioned in other chapters of this book, there is a significant scope for infection prevention strategies and early patient involvement in risk reduction in order to prevent complications.

Perioperative PJI risk reduction is gaining traction. Zywiel et al.[67] devised a protocol where 82% chlorhexidine-impregnated washcloths were used (neck-chest-abdomen, arms, right leg, left leg, back, surgical site) the evening before surgery and the morning of surgery. No SSI was found in the patient cohort who followed the protocol in comparison to 3.0% in patients who did not. Reduction of presurgical hospital stay, hair removal just before the surgery, usage of providone-iodine impregnated film drapes for the incision, and reduction in operating room traffic help in reducing PJI.[68] Antibiotic prophylaxis reduces the absolute risk of wound infection by 8% and the relative risk by 81% as compared with no antibiotic prophylaxis.[69] Laminar airflow and space suits are used regularly in TKA, but their usage is controversial. The New Zealand Joint Registry has shown a 6-month revision rate for deep infection of 0.17% in conventional theaters versus 0.33% in laminar airflow theaters; it similarly found 0.28% for space suits versus 0.22% for no suits during TKA.[70] Intraoperative joint lavage with dilute povidone-iodine 0.35% for

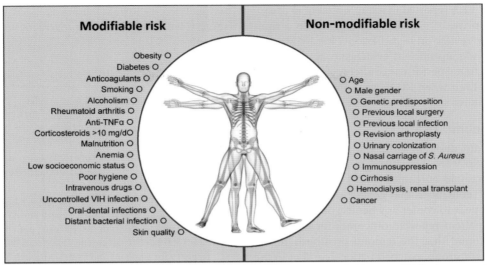

Fig. 13.1 Risk factors for prosthetic joint infection. (From Marmor S, Kerroumi Y. Patient-specific risk factors for infection in arthroplasty procedure. *Orthop Traumatol Surg Res.* 2016;102(1 Suppl):, S113–S119.)

3 minutes reduced the risk of postoperative PJI from 0.97% to 0.15%.[71] The role of antibiotic-loaded bone cement (ALBC) has been controversial in primary TKA. In a registry data of 731, 214 patients in the National Joint Registry of England and Wales, it was found that ALBC was associated with a lower risk of revision for all aseptic causes (hazard ratio [HR] = 0.85; 95% CI, 0.77 to 0.95; $P < .001$) and revisions for infection (HR = 0.84; 95% CI, 0.67 to 1.01; $P = .06$).[72] Whereas, in a study by Gutowski et al.,[73] ALBC increased the rate of infection from 0.75% to 0.83% within 2 years of TKA.

SURGEON EXPERIENCE AND TKA OUTCOMES

Many patients are rightfully worried about the surgeon's experience and its influence on the outcome. In a 12-year study on 2646 TKA Wilson et al.[74] determined that there were no associations between the measured complications, transfusion rates, or surgical readmissions and trainees and consultants. Weber et al.[75] also determined that there was no difference in complications and PROM in surgical trainees and senior consultants and concluded that supervised TKA is a safe procedure during the learning curve of young orthopedic surgeons. In

a systematic review Lau et al.[76] analyzed 11 published studies across various geographies of North America, Europe, and Asia comprising 286,875 patients. They defined low surgeon volume as fewer than 3 to 52 surgeries per year and high surgeon volume as more than 5 to 70 TKA per year. Lau et al. also determined that there was a significant association between low surgeon volume and a higher rate of infection (0.26% to 2.8% higher), procedure time (165 vs. 135 minutes), longer length of stay (0.4 to 2.13 days longer), and transfusion rate (13% vs. 4%), and worse patient-reported outcomes were found.[76] Furthermore, they concluded that higher volume surgeons had better outcomes.

IMPLANT DESIGN AND TKA OUTCOMES

High-Flexion TKA

To improve flexion and facilitate activities such as squatting and kneeling, high-flexion designs were introduced in TKA. In a review of the institutional registry of a 64,000 community-based sample of primary TKA Namba et al.[77] noted high-flexion components had a higher risk of revision compared with conventional components. A metaanalysis by Sumino et al.[78] comparing posterior-stabilized knee design of high-flexion versus conventional TKA reported that improvement of preoperative flexion was similar in both cohorts. In a similar systematic review on high-flexion TKA by Murphy et al.[79] there was insufficient evidence of an improved ROM or functional performance after high-flexion knee arthroplasty. Even when ROM was superior, there was no change in knee scores in those studies.

Gender-Specific TKA

Female-specific designs with changes in the femoral aspect ratio were introduced to improve anatomical and functional outcomes. In a systematic review Cheng et al.[80] concluded that gender-specific prostheses do not appear to confer any benefit in terms of clinician- and patient-reported outcomes for the female knee. They found that the femoral prosthesis in the standard unisex group matched better than that in the gender-specific group. In a prospective randomized controlled trial of 138 female patients and a mean follow-up of 3.25 years Kim et al.[81] determined that there were no significant differences between the two groups in clinical and radiological results, patient satisfaction, or complication rate.

SUMMARY

In conclusion, 75% to 89% of patients who received a TKA are satisfied, and the TKA met their expectation for relief of symptoms. Preoperative health optimization is imperative to reduce postoperative complications of TKA, and universal protocols with care pathways for perioperative management reduce complications of TKA. Certain controversies still exist in TKA, as summarized in Box 13.3; however, TKA is a successful surgery with significant improvement in the QOL of patients.

BOX 13.3   **Current Controversies in Total Knee Arthroscopy**

a. Space suits and laminar airflow
b. Surgeon volume and experience
c. Antibiotic-loaded bone cement and postoperative infection
d. Highly cross-linked polyethylene liners
e. Patellar resurfacing
f. Deep venous thrombosis chemoprophylactic medications
g. Mechanical versus kinematic alignment
h. Robotic, navigation, and patient-specific instrumentation in routine total knee arthroscopy

---

REFERENCES

1. Pg. 110. The New Zealand Joint Registry. Twenty Year Report: January 1999 to December 2018. 2019. https://nzoa.org.nz/system/files/DH8328_NZJR_2019_Report_v4_7Nov19.pdf
2. Pg. 63. http://connect.ajrr.net/2019-ajrr-annual-report.
3. Pg. 70. The Swedish Knee Arthroplasty Register- Annual Report 2019-PartII.
4. Baker PN, van der Meulgen JH, Lewsey J, Gregg PJ. National Joint Registry for England and Wales. The role of pain and function in determining patient satisfaction after total knee replacement. Data from the National Joint Registry for England and Wales. *J Bone Jt Surg Br.* 2007 Jul;89(7):893–900.
5. Kahlenberg CA, et al. Patient satisfaction after total knee replacement: A systematic review. *HSS J.* 2018;14(2):192–201. https://doi.org/10.1007/s11420-018-9614-8.
6. Bourne RB, et al. Patient satisfaction after total knee arthroplasty: Who is satisfied and who is not? *Clin Orthop Relat Res.* 2010;468(1):57–63. https://doi.org/10.1007/s11999-009-1119-9.
7. Losina E, Walensky RP, Kessler CL, et al. Cost-effectiveness of total knee arthroplasty in the United States: Patient risk and hospital volume. *Arch Intern Med.* 2009;169(12):1113–1122. https://doi.org/10.1001/archinternmed.2009.136.
8. Kamaruzaman H, et al. Cost-effectiveness of surgical interventions for the management of osteoarthritis: A systematic review of the literature. *BMC Musculoskelet Disord.* 2017 May;18(1):183. https://doi.org/10.1186/s12891-017-1540-2.
9. Healy WL, Della Valle CJ, Iorio R, et al. Complications of total knee arthroplasty: Standardized list and definitions of the Knee Society. *Clin Orthop Relat Res.* 2013;471(1):215–220. https://doi.org/10.1007/s11999-012-2489-y.
10. Jacob AK, Mantilla CB, Sviggum HP, Schroeder DR, Pagnano MW, Hebl JR. Perioperative nerve injury after total knee arthroplasty: Regional anesthesia risk during a 20-year cohort study. *Anesthesiology.* 2011;114(2):311–317. https://doi.org/10.1097/ALN.0b013e3182039f5d.
11. Abularrage CJ, Weiswasser JM, DeZee KJ, Slidell MB, Henderson WG, Sidawy AN. Predictors of lower extremity arterial injury after total knee or total hip arthroplasty. *J Vasc Surg.* 2008;47:803–807. https://doi.org/10.1016/J.JVS.2007.11.067.

12. Leopold SS, Mcstay C, Klafeta K, et al. Primary repair of intraoperative disruption of the medial collateral ligament during total knee arthroplasty. *J Bone Jt surg Am*. 2001;83-A:86–91.

13. Schoderbek Jr RJ, Brown TE, Mulhall KJ, Mounasamy V, Iorio R, Krackow KA, et al. Extensor mechanism disruption after total knee arthroplasty. *Clin Orthop Relat Res*. 2006;446:176–185.

14. Idusuyi OB, Morrey BF. Peroneal nerve palsy after total knee arthroplasty. Assess predisposing prognostic factors. *J Bone Jt Surg Am*. 1996;78:177–184.

15. Lin YC, Chang CH, Chang CJ, Wang YC, Hsieh PH, Chang Y. Vascular injury during primary total knee arthroplasty: A nationwide study. *J Formos Med Assoc*. 2019 Jan;118(1 Pt 2):305–310. https://doi.org/10.1016/j.jfma.2018.05.009.

16. Nam D, Abdel MP, Cross MB, LaMont LE, Reinhardt KR, McArthur BA, et al. The management of extensor mechanism complications in total knee arthroplasty. AAOS exhibit selection. *J Bone Jt Surg Am*. 2014;96:e47.

17. Dobbs RE, Hanssen AD, Lewallen DG, Pagnano MW. Quadriceps tendon rupture after total knee arthroplasty. Prevalence, complications, and outcomes. *J Bone Jt Surg Am*. 2005;87:37–45.

18. Menendez ME, Lu N, Huybrechts KF, Ring D, Barnes CL, Ladha K, Bateman BT. Variation in use of blood transfusion in primary total hip and knee arthroplasties. *J Arthroplasty*. 2016;31(12):2757–2763. https://doi.org/10.1016/j.arth.2016.05.022. e2752.

19. Slover J, Lavery JA, Schwarzkopf R, Iorio R, Bosco J, Gold HT. Incidence and risk factors for blood transfusion in total joint arthroplasty: Analysis of a statewide database. *J Arthroplasty*. 2017;32(9):2684–2687. https://doi.org/10.1016/j.arth.2017.04.048. e2681.

20. Helder CW, Schwartz BE, Redondo M, Piponov HI, Gonzalez MH. Blood transfusion after primary total hip arthroplasty: National trends and perioperative outcomes. *J Surg Orthop Adv*. 2017;26(4):216–222.

21. Noticewala MS, Nyce JD, Wang W, Geller JA, Macaulay W. Predicting need for allogeneic transfusion after total knee arthroplasty. *J Arthroplasty*. 2012;27(6):961–967. https://doi.org/10.1016/j.arth.2011.10.008.

22. Maempel JF, Wickramasinghe NR, Clement ND, Brenkel IJ, Walmsley PJ. The pre-operative levels of haemoglobin in the blood can be used to predict the risk of allogenic blood transfusion after total knee arthroplasty. *Bone Jt J*. 2016;98-B(4):490–497. https://doi.org/10.1302/0301-620X.98B4.36245.

23. Alshryda S, Sarda P, Sukeik M, Nargol A, Blenkinsopp J, Mason JM. Tranexamic acid in total knee replacement: A systematic review and meta-analysis. *J Bone Jt Surg Br*. 2011 Dec;93(12):1577–1585. https://doi.org/10.1302/0301-620X.93B12.26989.

24. Gibbons CE, Solan MC, Ricketts DM, Patterson M. Cryotherapy compared with Robert Jones bandage after total knee replacement: A prospective randomized trial. *Int Orthop*. 2001;25:250–252. https://doi.org/10.1007/s002640100227.

25. Juelsgaard P, Larsen UT, Sørensen JV, Madsen F, Søballe K. Hypotensive epidural anesthesia in total knee replacement without tourniquet: Reduced blood loss and transfusion. *Reg Anesth Pain Med*. 2001;26:105–110. https://doi.org/10.1053/rapm.2001.21094.

26. Galat DD, McGovern SC, Larson DR, Harrington JR, Hanssen AD, Clarke HD. Surgical treatment of early wound complications following primary total knee arthroplasty. *J Bone Jt Surg*. 2009;91(1):48–54. https://doi.org/10.2106/JBJS.G.01371.

27. Yang G, Zhu Y, Zhang Y. Prognostic risk factors of surgical site infection after primary joint arthroplasty: A retrospective cohort study. *Medicine (Baltimore)*. 2020;99(8):e19283. https://doi.org/10.1097/MD.0000000000019283.

28. Siqueira MBP, Haller K, Mulder A, Goldblum AS, Klika AK, Barsoum WK. Outcomes of medial collateral ligament injuries during total knee arthroplasty. *J Knee Surg*. 2016;29(1):68–73. https://doi.org/10.1055/s-0034-1394166.

29. Dalury DF, Pomeroy DL, Gorab RS, Adams MJ. Why are total knee arthroplasties being revised? *J Arthroplasty*. 2013;28:120–121. https://doi.org/10.1016/j.arth.2013.04.051.

30. Pg. 55 Australian Orthopaedic Association National Joint Replacement Registry (AOANJRR). Hip, Knee & Shoulder Arthroplasty: 2019 Annual Report. Adelaide: AOA, 2019.

31. Hadi M, Barlow T, Ahmed I, et al. Does malalignment affect revision rate in total knee replacements: A systematic review of the literature. *SpringerPlus*. 2015;4:835. https://doi.org/10.1186/s40064-015-1604-4.

32. Valkering KP, Breugem SJ, van den Bekerom MP, Tuinebreijer WE, van Geenen RC. Effect of rotational alignment on outcome of total knee arthroplasty. *Acta Orthop*. 2015;86(4):432–439. https://doi.org/10.3109/17453674.2015.1022438.

33. Insall JN, Binazzi R, Soudry M, Mestriner LA. Total knee arthroplasty. *Clin Orthop Relat Res*. 1985 Jan-Feb;(192):13–22.

34. David H, Krackow S, Kenneth A. Total joint arthroplasty of the knee. *Clin Orthop Relat Res*. 1985;192:23–33.

35. Cho KJ, Seon JK, Jang WY, et al. Robotic versus conventional primary total knee arthroplasty: Clinical and radiological long-term results with a minimum follow-up of ten years. *Int Orthop*. 2019 Jun;43(6):1345–1354.

36. Kayani B, Konan S, Ayuob A, Onochie E, Al-jabri T, Haddad F. Robotic technology in total knee arthroplasty: A systematic review. *EFORT Open Rev*. 2019;4:611–617. https://doi.org/10.1302/2058-5241.4.190022.

37. Brin YS, Nikolaou VS, Joseph L, Zukor DJ, Antoniou J. Imageless computer assisted versus conventional total knee replacement. A Bayesian meta-analysis of 23 comparative studies. *Int Orthop*. 2011;35(3):331–339. https://doi.org/10.1007/s00264-010-1008-6.

38. Kizaki K, Shanmugaraj A, Yamashita F, et al. Total knee arthroplasty using patient-specific instrumentation for osteoarthritis of the knee: A meta-analysis. *BMC Musculoskelet Disord*. 2019;20:561. https://doi.org/10.1186/s12891-019-2940-2.

39. Kim J, Nelson CH, Lotke PA. Stiffness after total knee arthroplasty: Prevalence of complication and outcome of revision. *J Bone Jt Surg*. 2004;86-A:1479–1484.

40. Yercan HS, Sugun TS, Bussiere C, Ait Si Selmi T, Davies A, Neyret P. Stiffness after total knee arthroplasty: Prevalence, management and outcomes. *Knee*. 2006;13(2):111–117.

41. Schiavone Panni A, Cerciello S, Vasso M, et al. Stiffness in total knee arthroplasty. *J Orthopaed Traumatol*. 2009;10:111–118. https://doi.org/10.1007/s10195-009-0054-6.

42. Scuderi GR. The stiff total knee arthroplasty: Causality and solution. *J Arthroplasty*. 2005;4(Suppl 2):23–26.

43. Dennis DA. Periprosthetic fractures following total knee arthroplasty. *Instr Course Lect*. 2001;50:379–389.

44. Aaron RK, Scot R. Supracondylar fracture of the femur after total knee arthroplasty. *Clin Orthop Relat Res*. 1987;219:136–139.

45. Felix NA, Stuart MJ, Hanssen AD. Periprosthetic fractures of the tibia associated with total knee arthroplasty. *Clin Orthop Relat Res*. 1997;345:113–124. https://doi.org/10.1097/00003086-199712000-00016.

46. Chalidis BE, Tsiridis E, Tragas AA, Stavrou Z, Giannoudis PV. Management of periprosthetic patellar fractures. A systematic review of literature. *Injury*. 2007;38:714–724. https://doi.org/10.1016/j.injury.2007.02.054.

47. Whitehouse MR, Mehendale S. Periprosthetic fractures around the knee: Current concepts and advances in management. *Curr Rev Musculoskelet Med*. 2014;7(2):136–144. https://doi.org/10.1007/s12178-014-9216-0.

48. Stulberg BN, Insall JN, Williams GW, Ghelman B. Deep vein thrombosis following total knee replacement. *J Bone Jt Surg*. 1984;66A(2):194–201.

49. Westrich GH, Haas SB, Mosca P, Peterson M. Meta-analysis of thromboembolic prophylaxis after total knee arthroplasty. *J Bone Jt Surg [Br]*. 2000;82-B:795–800.

50. Memtsoudis SG, Besculides MC, Gaber L, Liu S, González Della Valle A. Risk factors for pulmonary embolism after hip and knee arthroplasty: A population-based study. *Int Orthop*. 2009;33(6):1739–1745. https://doi.org/10.1007/s00264-008-0659-z.

51. National Institute for Health and Clinical Excellence Venous thromboembolism in over 16s: reducing the risk of hospital-acquired deep vein thrombosis or pulmonary embolism. *NICE Guidel (NG89)*. 2018 https://www.nice.org.uk/guidance/ng89.

52. Falck-Ytter Y, Francis CW, Johanson NA, et al. Prevention of VTE in orthopedic surgery patients: Antithrombotic Therapy and Prevention of Thrombosis, 9th ed: American College of Chest Physicians Evidence-Based Clinical Practice Guidelines. *Chest*. 2012;141(2 Suppl):e278S–e325S. https://doi.org/10.1378/chest.11-2404.

53. American Academy of Orthopaedic Surgeons. Preventing venous thromboembolic disease in patients undergoing elective hip and knee arthroplasty. Evidence-based guidelines and evidence report. https://www.aaos.org/globalassets/quality-and-practice-resources/vte/vte_full_guideline_10.31.16.pdf.

54. Berstock JR, Beswick AD, López-López JA, Whitehouse MR, Blom AW. Mortality after total knee arthroplasty. *J Bone Jt Surgery*. 2018 Jun;100(12):1064–1070. https://doi.org/10.2106/JBJS.17.00249.

55. Parvizi J, Sullivan TA, Trousdale RT, Lewallen DG. Thirty-day mortality after total knee arthroplasty. *J Bone Jt Surg Am*. 2001 Aug;83(8):1157–1161.

56. Collier JP, Mayor MB, McNamara JL, Surprenant VA, Jensen RE. Analysis of the failure of 122 polyethylene inserts from uncemented tibial knee components. *Clin Orthop Relat Res*. 1991;273:232–242.

57. de Steiger RN, Muratoglu O, Lorimer M, Cuthbert AR, Graves SE. Lower prosthesis-specific 10-year revision rate with crosslinked than with non-crosslinked polyethylene in primary total knee arthroplasty. *Acta Orthop*. 2015;86(6):721–727. https://doi.org/10.3109/17453674.2015.1065046.

58. APA Partridge TCJ, Baker PN, Jameson SS, Mason J, Reed MR, Deehan DJ. Conventional versus highly cross-linked polyethylene in primary total knee replacement. *J Bone Jt Surg*. 2020 Jan;102(2):119–127. https://doi.org/10.2106/JBJS.19.00031.

59. Naudie DDR, Ammeen DJ, Engh GA, Rorabeck CH. Wear and osteolysis around total knee arthroplasty. *J Am Acad Orthopaedic Surg*. 2007 Jan;15(1):53–64.

60. Won CH, Rohatgi S, Kraay MJ, Goldberg VM, Rimnac CM. Effect of resin type and manufacturing method on wear of polyethylene tibial components. *Clin Orthop Relat Res*. 2000;376:161–171.

61. Khan M, Osman K, Green G, Haddad FS. The epidemiology of failure in total knee arthroplasty. *Bone Jt J*. 2016;98-B(1_Supple_A):105–112.

62. Australian Orthopaedic Association National Joint Replacement Registry. Hip, Knee & Shoulder

Arthroscopy Annual Report: Lay Summary. 2019. Pg. 55. https://aoanjrr.sahmri.com/annual-reports-2019

63. Abu-Amer Y, Darwech I, Clohisy JC. Aseptic loosening of total joint replacements: Mechanisms underlying osteolysis and potential therapies. *Arthritis Res Ther.* 2007;9(Suppl 1). https://doi.org/10.1186/ar2170. (Suppl 1):S6.

64. Sundfeldt M, Carlsson LV, Johansson CB, Thomsen P, Gretzer C. Aseptic loosening, not only a question of wear: A review of different theories. *Acta Orthopaedica.* 2006;77(2):177–197. https://doi.org/10.1080/17453670610045902.

65. Lenguerrand E, Whitehouse MR, Beswick AD, et al. Risk factors associated with revision for prosthetic joint infection following knee replacement: an observational cohort study from England and Wales for England NJR, Wales N. *Lancet Infect Dis.* 2019;19(6):589–600.

66. Pruzansky JS, Bronson MJ, Grelsamer RP, Strauss E, Moucha CS. Prevalence of modifiable surgical site infection risk factors in hip and knee joint arthroplasty patients at an urban academic hospital. *J Arthroplasty.* 2014;29(2):272–276.

67. Zywiel MG, Daley JA, Delanois RE, et al. Advance pre-operative chlorhexidine reduces the incidence of surgical site infections in knee arthroplasty. *Int orthop.* 2011;35:1001–1006.

68. Solarino G, Abate A, Vicenti G, Spinarelli A, Piazzolla A, Moretti B. Reducing periprosthetic joint infection: What really counts? *Joints.* 2016;3(4):208–214. https://doi.org/10.11138/jts/2015.3.4.208. Published 2016 Jan 31.

69. AlBuhairan B, Hind D, Hutchinson AJ. Antibiotic prophylaxis for wound infections in total joint arthroplasty: A systematic review. *Bone Jt surg Br.* 2008;90:915–919.

70. Pg.99. https://nzoa.org.nz/system/files/DH8328_NZJR_2019_Report_v4_7Nov19.pdf

71. Brown NM, Cipriano CA, Moric M, Sporer SM, Della Valle CJ. Dilute betadine lavage before closure for the prevention of acute postoperative deep periprosthetic joint infection. *J Arthroplasty.* 2012;27(1):27–30.

72. Jameson SS, Asaad A, Diament M, et al. Antibiotic-loaded bone cement is associated with a lower risk of revision following primary cemented total knee arthroplasty: An analysis of 731,214 cases using National Joint Registry data. *Bone Jt J.* 2019 Nov; 101-B(11):1331–1347. https://doi.org/10.1302/0301-620X.101B11.BJJ-2019-0196.R1.

73. Gutowski CJ, Zmistowski BM, Clyde CT, Parvizi J. The economics of using prophylactic antibiotic-loaded bone cement in total knee replacement. *Bone Jt J.* 2014;96-B(1):65–69. https://doi.org/10.1302/0301-620X.96B1.31428.

74. Wilson MD, Dowsey MM, Spelman T, Choong PFM. Impact of surgical experience on outcomes in total joint arthroplasties. *ANZ J Surg.* 2016;86:967–972.

75. Weber M, Worlicek M, Voellner F, Woerner M, Benditz A, Weber D, et al. Surgical training does not affect operative time and outcome in total knee arthroplasty. *PLoS ONE.* 2018;13(6):e0197850. https://doi.org/10.1371/journal.pone.0197850.

76. Lau RL, Perruccio AV, Gandhi R, et al. The role of surgeon volume on patient outcome in total knee arthroplasty: A systematic review of the literature. *BMC Musculoskelet Disord.* 2012;13:250. https://doi.org/10.1186/1471-2474-13-250.

77. Namba RS, Inacio MCS, Cafri G. Increased risk of revision for high flexion total knee replacement with thicker tibial liners. *Bone Jt J.* 2014;96-B:217–223.

78. Sumino T, Gadikota HR, Varadarajan KM, Kwon YM, Rubash HE, Li G. Do high flexion posterior stabilised total knee arthroplasty designs increase knee flexion? A meta analysis. *Int Orthop.* 2011;35(9):1309–1319. https://doi.org/10.1007/s00264-011-1228-4.

79. Murphy M, Journeaux S, Russell T. High-flexion total knee arthroplasty: A systematic review. *Int Orthop.* 2009;33(4):887–893. https://doi.org/10.1007/s00264-009-0774-5.

80. Cheng T, Zhu C, Wang J, et al. No clinical benefit of gender-specific total knee arthroplasty. *Acta Orthop.* 2014;85(4):415–421. https://doi.org/10.3109/17453674.2014.931194.

81. Kim YH, Choi Y, Kim JS. Comparison of standard and gender-specific posterior-cruciate-retaining high-flexion total knee replacements. A prospective, randomised study. *J Bone Jt Surg Br.* 2010 May;92(5):639–645. https://doi.org/10.1302/0301-620X.92B5.24129.

INDEX

Page numbers followed by *f* indicate figures; *t*, tables; *b*, boxes.